Body Foods
for Life

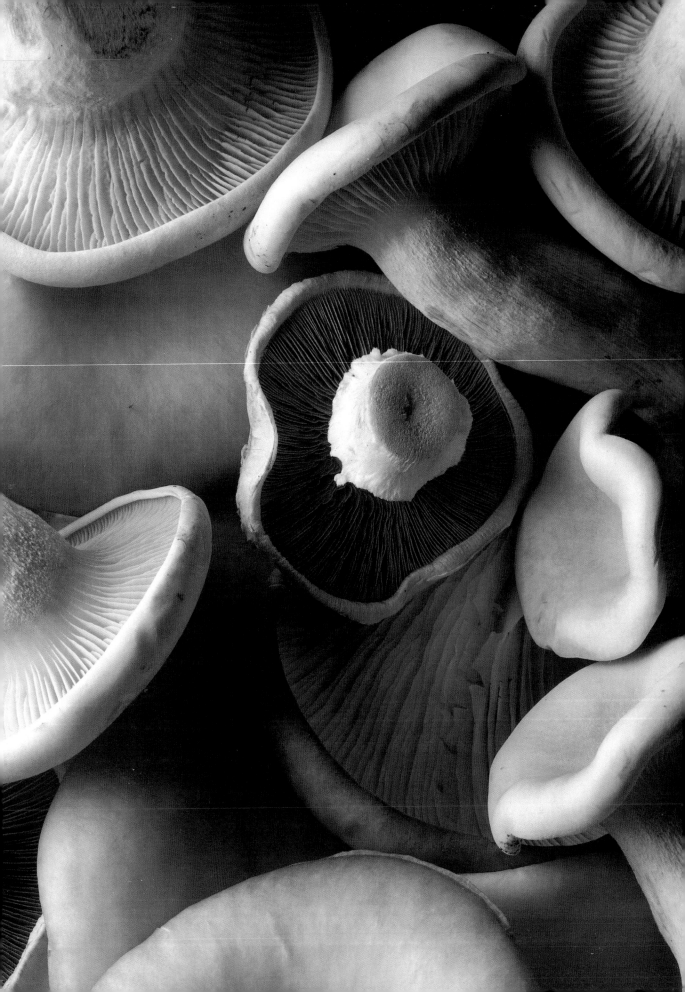

Body Foods for Life

Feel good, look good, stay good

Jane Clarke

*Photographs
by Jess Koppel*

SEVEN DIALS

for boats, butterflies and rainbows

First published in Great Britain in 1998
by Weidenfeld & Nicolson Ltd

This paperback edition first published in 1999 by
Seven Dials, Cassell & Company
The Orion Publishing Group
Wellington House, 125 Strand
London, WC2R 0BB

A CIP catalogue record for this book is available
from the British Library

ISBN 1841880345

Designed by Lucy Holmes
Colour photographs by Jess Koppel
Food styling by Lyn Rutherford
Illustrations by Emily Hare
Typesetting by Tiger Typeset
Author photograph by Victoria Blackie
Index by John Noble
Printed in Italy by Printer Trento srl

Contents

Introduction

We all want good health and vitality, so much so that hundreds of hours and pounds are spent reading advice or buying so-called 'health foods' and pills which promise the elixir of life. But how many 100 per cent healthy people do you know? Very few, I suspect. Most of us have a few little niggles such as tiredness, headaches, problems sleeping, colds or digestive problems. This is because modern-day living is a disease. From birth our bodies are exposed to environmental stresses and toxins. A body that is continually drained through working too hard, cutting corners, not resting and eating inappropriately is much more likely to have a suppressed immune system and therefore be susceptible to viruses and bacteria. In more extreme, but not uncommon, circumstances the cells can be battered into behaving abnormally and eventually develop life-threatening conditions such as heart disease and cancer. These days we push ourselves to the absolute limits, both in terms of work pressure and bad eating habits. We have to acknowledge that our bodies need respect, and nourishment.

It is not an impossible goal to expect your body to wake up feeling refreshed, to be able to get through a day without energy swings and headaches. Men can eat dinner without having indigestion. Children have the right to run around fit and healthy, growing strong with the knowledge that their bodies, if treated well, should remain so for many years. Elderly people should still enjoy their meals despite having health problems that alter the way the body reacts to foods. People suffering from life-threatening illnesses can eat real food, without having to resort to chemically produced supplements. Families can sit down together and eat something easy to prepare: shopping for and cooking nutritious food doesn't need to be a military exercise that sucks all your energy. The trick is knowing which are the health-giving foods and how to turn them into something simply delicious.

Disease is not as inevitable as it appears in today's society. Good eating habits reduce your likelihood of developing the major killers: heart diseases and cancer. They also help you get through life more enjoyably. Children are less likely to be overweight and irritable. Adults are less likely to swing from cold to cold, one tired day to another. Take the time to think about the food you put in your mouth and how you expect your body to cope with it and you will receive the dividends for many years.

The food you need – real, tasty, nutritious food – is out there, somewhere. The shops and markets are flooded with thousands of different food products, some supposedly 'fresh', others whose packaging promises life-enhancing properties: low-fat spreads that lower your cholesterol levels; breakfast cereals that boost your vitamin and mineral intakes; yoghurts that help stave off hunger cravings. I ask why should we need these foods, when nature has provided such a wonderful choice?

Thankfully we are coming to realize that just because something sounds good on the label, doesn't mean it is good. Equally, when a food tastes good it doesn't mean it is bad for you. As world health professionals are slowly recognizing, if society is to feel well and not just survive, we need to find health-giving rather than health-hindering foods.

I am not saying that this is easy. You will be up against the powerful marketing machines of the food industry, which have not only confused us as to what is in food, but are also not entirely trustworthy. The food marketing engine has also caused many people to lose confidence in their own ability to find and cook simple nutritious foods; they would rather take the word of a ready-made meal than try to work out something simpler and cheaper.

Today's society does not suffer from lack of variety in food, but from the difficulty of finding foods that taste good: tomatoes that taste like tomato, milk that truly tastes like milk, not a white watery liquid.

Eaten correctly, food can give you the greatest boost to energy and health. If consumed incorrectly, gulping down a sandwich while on the telephone or if you're in a permanent state of stress, it can aggravate disease and predispose you to developing health problems far too early in life. *Body Foods for Life* will help you choose foods that will help rather than hinder your body, and will inspire you to put food back in its rightful place as both a pleasure and one of the greatest healers on earth.

'A good cook is half a physician.' Although Andrew Boorde (1490–1549) said this 500 years ago, it still epitomizes how food can be used to help our bodies. Natural medicines exist, and by looking at the food you put into your body you should be able to save it from artificial supplements, pain relievers, antibiotics and other drugs. You can stimulate the body to become primarily self-sufficient, reducing its need for unnatural, symptom-masking drugs.

- The executive who takes his indigestion remedies on every trip could protect his health by drinking ginger tea and avoiding the traditional 'cooling' milk.
- The child with constipation could be saved from laxatives if he drank more fresh fruit juices and sparkling mineral water, instead of cola drinks.
- The woman with period pain could prevent monthly stomach cramps if she boosted her intake of oily fish such as salmon or tuna.

The Body Foods philosophy promotes good health by understanding the simple way food behaves in your body and how your life can be enhanced with the 'fruits' Mother Nature provides. The 8,000 or so patients I have seen over the years, ranging from babies with colic to elderly people with Alzheimer's disease or osteoporosis, can hardly believe how good health is compatible with eating delicious food. With Body Foods you can eat anything (as long as you eat it right) and so you can eat your way to good health.

The Body Foods concept is very different from the traditional nutritional advice dished out in GPs' surgeries and health clubs. For instance, the traditional advice to someone who is allergic to cows' milk would be to avoid all dairy products. The Body Foods answer is to consider creating delicious dishes with goats' or sheep's cheese. Instead of immediately dismissing chocolate as unhealthy, Body Foods considers how we can eat chocolate healthily: I recommend that you choose a good-quality chocolate, with a high cocoa bean content, rather than a cheap, sugar-loaded bar, and eat it after a meal, rather than on an empty stomach.

Body Foods inspire you to work towards reachable goals

Food has to fit into your lifestyle.

- A mother with children doesn't want to be told to count calories or to check the fat content on every food label. All she needs to do is to take simple steps. For instance, instead of baking a cake with white flour and lots of sugar she could follow a recipe with wholewheat flour and sweetened with sultanas or dates soaked in fresh orange juice.
- Businessmen and women need to be better informed about 'working' lunches. They frequently feel that it's not worth the effort trying to lose weight unless they sign themselves into a health farm. But small steps mount up. By following the Body Foods philosophy even 80 per cent of the time, for example by choosing a fresh vegetable soup or spinach and orange salad, and cutting down on coffee, they will not only look good, but also feel good.

Body Foods are quick and easy foods

Lack of time is one of the main reasons people give for not cooking or looking after their bodies. They think that it is much quicker to pop a convenience meal in the microwave than to start from scratch. Unfortunately, convenience foods contain many substances we would do well to avoid. Sugar, salt, fat and preservatives don't help our bodies to feel well and if taken in excess can lead to a myriad of health problems. Nutritious meals can be achieved as easily as popping a meal in the microwave, but are twice as delicious and much more satisfying. *Body Foods for Life* contains plenty of simple suggestions for meals in minutes.

Body Foods are good value

Healthy eating does not make your shopping bills more expensive. Not only are simple foods usually less expensive weight for weight, but if you value your body, just count up the cost of sickness leave and productive hours lost from feeling sleepy and exhausted during the day. Prescriptions for medicines and the cost of vitamin and mineral supplements soon add up. We were designed to savour food, quaff refreshing beverages, not swallow jars of pills!

Body foods are sensual foods

As we struggle with the stress of modern living, we often lose sight of the sensory aspect of eating. The mouth, eyes, ears and nose need titillating if we are to be healthy. We glean the most satisfaction from foods with a high organoleptic quality, in other words they stimulate more than one sense – think of sizzling bacon, the pop of champagne, the bubbling of thick soup. Banish the tasteless boring foods you feel obliged to eat. Replace them with gorgeous, tasty foods that you really want to eat.

Body Foods are habit-forming

To break old eating habits and form new healthy ones, *Body Foods for Life* teaches you how to respect your body; to get into the habit of feeding it good food and allowing it to perform well.

Many people think they know all there is to know about healthy eating, low fat and high fibre diets. But I find that they run into problems simply because they are so fed up with hearing what they can't eat that their mouth and brain sensors switch off. Food becomes the enemy. By focusing on all the marvellous foods they can enjoy and how they can re-educate their body to use foods efficiently, they feel able to achieve their health goal.

Body Foods set you up for life

Eating well allows the body to build up a reserve of nutrients for those moments when there simply isn't the time to eat properly. If you manage for 80 per cent of the time to eat well, your body will be able to withstand the odd period of nutrient strain.

Eating the Body Foods way helps prepare your body for the future. Men whose fathers died at an early age from a heart attack need to channel their worry into positive eating strategies. Women who fear cancer want to learn how they can build a strong immune system. Parents want to know how they can set their child on the right path for building a strong, healthy body. The last thing anyone wants is to suffer from avoidable ills.

This book will help you find the foods that not only help you and your family think good, look good, feel good and stay good, but most importantly those that taste good.

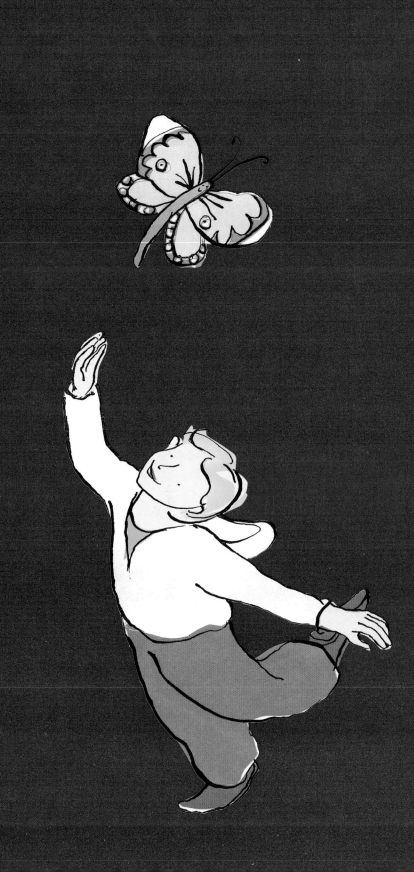

1

think good

Respect your body

The body is like a finely tuned engine which can work amazingly well if maintained and fuelled appropriately. It needs to be respected and not abused, and this means meeting its requirements to develop a healthy skeleton, muscles and the organs that enable it to support itself effectively.

In school we should be made more aware of the importance of the digestive system, since it provides the body with all its nutrients: the 'fuel' we need for life and health. Many of my patients find that their lives are greatly improved simply by thinking of the stomach as the centre of the body and not just something that takes whatever we throw at it. Keeping a food diary (see page 85) can tell us a great deal; being aware of what we are putting in our body and how it can be improved can cure many common ailments before any active treatment is undertaken. In many cases our bodies are reacting badly because we are not offering them the respect they deserve.

Yet man has long since recognized that food nourishes not only the body but also the mind. 'Food is better than power,' advised the Indian Upanishads in the third century BC. 'If a man abstain from food for ten days, though he lives, he would not be able to see, hear, perceive, think, act, and understand.' Back then people knew how important it was to eat well, but in some cultures we have lost sight of the potential healing power of food.

Why are so many people abusing their bodies by eating too many health-hindering items? If we ate only the easily available 'fast' food, we would end up consuming vast amounts of fat, sugar and grossly overprocessed ingredients. In time we would not only feel lousy, but also develop disease. Some people think, 'well, it's only food and not drugs you are taking or abusing.' They forget that 'drugs' are not just dangerous chemicals, but any substance that alters the way the body reacts; many drugs are derived from plants, such as opium from a type of poppy. Think how small a tablet is needed to make you feel well and extrapolate that to the volume of food you eat. If you get the combination of foods right you can feel marvellous, but if you get it wrong your body complains. For example, liquorice sweets look innocuous, but in some people liquorice can cause high blood pressure and swollen feet.

It is not only lay people who fail to realize the importance of eating well. Doctors often tell patients that their health problem has little to do with their eating habits, but this is only partly true; many of the patients I see are able to cope without medication or at least reduce their dependency on it once they learn to respect their bodies and eat good, nutritious foods that encourage optimum health.

Developing a positive relationship with food

Food imaginatively and lovingly prepared, and eaten in good company, warms the being with something more than the mere intake of calories.
Marjorie Kinnan Rawlings (1896–1953)

Every day of my working life I confront the issues of eating behaviour with patients of all ages. Adults wish they had started life with better eating habits or regret veering off the path at a later date. Parents wonder how they can give their child the best start in life, not only in terms of a well-nourished body, but also a healthy attitude towards eating. It's not just what you eat that matters, but also how you eat.

As a society our eating habits have become very confused. Every day we hear reports and read articles telling us to change our diet in some particular way. On top of this, so many emotions are bound up in the business of preparing and eating food; it goes far beyond taking enough fuel on board to get us through the day. While food can play a major role in the giving and receiving of love and affection, children should not be made to feel guilty about not eating their mother's food or eating too much. I see children as young as seven or eight suffering from constipation and stomach pains, which can be traced back to stress at the meal table. Overweight adults battle with diet after diet, desperately trying to find a food cure for the underlying destructive relationship between food and their body.

Approached positively, food can provide you with the most amazing foundation to life, but if caught up in guilt and angst, it can become a source of discontent. We must learn to separate food and affection if we are to prevent more and more children and adults from being trapped within an anorexic, bulimic or overweight body.

Setting the thermostat
To understand the best way to build a healthy relationship with food, let us look at how feeding begins. The first big decision when you have a baby is whether to breast or bottle feed. Remember, the most important goal is to relax and enjoy feeding your baby in a way that gives you both the greatest pleasure. Breast milk is the perfect food for a baby. It has properties that can never be copied in formula milks, and the physical act of breastfeeding helps to build a strong emotional bond between mother and baby. But if breastfeeding is not for you, rest assured that bottle-fed babies can grow up just as happily as breast-fed infants; cuddle them while you feed them, enjoying skin to skin contact as you hold your baby against your chest.

Whether you feed your baby when she or he is hungry or whether you try to feed according to a structure is ultimately up to you. I am in favour of demand feeding as I feel this starts the child off on a positive footing of having food when they are hungry. I believe that the sooner we start to teach our children about

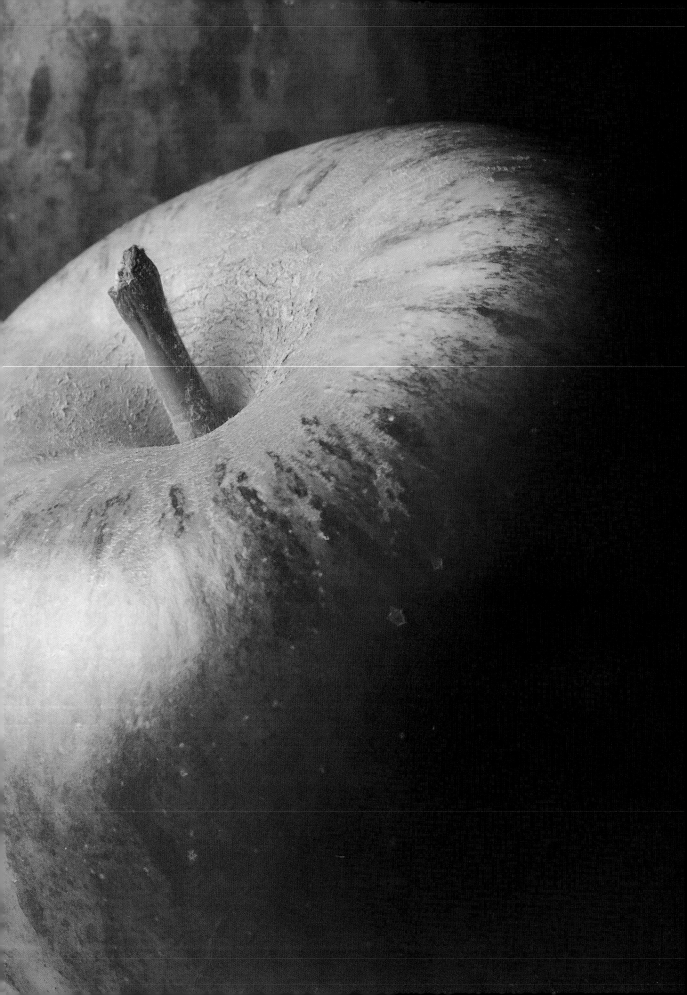

the way the appetite works, the more likely they are to grow up into adults who have a good relationship with food. I frequently see men and women who have problems with their eating habits because they haven't got used to responding appropriately to their hunger impulses. They are much more likely to eat at irregular, unsuitable intervals and eat foods which their body finds unacceptable.

Sweets and treats

There is a school of thought that your food preferences can be directly attributed to your mother's eating habits during pregnancy and breastfeeding. You may believe it is not as simple as that, but few would disagree with the observation that cravings for sweet foods are generally established in early childhood. You have only to look at the attitude of so many parents; that children have to finish the savoury part of the meal before they can have the sweet treat. In the majority of cultures sweets are given as rewards or gifts of affection. Children soon learn to associate sweets with rewards, which can cause problems in later life, when these children grow into adults who grab a chocolate bar 'to cheer themselves up' and feel deprived when they don't round the meal off with a dessert. Serious conditions such as irritable bowel, hypertension, diabetes and weight-related disorders can plague us if we place too much emphasis on sweet foods. Parents should try to reward their child with non-food activities, or if food is used, treat them with a special fruit or a savoury food.

The appetite mechanism

It is never too late in life to change the way you eat. Every day I spend time explaining to adults how the appetite mechanism works and how they can use it to help them achieve a body they feel happy with. Astonishingly, only ten percent of the people who walk through my door eat correctly.

By understanding hunger and satiety (the feeling you get when you are happily full) you will be able to feel well after eating, both physically and mentally. Satiety, or sensory satisfaction, encompasses physical properties such as smell, taste, texture and temperature, and the emotional and psychological aspects of eating. The greater the degree of satiety, the more we enjoy what we eat and drink.

Appetite is coordinated in an area of the brain called the hypothalamus; this same area controls a lot of our emotions, which is why food is far more than mere body fuel. The 'feeding' centre within the hypothalamus is sub-divided into 'hunger' and 'satiety' centres. The signals reaching these centres dictate whether you feel hungry or full. If you feel pleasantly full and contented after your meals you'll be less likely to binge or pick on inappropriate foods. There are basically four key signals recognized by the satiety centre.

- Chew your food, don't gulp! Within the jaw are stretch receptors, which respond when you chew. The more you chew and the more time you take over eating, the greater the feeling of fullness.

- Keep your taste buds on their toes. If you have exciting flavours, varying temperatures and textures within a meal, your mouth has a greater opportunity to register satisfaction. The foods with the highest satiety value are those with several organoleptic properties, in other words they stimulate more than one sense: they look good, smell good, feel good in the mouth, taste good and even sound good – the bubbling of thick soup on the stove or the smell of freshly baked bread straight from the oven. Think about stimulating as many of the senses as possible when planning your meals. If you eat similar foods all the time, mouthful after mouthful of soup, your mouth gets used to the taste and texture, and to some extent 'switches off'. Eating croûtons or a slice of toast with the soup will stimulate other nerves in the mouth and juggle the signals which go to your brain, and will help the fullness centre to tell you when you have eaten enough. The production of saliva and other digestive juices increases when you choose food you love, and both your body and your mind recognize the experience of eating. It is hopeless to place yourself in a situation you're not going to enjoy, as your sensory recognition mechanism will switch off and you won't feel as if you've eaten. Notice your food, concentrate on eating and avoid needless consumption when your mind is distracted.
- The more often you lift your hand to your mouth, delivering food, the greater the satiety. Take smaller mouthfuls and pause between each one. Eat slowly and cut food into smaller pieces using a knife and fork. For example, rather than holding a sandwich to your mouth while you are doing something else, cut it into quarters and appreciate each piece.
- Within the stomach wall are stretch receptors, which send signals of fullness to your brain when there is food in your stomach. If you take in foods that are low in fibre, such as sweets or fatty foods, they pass through the stomach very quickly, so it can't send many signals to the satiety centre, therefore you don't feel full for very long and you are likely to take in more food before feeling full. The converse occurs when you eat high-fibre foods, such as fresh fruit and vegetables, pulses and wholegrain bread, pasta and rice. These foods have thick cell walls and are more difficult for the body to break down; they stay in the stomach a lot longer, swell in the presence of water and send lots of signals back to the satiety centre in the brain, making you feel full and contented. Note that is important to drink plenty of water.

Relax

One of the most important aspects of allowing your body to glean the most from its food is learning to relax when you are eating. Sitting calmly allows your body to concentrate its blood supply and fully acknowledge the stomach, so you gain satiety from the eating experience. On the other hand, when there are stress hormones in your bloodstream the majority of blood goes to your limbs; stress hormones are sometimes called 'fight or flight' hormones because they prepare the body to run.

The digestive system is a collection of glands and muscles. It needs a plentiful supply of oxygen (brought in by the blood) and the appropriate hormones to enable it to work efficiently. If you get up and rush around immediately after eating, or worse still, eat 'on the run', oxygen is diverted away from the stomach to other muscles, which hinders digestion and can double you up with indigestion, stomach cramps and bloating half an hour later.

Mother Nature tries to help us by releasing hormones that make us feel sleepy immediately after a meal. You don't have to sleep, just rest for 10–15 minutes before rushing off – make a few phone calls, read letters, as long as you keep your body stationary for this short time. City traders and mothers are a few of the people who tell me they haven't got time to sit down and eat and relax, three times a day, but I point out that if they give themselves these few minutes they will feel better and be more efficient afterwards.

Position of eating
Sitting upright allows gravity to help rather than hinder your stomach. To establish a good eating posture early in life, sit your child in a supportive chair which is the correct height for the table. If you are eating in bed make sure that you have plenty of pillows propped behind you. Elderly people who eat in a soft lounge chair may find it difficult to eat much because their stomach is scrunched up. They also risk indigestion because the acid contents of the stomach can more easily leak up into the oesophagus.

When should we eat?
To say that humans need to eat three times a day doesn't give an accurate picture of what each person needs to feel well. In different periods of history and in other cultures, two meals a day was or still is the norm. Some people cannot function after eating a large breakfast, let alone a substantial lunch, whereas others need a hearty breakfast and a snack every two hours to keep up their energy levels. There's no hard-and-fast rule, it's just a question of working out how your body responds to foods and how you can eat to maximize your performance and overall health.

People are likely to run into problems when they keep the stomach empty during the day. They feel more alert when they don't eat, and keep themselves going by drinking endless cups of coffee. By the evening they are desperate for food, which has to be ready in an instant. Not only do they place their body under a huge strain, expecting it to digest a lot of food having had nothing for hours, but it is also unlikely that in the course of one meal they will manage to eat the five portions of fresh fruits and vegetables and other health-giving foods we know our bodies need. These people set themselves up for heart disease, digestive problems and even an increased risk of cancer.

It is much better to take a little time to think about what your daily schedule demands and how you can choose foods to meet your body's needs. The best way to do this is to keep a diary. Write down how you feel in the morning, after lunch, evening. Is your busiest time – when your mind needs to be sharpest – late afternoon? If you don't have a snack at this time, do you end up ravenously hungry, feeling ratty and shattered by the time you reach the evening meal table? Before changing your eating habits you need to consider all the evidence.

The time food takes to be broken down, absorbed and passed through your digestive system differs in everyone, taking anything from twelve to thirty-six hours. This is partly why some people find they have to have a little something every two to three hours, while others are content with three meals a day. Whatever you feel, you shouldn't go for long periods without eating. Not only can this harm the digestive system by leaving it exposed to acids produced by the stomach, it also makes you more inclined to eat inappropriately or overeat. Overeating after a period of starvation can take your digestive system by surprise: the production of digestive juices slows down when you don't eat; if you then eat a lot there aren't enough juices to digest the food properly. The food may then sit undigested in your stomach, making you feel uncomfortable and bloated, or it can pass through the system partly digested, which can cause other gut problems such as diarrhoea or constipation. Regular snacks are therefore preferable to starving and then eating a large meal.

Drink to complement the food

Wine can be a perfect digestive partner to food, and it has now been found to have health-giving properties of its own (see page 48). If you aren't able to drink alcohol with your meal, think about an alternative, such as apple juice or pure water. Drinking water with meals does not interfere with digestion. Some people find that drinking large volumes of water with meals increases the likelihood of indigestion and bloating. I recommend that you take small sips of water between mouthfuls of food as this not only helps the fibre within the food to swell and hence stimulate the stretch receptors in your stomach (see page 16), it also refreshes the palate.

Make food worth looking at

To get the digestive process off to a good start, taking time to think about the presentation of the food can start the saliva flowing even before a morsel has passed your lips. It is not just how food tastes, but also how it stimulates our eyes that helps us decide whether we want to eat. Think about contrasting colours, shapes and textures. A small bunch of juicy green grapes with a creamy cheese and a few rustic oat biscuits, served on a plate, is much more appealing and satisfying than a lump of cheese squashed between two slices of bread, eaten off the kitchen surface. The size of the plate is important too; food should neither be lost nor crowded on its plate.

Overweight people often find it difficult to leave food on their plate; they may well have acquired this habit in childhood when their parents refused to let them leave the table until they had 'cleared their plate'. Serving smaller portions can make you stop and question whether you need a second helping. Allowing children to leave some of their food rather than forcing them to finish everything can teach the child to recognize when they are hungry or full.

Special diets

It is particularly important that anyone on a special diet, be they a hyperactive child who needs to avoid sugary and additive-laden products or a diabetic adult who needs to regulate their intake of carbohydrates, should not feel deprived of 'normal' food. As far as possible they should enjoy the same food as their friends or family. For example, rather than telling a child that they can't have ice lollies you could make lollies for all the children, using freshly squeezed orange and grapefruit juice, a lolly mould and lolly stick. Baking a date and walnut cake made with wholemeal flour to eat at tea time instead of sugar-loaded Madeira cake will make a diabetic feel much happier and less isolated.

If you don't make a big issue of avoiding ingredients there will be less aggravation at the meal table. If you have a wheat intolerance, don't feel you need to cook one dish for your family and something different for yourself. There will be lots of dishes you can all enjoy: risottos, buckwheat pancakes, sauces thickened with potato flour instead of wheat flour.

Be positive about the prospect of foods helping to improve your body and your life. Patients who feel deprived and angry towards any nutritional therapy rarely achieve the results they want. Just think how much better it is to manage your body with wonderful food rather than bombarding it with drugs, and potentially suffering from their adverse side effects. Empower yourself through food.

Eat without guilt

So many people, even children, think of foods as bad and good foods. Of course there are foods that have more beneficial qualities than others, but we set ourselves up for other problems if we build a barrier around foods that taste delicious but we think are bad for us. I've heard children as young as six or seven years old say, 'chocolate is bad for me...I shouldn't be eating bread, it's fattening.'

I spend hours trying to explain that all foods, including chocolate, can be incorporated in a healthy eating lifestyle, unless there is a proven negative reaction such as an allergy. Even then you should be able to find equally delicious alternatives. Denying yourself or your family will only make the likelihood of bingeing on the foods more likely.

Eating without guilt is my most important doctrine. If you fill yourself with guilt you will also tie yourself up in knots, swinging from a 'virtuous' healthy meal which makes you feel deprived to a guilt-ridden overindulgent meal. Establishing a balance, basing 90 per cent of your meals around healthy foods which you like, allows you to indulge in foods which you know are a little over the top on occasions. Eat and enjoy, just get back on track the next day.

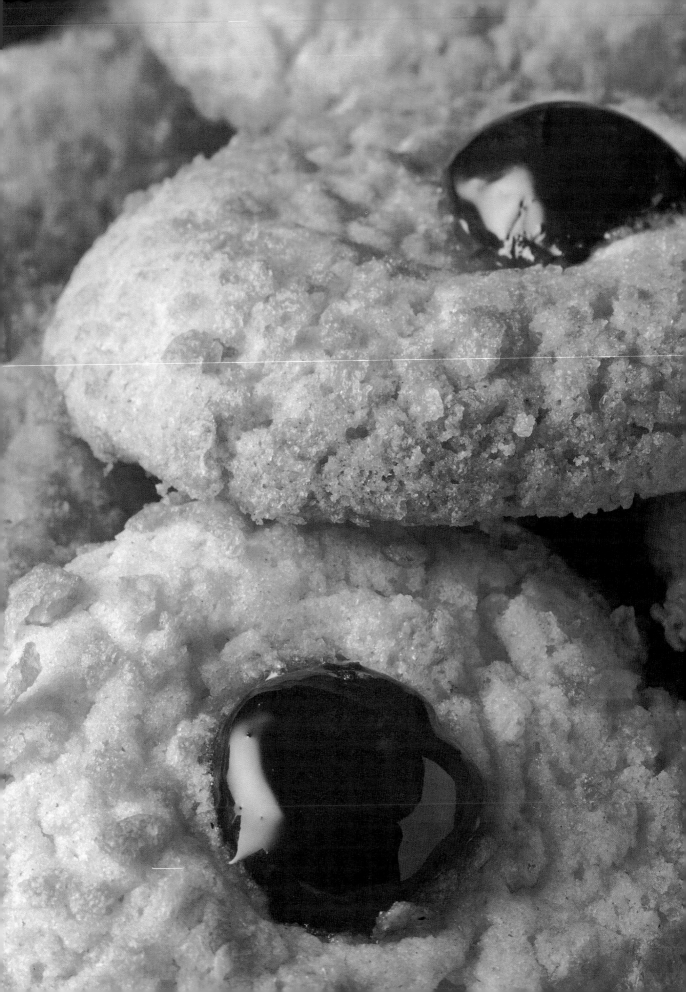

Children's eating habits

How to deal with fussy and erratic eaters

Your child will imitate your eating habits, along with your likes and dislikes. This may seem an obvious point to make, but many parents try to force their children to eat things they don't actually eat themselves. According to some recent research a child may even develop a penchant for certain types of food while still in the womb. As they grow older, children tend to veer towards the foods their mothers ate, whether this be chocolate ice cream or a spicy curry!

Another common problem is the child who just won't sit still to eat – again, they are only mimicking mum, who nibbles at her food while she is doing something else. Many children have erratic eating habits: they eat very little on occasions and then make up for it later. Some children develop a pattern of just having one meal when they really seem to 'tuck in', commonly breakfast, while at other meal times they hardly bother to eat. Other children develop fads such as eating only jam sandwiches, which can drive their parents mad as they battle to make their diet more varied.

The best way to deal with any such fad is to ignore it. If you make a fuss the child will associate food with conflict: meal times can become a 'war zone' and children may develop a lifelong dislike of certain foods. Try to keep things in perspective. If your child is happy and healthy, let the issue of their eating habits sit on the back burner. On the other hand, if they are not growing or are often unwell you should seek the help of your doctor or dietitian.

Establishing good eating habits within a young family

- Sit down to eat with your children whenever possible. Even if you want to eat your main meal with your partner later, sit and have a drink, a piece of fruit or a bowl of soup.
- Eat slowly. Rushed children frequently become obese adults, who don't notice what they eat. Rushing their meals can also set them up to develop stress-induced indigestion in their twenties.
- Eat a varied diet. If you serve the same things every day, boredom will set in and children will not learn to enjoy their food. A variety of foods is also more likely to fulfil your family's nutritional needs (see pages 25 – 47).
- Use convenience foods wisely. Don't dismiss all tinned and frozen foods and packets as nutritionally inferior to fresh. It's much more important for you to be relaxed at the meal table than to turn the whole thing into a military exercise, ending with you sitting down exhausted, having done your culinary duty. With careful shopping you can build up a store of nutritious convenience foods, such as canned pulses, pizza bases, and frozen vegetables.

- Try to get into the habit of cooking more than one meal's worth at a time and freezing the rest for another day. For the same amount of effort you could cook two large pies – and just think of the time it will save.
- Remember to make food fun. Learning about food is a valuable activity, so encourage your child to spend time with you while you're cooking.
- Spend time with your child when you go shopping. Knowing where produce comes from is a very important tool in food appreciation – a little enthusiasm from you will rub off on your child. Herb gardens and markets are good places to start, but even if you can only get to supermarkets, talk to your child about the different foods and their seasonality.

  Some scientists believe that if you eat foods in season throughout the year you will have a good cycle of nutrient intakes. Looking forward to the first new potatoes of spring, I'm sure, makes them taste far better than they would at any other time of the year. I remember my father proudly presenting his first crop of runner beans at the Sunday lunch table; the only problem was that there were only half a dozen of them!
- Eat your meals without any distractions. This will allow children to concentrate on the flavours and foods, as well as relax and communicate. Switch off the TV and switch on to the meal.
- Try not to give the impression that the dessert is the best part of the meal, something to be enjoyed after forcing down the savouries and vegetables. The relationship between food and reward does not have to be sweet-based.

Children and their weight

The most important thing in this weight-obsessed society of ours is not to over-play the issue with children. The more fuss you make the more problems they will have, and they will either eat even more or they will go the other way, down the road to anorexia. Remember that all children have some puppy fat and you should let them grow into their height. If your child is growing proportionately in height and weight it is unlikely that there is a real problem. They will find the right time in their lives to tackle their appearance. Your doctor or practice nurse will have growth charts to check whether your child is the correct weight for his height, or whether he is carrying too little or much weight.

If there is a problem, think about the weight you were as a child and relate it to the current situation. For example, some ex-anorexic mothers, who recognize and exaggerate the link between food and affection, overcompensate for denying themselves the delights of food by overfeeding their child. Conversely, a parent who had problems as a slightly overweight child may force their own child to become obsessed with calories and their body shape.

What to do if a child is not eating much at the meal table

- Check that they are not filling up with drink. Children frequently prefer to drink rather than eat. Changing from a bottle to a beaker can help, as it is slightly more difficult to manage. Ideally leave an least an hour after a drink before starting to eat, then encourage children to have a few sips of drink at the end of the meal.

- Introduce unfamiliar foods without comment. A little quip about a food being something they've not had before can prompt children to say they don't like it, even before they've tried it. Introduce new foods within familiar dishes, such as spinach in a soup or as a layer in lasagne.
- Use the same technique when they leave something on their plate, saying that they don't like it. Without comment, try it again a few days later served in a different way: carrots could be cooked or raw, cut into rounds, sticks or dice, puréed or served in a sauce.
- Use different textures in foods. For instance if you are encouraging children to have a little bit of meat and you know that they don't like the texture or the look of it, make it into a pâté. Liver pâtés are an excellent source of iron for children, which is useful if they are anaemic. Making lean minced meat into sausages with different herbs and spices is another way to make meat more tempting, and children can help with mixing and shaping.
- Try to avoid snacking between meals. Even if a child hasn't eaten much at the table, don't feel that you need to give him or her a snack; this can lead to erratic eating patterns and manipulation by the child. They will learn that they can fill the hungry space at the next meal time; just remember to make it a good, nutritious meal. Encourage your relatives and nannies to do the same, so that the child knows where they stand.
- Conjure up novel ways of eating. Arrange theme meals and picnics, even if they take place on the kitchen floor or in the back garden.
- Involve your child in the preparation of the meal. However small their involvement, it can help them feel like eating more. Even setting the table can act as an appetizer (or so my father often told me!), or doing the washing up. It's strange that we really look forward to splashing those dishes in the water as children and then spend the rest of our lives trying to avoid it.

What to do if your child is overweight
Whatever you do, do not put your child on a restricted diet. It is vital that they eat a variety of healthy foods to provide plenty of calcium, protein, iron and all the other essential nutrients. A well balanced diet, a healthy lifestyle and a positive relationship with food are the best gifts you can give your child. If you are worried or your child is uncomfortable with their weight, read the chapter on Achieving your ideal weight. Remember that a high fibre diet gives a great deal of satiety – in other words a full and contented feeling.

- Look at the eating habits of the whole family. I suggest that you organize a family health day (see page 81) to see whether there are changes you can all make that will not only help your child to find their right weight, but also encourage the family to eat more healthily.

- Make main meals delicious, fun and nourishing. Your child should not feel hungry, and neither physically nor psychologically deprived between meals.
- Choose a high fibre breakfast cereal, rather than the sugar-coated ones.
- Eat plenty of vegetables and fruits, including special fruits such as little tangerines, slices of mango, papaya and kiwi fruits. Add fruits or fruit purée to breakfast cereals, serve fruit on sticks. Vegetables can be tucked into pies, or made into soups or purées of different colours. High fibre jacket potatoes can be served with all manner of fillings, instead of always having chips or other fried potato dishes.
- Choose a variety of breads, mainly wholemeal, but also including olive, fruit and tomato breads (watching the nut varieties with young children). But don't fill your child up with wholemeal bread; white bread can also be part of a healthy diet, as it is often fortified with calcium.
- Have desserts as a treat, rather than the norm. Resist giving high-sugar biscuits and cakes, and choose fruit-based desserts rather than cream, pastry or sponge-based puddings. Make your own cakes and biscuits using wholemeal flour, oats and other high-fibre ingredients such as dried fruit.

Provide healthy school snacks

Children are frequently expected to take a snack for the break time, so don't let your child feel left out. But instead of sweets or crisps, pack a yoghurt, some fresh fruit or a high-fibre oaty biscuit like apple flapjacks (see page 331). These are higher in calories than fruit, but they are also high in 'filling' fibre, therefore the likelihood is that the child won't need as much to eat at the following meal.

Crisps, even '25% less fat' types, are high in fat and don't contain much fibre, therefore they don't fill you up for very long. However, since most children love them, remember that it is the overall picture of a healthier way of eating and more exercise that will help your child lose weight, not 'filling' them (excuse the pun) with fears over an occasional packet of crisps.

Try different forms of exercise

These could be as simple as walking to school. It's all too easy to pop along in the car, but a little time invested in walking to school can provide exercise for both you and your child, and can also give you time together, noticing objects, smells and sounds that go unnoticed when travelling by car.

Overweight children often feel embarrassed and self-conscious taking part in sports and games sessions at school, so try to find a form of exercise that they enjoy. Take them swimming, or for long walks at weekends. Encourage them to do something active rather than watching television or playing with computers for prolonged periods.

Keep the emphasis away from food, explaining that exercise will help them get fitter, making it easier for them to run without feeling out of breath. Above all, try not to make them feel different in a negative way, either at home or school.

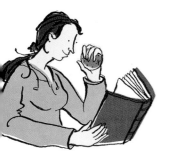

Understanding your nutritional needs

In the grand plan of looking, feeling and staying good, one of the first things to consider is how you can give your body the nutrients it needs. We all need a combination of foods from the main groups: carbohydrates, proteins and fats. Within these foods are found vitamins, minerals and other compounds which are important to our health and well-being. Some people hesitate when I use the words carbohydrate and protein, as they seem to feel the concept is too complicated to grasp. But if you take a little time to read the following text, you should feel more confident at the end of it. Once you have identified the sources of nutrients you really enjoy eating, the slightly easier part is to think how these foods can feature in your day to day life.

Carbohydrates

Carbohydrates in the diet, along with fats, provide our bodies with energy vital for our survival; not just 'visible' energy that we use in moving about, but also for the many processes that are going on within our bodies. There is a great deal of evidence to show that children need the right balance of carbohydrates: too little can stop them from growing and bounding with energy; too much refined carbohydrate can cause dental cavities, hyperactivity, obesity and health problems (both in infancy and in later life); too much of certain types of fibre (found in unrefined carbohydrates) can inhibit the absorption of nutrients and the release of energy. It is all a question of balance.

There are two types of carbohydrate: sugar and starch. Sugar and starch can be refined or found in a more natural form:
- Natural sugars are found in fruits and vegetables.
- Refined sugars (which include honey and both white and brown sugar) are found in soft drinks, cakes, biscuits, jams, jellies and sweets.
- Natural starches are found in wholegrain and wholemeal breakfast cereals, wholemeal flour and breads (from the dark, dense pumpernickel types to the lighter, seeded wholemeal loaves), wholewheat pasta, brown rice, potatoes and yams, lentils, chickpeas and beans, bananas and plantains, nuts, sweetcorn, parsnips and other root vegetables.
- Refined starches are found in sugary processed breakfast cereals, white flour and white bread, white pasta, white rice, biscuits and cakes.

While refined carbohydrates are not in themselves bad for us, they don't enable the body to work as efficiently as the unrefined or natural types. All carbo-hydrates taken in by the body have to be digested and converted into glucose, a type of sugar that the body can use. This is absorbed into the blood, and an

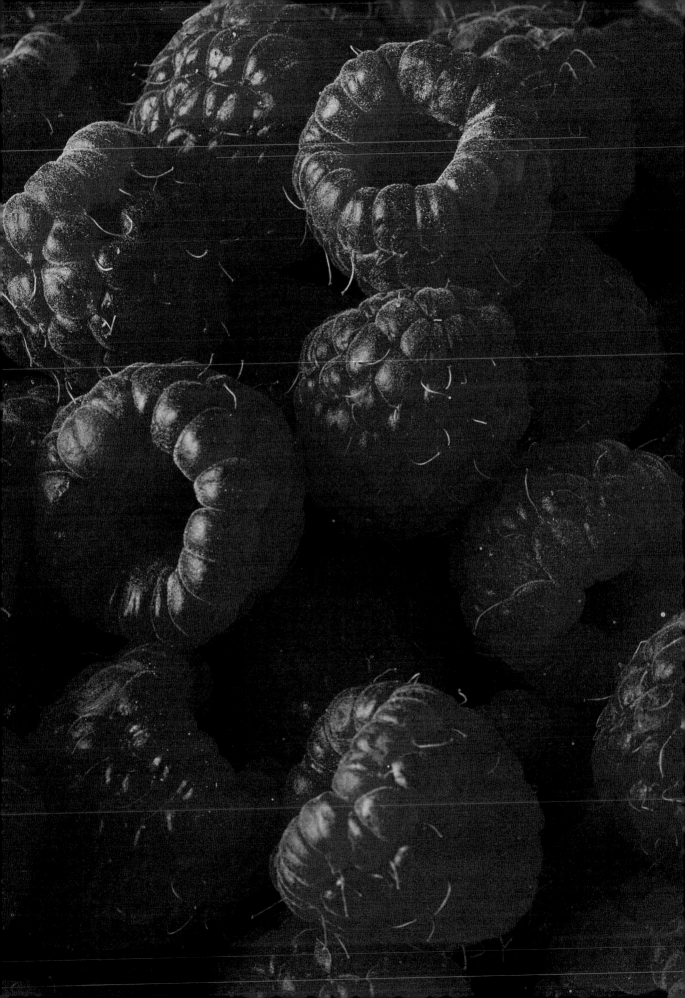

organ called the pancreas secretes insulin, a hormone that helps take the sugar into the cells for them to use. If the cells receive more sugar than they need, the body stores some of the sugar as glycogen, either within the liver or in the fat around the body. Then when you do need energy, a hormone called glucagon breaks down the glycogen to be used by the cells. So sugar metabolism is a cycle of sugar, insulin and glucagon reactions.

The gentler those reactions are, in other words the slower the release of the sugar and hormones, the more stable you will feel. Rapid changes adversely affect your energy and mood levels and can cause hyperactivity, depression, chronic fatigue, the mid-afternoon shakes and after-work rattiness.

The refining of carbohydrates (for example when brown rice has its outer husk removed to become white rice) involves breaking them down into simpler parts, doing work that in natural carbohydrates is done at a steady pace within the body. When making up your daily eating plan you should base each of your meals on a starch food such as potato, rice, beans, pasta or bread. These provide energy at a slower, steadier rate than sugary foods. If you can include some wholegrain versions, so much the better for your body, as the fibre helps slow the digestion process further and enables the gut to work effectively; it has the added benefit of reducing 'bad' cholesterol levels in your blood (see page 255).

If you are worried about putting on weight, remember that starchy foods in themselves are not fattening; problems arise when you load them up with butter or deep-fry them – or, like most foods, when you eat them to excess.

Sometimes starchy foods can make you feel exceedingly sleepy, which can of course be used to your advantage in the evenings; a bowl of pasta can provide a natural alternative to sleeping pills or can help children to settle at night. The best way to test your body's reaction to carbohydrate-rich foods is to keep a food and symptom diary (see page 85).

The natural sugars found in fruits and vegetables come as a complete package with fibre, vitamins and minerals, but refined sugary foods are of very little nutritional benefit and can aggravate a host of health problems; you should keep your intake of them low.

FIBRE

In simple terms fibre is needed to:

- Stimulate the bowel to excrete waste products on a regular basis.
- Ensure that the absorption of nutrients from our foods occurs in a controlled and gradual fashion, thereby avoiding energy and mood crashes.
- Stimulate the body to produce substances that limit free-radical damage. Free radicals are highly reactive molecules produced in the body, but increased as a result of stress, pollution, including cigarette smoke, and too much sun. They increase the risk of developing cancers, heart disease and other health problems, and are a major factor in ageing.

Avocado is one of the best foods for vegetarian children; it can be introduced from the age of six months. It contains 10–15% unsaturated fat, 1–2% protein, no starch and very little sugar, a small amount of vitamin C, but useful quantities of B vitamins and vitamin E.

Five things to do with an avocado
- *Mash with a little lemon juice and seasoning. Serve on toast*
- *Slice and serve with sliced tomatoes, basil, and mozzarella cheese. Drizzle with olive oil and lemon juice*
- *Liquidize with banana and orange to make an energizing drink*
- *Fill halved avocados with a mixture of diced tomato, chopped spring onion, yoghurt and seasoning. Place in an ovenproof dish and grill for 5–10 minutes, until turning golden*
- *Mash with garlic, chopped chillies, diced tomato, lemon juice and seasoning. Serve as a dip*

Fibre is one of the most exciting areas of nutritional research, and the messages are nearly all positive. In addition to the above benefits, soluble fibre (found in fruit and vegetables, oats and pulses) is able to reduce the amount of cholesterol you absorb from food. Eating a highfibre diet can decrease your risk of developing digestive disorders, constipation, certain types of cancer and heart disease. Vibrant salads, exotic fruits, vegetable crumbles and stir-fries are just some of the delicious ways to boost your fibre in take.

The main providers of fibre in our diet are cereals (edible grains) such as wheat, corn (maize), oats and rice and foods made from them, preferably wholegrain or wholemeal types, including bread, pasta and breakfast cereals. The other great fibre providers are vegetables (including fresh or dried beans and lentils, otherwise known as pulses) and fruits.

It is important to know that if fibre is going to work efficiently in your body you need to drink at least two litres/four pints of water every day. That is the adult requirement; you should generally respond to your child's thirst and encourage them to drink a lot of fluid. Water helps the fibre to swell and carry out its functions; without water the fibre will just lie in your stomach, doing very little apart from possibly causing constipation and a clogged-up, heavy feeling.

It is generally from the teenage years onward that our bodies need to eat plenty of fibre. However, some people with digestive disorders such as Crohn's disease and some forms of irritable bowel have problems digesting certain fibrous foods. If this is the case, I suggest you keep a detailed food and symptom diary (see page 85) to try to identify which foods upset you, as I often find that patients can cope with one but not another fibrous food.

Young children generally don't need much fibre. They will receive sufficient from eating fruits and vegetables, along with small amounts of wholegrain breads and pulses. It is important not to overface children with mounds of fibre at the expense of lean proteins, some fats and foods containing natural sugars. Children under the age of six months should be given rice and potato in preference to bread, as the gluten could overload your child's immune system and cause them to develop a food allergy. See the chapter on Managing allergies.

ENERGY

The only drawback is that an excess of fibre can hinder the release of energy. This can be advantageous if you are overweight, but if you are underweight or of normal body weight and don't want to go any lower you may find that if you fill yourself up with cereal foods, pulses, vegetables and fruits you might begin to lack energy and lose a little too much weight. This can be a particular problem for vegetarians, especially vegetarian children, who can be slow to develop and grow or just tetchy and forever tired.

In order to keep your energy level up you need to include some lower fibre starches (bread, pasta, rice and other cereals); cheeses, nuts (and peanut butter), olive oil, bananas and avocados.

Pears are good weaning foods for babies, and are excellent for people with sore mouths or swallowing difficulties.

Five things to do with a pear
- *Serve with crumbly white cheese such as Wensleydale, or blue cheese such as Stilton or Roquefort*
- *Purée and serve with yoghurt*
- *Poach in red wine*
- *Slice and dip into melted plain high-quality chocolate*
- *Stew with apples and serve with vanilla custard*

In order to gain the maximum benefit from the fibre, vitamins and minerals so beautifully abundant in fruit and vegetables, it is recommended that you eat five good-sized portions of fresh fruits or vegetables every day. The type of fruit or vegetable is up to you, but you should aim to get plenty of variety. It doesn't really matter whether they are raw or cooked; a combination of the two is best.

Five portions may sound a lot, but I have plenty of ideas to make it easy to achieve. Liquidize oranges and mango to make a delicious fruit shake; mix some freshly chopped fruit in with your yoghurt; slice some ripe, flavoursome tomatoes and peppers into your sandwich; always include vegetables with your main meals, whether you choose a vegetable-based main course or soup, a starter of asparagus or artichokes, a salad for your first or main course, char-grilled or roasted vegetables, or lightly cooked vegetables tossed in a healthy dressing (see page 312). Round off each meal with a piece of fresh fruit or a portion of poached pears or fruit compote, and you've easily had five portions throughout the day.

Don't worry that vegetable hot pots and similar slow-cooked dishes may not provide much in terms of beneficial nutrients. Although some vitamins and minerals are lost with long cooking times, the benefits of the nutrients and fibre that remain outweigh the losses.

Protein

Protein is needed to help the body build strong muscles, repair tissues and maintain an effective immune and hormonal system. Proteins in the diet are broken down by digestive enzymes and absorbed into the blood as amino acids, often called the 'building blocks' of protein. These are then taken to build and repair cells, as needed. Any extra may be used for energy or stored as fat.

As far as quantity is concerned, astonishingly we only need approximately 1 gram of protein per kilo of body weight, per day. If you have a very physically active job or are involved in rigorous sports training, you may need more protein in your daily diet. Too little protein can compromise your health by stunting growth in children or losing muscle mass as we get older. A more common problem for adults in Western societies is too much protein; as with carbohydrates and fats, if you eat too much protein your body stores it as fat.

For the average adult, you need a piece of lean protein about the size of a breast of chicken for your main meal, plus an additional portion, half this size, in a smaller meal or snack. For a number of health reasons, it's best to choose a lean protein (one without noticeable fat) rather than fatty meats or products such as sausages and pies.

Vegetarians should also aim to have one portion of protein-rich food as a main meal and half a portion in a smaller meal. A portion could be 2 eggs, about 150 g/5 oz (cooked weight) of pulses, 90 g/about 3 oz of nuts or 225 g/8 oz of tofu. Vegetarians should aim to include a cereal food (such as pasta, bread and

Rice is a good source of protein for vegetarians as it contains a wide spectrum of amino acids. White rice has had its outer husks removed, consequently it has much less fibre and has also lost a proportion of its B vitamins. Brown rice contains a significant amount of both fibre and B vitamins, particularly vitamin B1 (thiamin). Don't rely on brown rice for all your protein, however, as the fibre can prevent some of the protein from being absorbed. There are many different types of rice, from long-grain, basmati and Thai rice to round-grain Italian arborio rice and pudding rice. Wild rice, although a grass and not a member of rice family, is rich in both protein and B vitamins, so it is a good plant to use within a vegetarian diet.

Another major advantage of rice over many other cereals is that it doesn't contain gluten, the protein found to upset many people. For this reason rice is a good first food for weaning children.

rice, all of which contain protein) together with another protein food (such as eggs, cheese, pulses and nuts) in both main meals and other meals/snacks.

A good intake of milk and other dairy products provides protein, calcium, vitamins B2 and B12, among other nutrients. In a typical day adults should try to include 600 ml/1 pint of milk or its equivalent.

SOURCES OF AMINO ACIDS

There are two types of amino acids: essential and non-essential. The body can produce non-essential amino acids from other sources, but essential amino acids must be obtained directly from food. You therefore need to make sure that your daily diet contains an adequate supply of essential amino acids.

Meat, poultry, game, fish and shellfish, eggs and dairy products, as well as soya products (soya milk, tofu), contain all the essential amino acids. Note that shellfish carries a high risk of setting off a food allergy in children under the age of two. Fish, however, is a good form of protein and can be given after a child is eight or nine months old.

Beans and other pulses, grains, nuts, seeds and manufactured vegetable protein foods contain protein, but don't contain all the essential amino acids. However, in combination – for example pulses with grains or pulses with nuts – they can be used by the body to meet its daily protein requirements. Some simple examples of meals that contain no animal foods include baked beans on wholegrain toast, lentil soup with wholegrain rolls, or vegetable kebabs with satay sauce (made with peanuts) and rice.

VEGETARIANS AND VEGANS

A potential problem for vegetarians lies in the way the body metabolizes carbo-hydrate and protein. If we don't eat enough carbohydrate, but eat some protein, the body can break down some of the protein into glucose, which would under normal circumstances be produced from carbohydrates. However, the body cannot make protein out of carbohydrate, so if you don't eat enough protein, it has to go without.

While some vegetarians have eggs, milk and cheese as protein sources, if you exclude all animal products you should make sure you eat a good quantity and variety of non-animal protein foods every day, to enable your body to use the proteins effectively. Don't think you have to eat beans on toast every day 'just to get your protein'; experiment with a wide range of the following foods – and above all, enjoy eating them.
- Pulses: chickpeas, lentils (red, green, brown, and the delicious Puy lentils), beans (a huge and colourful variety, including borlotti, black-eyed, haricot, cannellini, flageolet, aduki, broad, butter and kidney beans), split peas. Use them for pâtés and dips such as hummus, in soups, lentil bakes, bean burgers, curries, stews and salads.
- Soya products: soya beans, milk and cheese, tofu (bean curd).

Think good

- Cereal and grain foods: rice, pasta and noodles, bread, breakfast cereals, oatcakes, tabbouleh, millet, wheat flour or buckwheat pancakes, stuffed with sweet and savoury fillings.
- Seeds: sunflower, pumpkin and sesame seeds (including sesame seed paste, or tahini).
- Nuts: Brazils, cashews, peanuts, walnuts, hazelnuts, almonds (but see the information in the chapter on Managing allergies). Peanut butter can be spread on toast or stirred into vegetable casseroles.
- Other vegetable protein foods such as Quorn.

OILY FISH

Besides being a good source of protein, oily fish such as salmon, anchovies, mackerel, herring, trout, mullet and sardines contain beneficial oils called omega-3 fatty acid and omega-6 fatty acid, which help to prevent heart disease and some types of cancer. They have also been shown to improve skin conditions such as psoriasis. To gain maximum benefit, try to include oily fish once or twice in your weekly eating pattern.

Fat

Nearly every day we read an article or hear a discussion about fat, and rarely is it cast in a positive light. Excess fat has been linked to many health problems, from obesity to heart disease and certain types of cancer. However, some fat is essential in everyone's diet. Foods that contain fats provide not only a concentrated source of energy but also the fat-soluble vitamins A, D, E and K, which are vital in the development and maintenance of a healthy body and mind.

Fats are digested by enzymes secreted by the pancreas and gall-bladder, absorbed through the intestine and then carried to various parts of the body to fulfil specific functions such as energy production, hormone metabolism or tissue repair. The body needs to store some fat to prevent excessive loss of body heat, which is especially important with babies. People with very low fat levels, such as anorexics or serious athletes, can have problems keeping warm, which is one of the tell-tale signs that your body is struggling with your low weight. Fat is also needed to produce and carry the sex hormones testosterone, oestrogen and progesterone around the body. Too little body fat can interfere with your libido and can cause women to stop menstruating. It can also make you more prone to developing osteoporosis, a condition that causes brittle bones, particularly in women.

Some recent research suggests that fatty foods may not be quite as deadly as is sometimes claimed. American specialists proffer experimental evidence that a high-fat diet reduces the risk of ischaemic stroke. Ischaemic stroke is caused by a blockage in a blood vessel in the head or neck and accounts for about 80 per cent of all strokes. Deprived of blood, the brain is damaged, often leaving permanent impairment. In Great Britain more than 11,000 people a year suffer strokes; a third of all major strokes are fatal and another third result in disability such as paralysis. While the results of this research are not conclusive I would suggest that eating a moderate amount of fat within a healthy diet may reduce your risk of stroke. It seems that it is extremes – whether excessive use or obsessive avoidance of fat – that set your body up for disease.

The problem in Western society is that many people eat too much and very often the wrong type of fat. This is all too easily done, partly because fat carries a lot of flavour in food. Getting enough fat is rarely a problem. Besides the fats we use in cooking, there is a small amount of fat in most cereal foods, dairy products, meat and fish. The only people who expose themselves to lack of fat in their diets are those on permanent restricted diets, anorexics, and children forced to share their parents' healthy eating diets of all fruits, vegetables, whole-grain cereals and very little cheese, full-fat milk or yoghurt, or lean proteins – the 'muesli babies'. Remember that children need some fat in their diet. Cheese, butter and full-fat dairy products are perfectly healthy for children, as they can be for adults, it is just a question of quantity and balance. For adults, the balance is provided by making sure that you include plenty of fibre in your diet. It is people who grab a lump of cheese as a quick snack or needlessly put lashings of butter on vegetables who run into problems with excess body fat, high blood cholesterol and certain cancers.

Excess fat in our diet usually leads to an increase in the amount of fat deposited in the blood vessel linings; this can cause serious problems such as heart disease. Tragically, we are now starting to see early signs of heart disease in children as young as nine; their blood vessels are clogging up with fat. In the majority of cases this occurs when they live on fast food: burgers, crisps, pizzas, ready-made 'convenience' meals, chocolate bars; it is far too easy for them to over-consume the bad fats.

There are two main types of fat: saturated and unsaturated. Unsaturated fats can be further divided into mono- and polyunsaturated fats. The fact that they are metabolized in slightly different ways means that we can bring about positive health changes by choosing one type of fat in preference to another.

SATURATED FATS

These are generally considered to be the 'bad' fats. They are solid at room temperature, and come mainly from animal products such as butter, lard, suet and dripping, meat, eggs, full-fat milk, cheese and full-fat yoghurt. If you cut the soft bloomy rind off a cheese, you are effectively cutting the fat content of the cheese in half, as this is the part of the cheese with the highest percentage of fat.

Saturated fats are also found in hard margarines (hydrogenated vegetable oil), which contain trans-fatty acids (see next page). Therefore most cakes, biscuits and pastry, which are generally made with butter or hard margarine, are likely to be high in saturated fats.

Coconut oil and palm oil are also high in saturated fats.

UNSATURATED FATS

These fats are better for your body; they are generally liquid at room temperature, and come from vegetable sources, namely oils such as olive, sunflower, safflower, rapeseed, soya, grapeseed, peanut and sesame.

They are also found in soft margarines labelled 'high in polyunsaturates' and oily fish such as herring, sardines, mackerel and trout.

TRANS-FATTY ACIDS

The reason why I don't generally recommend margarines and low-fat spreads is that they often contain hydrogenated vegetable oil. Hydrogenation entails transforming the vegetable oil into a solid fat by changing its chemical structure, in other words it becomes a trans-fatty acid. It was once thought that all vegetable fats, solid or liquid, had fewer detrimental health effects than animal fats, but we now know that trans-fatty acids can cause free-radical damage within the body's cells (see page 46), linked with heart disease and cancer.

In preference to hard margarine, use a small amount of either olive oil or butter. Do keep the quantity small, though, and make sure that you have plenty of fibre and water in your diet to help your body deal with the fat.

REDUCING YOUR FAT INTAKE

We should all watch our total fat intake, whether it be from animal or vegetable sources, and keep the quantity low. When limiting your intake, don't fall into the trap of believing that just because something is sold as fat free it is healthy. This is very rarely the case with processed foods.

Unless you have a medically diagnosed cholesterol problem, choose the fat you like, whether it's butter or olive oil, but use it in small amounts. It is frequently through sheer force of habit that we use a certain quantity of fat for cooking; a small amount of fat is useful to prevent meat or vegetables from sticking and helping them to brown slightly, or for bringing out the aromas of spices, but halving the quantity will seldom reduce your appreciation of the final dish. Chargrilling, on a ridged pan or special slate that is heated to a high temperature, is a great way to cook with minimal oil; peppers, aubergines, courgettes, lean meat, breast of chicken, fresh prawns and salmon steaks all cook well this way. Steaming or microwaving produces very clean-tasting vegetables, which don't need lashings of butter. If you are frying, use a nonstick pan and add a splash of water to prevent the contents from sticking. Avoid using low-fat spreads in cooking as their water content frequently means they burn easily.

You can also keep the level of fat in your diet down by choosing lean sources of protein such as fish and shellfish, chicken, turkey, game, well-trimmed Parma, or honey roast ham, pulses and other non-meat protein sources. Trim the visible fat off beef, lamb and pork, and avoid cheap sausages and salami, pâtés and pies.

By actively cutting down on fat as much as possible, you will be able to enjoy occasional indulgences of good-quality cheese, cream or chocolate.

Water

People are often amazed at the quantity of water I suggest they drink, but when they try it they are amazed at how well they feel, once their body receives the water it so desperately needs.

While humans can survive for quite a time without food, we can only live for a few days without water. Dehydration is particularly serious in children, and must be treated urgently. In adults, a persistently dehydrated body may suffer from lethargy, poor skin, high blood cholesterol levels, urinary tract infections such as cystitis, and bowel problems such as constipation.

Water is needed to keep the body flushed of waste products; to keep the skin, hair and body organs healthy; to produce digestive enzymes; and to enable the body to glean all the essential nutrients from the food and drinks we consume. Water helps the vitamins, minerals, natural sugars and other nutrients to flow from the food into the body. In a healthy diet, water is closely associated with fibre; water helps the fibre to swell, stimulates the walls of the gut and helps to prevent constipation. If you suffer from constipation, look to water before you delve into the laxatives.

We lose water mainly through our skin and kidneys. We also lose a lot of water when we suffer from sickness, diarrhoea or any infection that causes fever. Since many of us live in centrally heated houses and work in offices with heating and air conditioning, we lose a lot more water through our skin than people in the past. Our diets also contain a lot more salt, additives and sugars than they once did, all of which place an extra strain on the body's water reserves.

Most adults should try to drink two or three litres (about four or five pints) of water every day. A two-year-old needs at least half a litre (about a pint) and a three-year-old at least three quarters of a litre (about a pint and a quarter), with more in hot weather. Urine is one of the best guides to the adequacy of fluid intake. Urine should be pale in colour and you should go to the loo regularly throughout the day. If the urine is dark, it suggests that you are not drinking enough water. If you have other symptoms such as a need to pass urine excessively, blood in the urine, pain or extreme itchiness or discomfort, it may mean that you have a urine infection which needs medical attention. When you boost your water intake the bladder will complain to begin with, and you will find yourself using the loo more frequently, but your body will soon adapt.

For people who have a poor appetite, or who need to put on weight or maximize their calorie intake, it is important not to drink large amounts of water at meal times. Water does not of itself disturb digestion, but if you fill yourself up with water it leaves less room for other foods. With digestive disorders such as a hiatus hernia or oesophagitis, when the stomach is poor at keeping in its acidic contents, having too much liquid can cause the stomach contents to leak up into the oesophagus, irritating the oesophagus walls and causing heartburn. In these cases, take small sips of water with your meal to refresh your palate, but make up your fluid requirement in between meals.

WHICH TYPE OF WATER SHOULD WE DRINK?

Mineral and spring water are ground waters, which means they landed as rain, seeped through rocks and collected in pools underground. When this water reaches the surface it can be bottled and labelled as spring water. 'Natural mineral water' is more rigidly defined and is better regulated. It has to come from a source which is naturally protected and of a constant composition and has to be free from all traces of pollution. A small amount is naturally sparkling, but most sparkling water has had carbon dioxide pumped into it. This poses no threat to health and provides a refreshing difference to still water.

Some people find the concept of paying for bottled water unnecessary and uneconomical, but others hate the taste of tap water. A water filter can remove some of the undesirable tastes, and has the advantage of producing water much lower in sodium than many bottled waters. Make sure your water filter is regularly serviced, otherwise you will be contaminating your water by passing it through an unclean filter. If you buy bottled water you should not open it then leave it in the refrigerator with the seal broken for a few days. This enables unwanted bacteria to grow, so use bottles within a day of opening.

Pure water is the best drink; it quenches thirst more effectively than other drinks. At work, choose water as a refreshing alternative to coffee or tea, and you will find that your ability to perform throughout the day is greatly enhanced.

There are many flavoured waters on the market; some of them have just a hint of flavour, which can help to add variety to the palate, but others are high in sugar and more like fruit squashes.

When you want a hot drink, there is a huge choice of herb and fruit teas and tisanes. Alternatively, make them yourself, using fresh mint leaves or a slice of root ginger (see page 343 for some ideas).

OTHER DRINKS

You should aim to drink the recommended amount of water every day, and then any fresh fruit juice or shake you drink on top of this will round up your fluid requirement. Don't overindulge on fruit juices as they contain large amounts of natural sugar, and therefore calories. A glass a day for adults and a couple of small glasses a day for children is a rough guide.

Although carbonated fizzy drinks are not bad in themselves, there are a number of traps you should look out for. First, many cola-based drinks contain caffeine, the intake of which should be restricted in any healthy eating plan (see page 50). Secondly, the majority of drinks on the market are high in sugar. The label might say dextrose, fructose, glucose or sucrose; these are all types of sugar, which can cause energy balance problems, headaches, mood swings, weight problems, tooth decay and hyperactivity in children. 'Diet' drinks contain artificial sweeteners and additives that, while not especially harmful in small amounts, unless you have an intolerance or allergy to a particular ingredient, are not as good or refreshing as simple water.

Vitamins and minerals

While I do not deny the possibility of vitamin and mineral deficiencies, it is a myth that everyone should be taking a vitamin or mineral supplement. In a few specific cases there are reasons why the body cannot receive enough of a particular mineral or vitamin, in which case there is a definite need for a supplement to be prescribed, but the common practice of taking a multivitamin just because you think it will do you good, or loading your body full of different pills, can potentially harm your body. Pills are so widely available that it is very easy to overdose. One lady carried twelve different calcium supplements into my practice, all of which she had been taking to help prevent osteoporosis. In this case, she was taking more than twelve times the recommended dose, which could have led to kidney stones and other metabolic problems.

For most healthy people there really is no need for vitamin and mineral supplements, as long as you are eating a wide range of fresh foods, eaten in a manner conducive to your body absorbing them, drinking sufficient water and not drinking excessive amounts of tea, coffee or cola-based drinks (the caffeine in these drinks inhibits the absorption and increases the excretion of vitamins and minerals). However, if you follow a restricted diet, such as avoiding dairy products, you should seek the advice of your doctor or dietitian to discuss whether you need to take a supplement.

Many people first become interested in vitamins and minerals when they have children. The current research surrounding vitamins such as folic acid alerts many women to the fact that they sometimes need to supplement their diet with a tablet. I shall discuss folic acid a little later, but generally speaking, if you are eating a well balanced diet and are healthy, you will have all the vitamins and minerals you need, and your breast milk will provide your baby with the same. Children fed on formula milk will also receive all their vitamins and minerals.

Many health professionals feel it is advisable for you to give children over six months and up to five years old a supplement that contains vitamins A, C and D. While I would not wish to criticize this, I feel it looks at a child's diet from the wrong perspective. It is so important to boost your child's intake of nutritious foods rather than be lulled into a false sense of security by giving them vitamin drops. While an orange doesn't have as much vitamin C as a mega supplement, eating an orange provides a complete package of nutrients, some natural fructose, fibre, and possibly other beneficial nutrients we will learn about in years to come. If your child is fussy I suggest you read pages 21–24; it may be necessary for you to give them a vitamin and mineral supplement to cover them while they grow out of an awkward eating stage. Never give a child more than one vitamin or mineral preparation at a time, as it can easily cause toxicity.

The suggestions that vitamin and mineral supplements can increase your child's intelligence are unfounded. As long as a child is eating a well balanced diet their brain will receive all the vitamins and minerals it needs to perform well. To check whether you, or your child, are receiving enough vitamins and minerals in your diet, draw up a vitamin check list. On the left hand side list all the vitamins and minerals this chapter talks about and then on the right hand side list foods rich in this particular nutrient that you regularly eat. In this way you will be able to highlight any shortfalls.

There are two types of vitamins: water-soluble vitamins (C and B complex) and fat-soluble (A, D, E and K). Water-soluble vitamins cannot be stored by the body, so foods containing these should be eaten daily. They can also be destroyed by overcooking, especially by boiling vegetables or fruits in lots of water. To preserve their vitamins you should try to eat these foods raw or lightly cooked.

VITAMIN A

This vitamin is essential for growth, healthy skin and hair, good vision and healthy tooth enamel. If you eat a well balanced diet you should easily receive enough vitamin A from your food. Adults need about 600–700 micrograms a day, increasing to 1000 micrograms if you are breastfeeding. Children need only 400 micrograms up to the age of four, increasing to 500 until they are eleven. At puberty it rises to the adult requirement, with men needing the higher figure. Vitamin A (also known as retinol) is found in animal products:

• liver and liver products such as pâté, kidneys; oily fish such as herring, mackerel and trout, and fish liver oils; milk, cheese (apart from low-fat cheese), butter, margarine and egg yolks.

Beta-carotene, a substance found in orange, yellow and green vegetables and fruits, is converted into vitamin A in the body. It is one of the important antioxidants (see page 46). Foods rich in beta-carotene include:

• carrots; dark green vegetables such as spinach, broccoli, cabbage, kale, Brussels sprouts and watercress; asparagus, peas and green beans, courgettes, leeks, lettuce (especially Cos lettuce), okra, parsley; tomatoes; red and yellow peppers; sweet potatoes; pumpkins; apricots and peaches (fresh and dried), mangoes, passion fruit, papayas, plums, watermelons and yellow-fleshed melons (such as cantaloupe).

Vitamin A preparations are sometimes used externally to treat skin conditions, but under no circumstances should you take a vitamin A preparation or supplement without medical supervision. Vitamin A from animal sources (retinol), if taken in excess, can build up in the liver and can cause serious damage. In the tiny liver of a baby, it does not take much to tip the delicate balance. For this reason it is best to avoid the vitamin A rich foods such as liver, pâté and cod liver oil when you are pregnant. However, plant sources have different effects and many positive health benefits; pregnant women can and should eat plenty of the orange, yellow and green vegetables and fruits.

VITAMIN B COMPLEX

The complex of B vitamins covers a group of substances including B1 (thiamin), B2 (riboflavin), B3 (nicotinic acid), folic acid, B5 (pantothenic acid), B6 (pyridoxine) and B12 (cobalamin). These vitamins are essential for the development and maintenance of a healthy nervous system. They also help digest food and convert it into energy, and are needed for the production of red blood cells. Some are used to maintain a healthy brain, immune system, skin, hair, teeth, gums, blood vessels and the lining of the nose and throat.

Several foods supply them in a package, so you don't need to become obsessed with them individually. Just for your information, recommended daily intakes (which vary depending on age, active or sedentary lifestyle, pregnancy and lactation) are as follows:

B1 (thiamin)	0.7–1.1 milligrams
B2 (riboflavin)	1.3–1.8 milligrams
B3 (nicotinic acid)	15–21 milligrams
B6 (pyridoxine)	1.2–1.4 milligrams
B12 (cobalamin)	1.5 micrograms
Folate (folic acid)	200–500 micrograms

B5 has no recommended allowance, but a suggested safe intake is 3–7 milligrams. In a regular, well balanced diet you should get enough of the B vitamins, but since B12 is found mainly in foods of animal origin (including milk and cheese), and lack of this vitamin may cause a form of anaemia, vegans may need to take a vitamin B complex supplement. The reason for taking a general B complex supplement is that B vitamins help each other to be absorbed. See your dietitian or doctor before you proceed. Some soya milks are fortified with vitamins B12 and B2; this can be very helpful for vegans and is one of the few instances where I support the action of food manufacturers. Many breakfast cereals are also fortified with B vitamins; these can be useful as long as they are not too sugary.

There has been a lot of interest in the role that the B vitamins, especially B6, play in the alleviation of pre-menstrual tension. Unfortunately the studies are inconclusive and can encourage women to take unnecessary vitamins, potentially causing toxicity. Vitamin B6 toxicity gives symptoms of extreme lethargy, numbness in the fingers and toes and lack of appetite, as well as liver problems.

Instead of taking supplements, I recommend that you eat foods rich in the B vitamins. The highest concentrations are found in liver, kidneys and yeast extract, but since the majority of us don't eat these in large quantities, I suggest you boost your intake of the following foods:

- meat, especially meat juices (so use them in sauce or gravy); milk, yoghurt, cheese; eggs; fish; brown rice, other wholegrain cereals, wheatgerm; green vegetables such as asparagus, broccoli, spinach; potatoes; nuts; pulses; bananas; dried fruits such as apricots, dates, figs.

FOLIC ACID

Folic acid is needed to create healthy blood cells, therefore if lacking in the diet it can cause anaemia. In addition it is needed to enable the body to absorb iron, itself a vital nutrient for strong blood; lack of iron results in the most common form of anaemia, iron-deficiency anaemia. Recent research has also shown an association between low levels of folic acid and an increased risk of athero-sclerosis, furring of the arteries.

Various medications such as aspirin and birth control pills hinder the absorp-tion of folic acid. This can slightly complicate things for people who take an aspirin a day to reduce the likelihood of heart disease, while women at risk of atherosclerosis, such as smokers, and those with anaemia should consider changing to another form of contraception; ask your doctor for advice.

Since it is such an important vitamin, you should concentrate on ensuring the foods you eat are rich in folic acid. The major sources of folic acid in the diet are:
• green leafy vegetables such as Savoy cabbage, spring greens, Brussels sprouts, curly kale, spinach, asparagus; fresh orange juice; wheatgerm (found in whole-meal bread and cereals).

One of the major concerns is that the folic acid content of food diminishes with time. It is at its highest when the food is first picked, but the majority of us rely on foods that have travelled from further afield than the garden, so that by the time we get them the folic acid content may be low. Eat folic acid rich foods as soon after buying as possible. In order to maximize the folic acid content we should keep cooking time to a minimum – think salads, stir-fries and lightly steamed vegetables rather than casseroles simmered in the oven for hours.

In pregnancy, when the body is rapidly producing new cells, your requirement for folic acid increases. Folic acid deficiency has been linked with birth defects, and this is another case where I concur with the advice that women should take a folic acid supplement for three months before and after conception. However, I do not believe that popping a pill is the only answer. Everyone should look to their diet, as the more folic acid we can get from natural sources the healthier our bodies will be.

VITAMIN C

Vitamin C is needed for growth and healthy body tissue, and is important in the healing of wounds. In addition, it helps the body to absorb iron, a very import-ant mineral (see page 43). Vitamin C (also known as ascorbic acid) is one of the best-known antioxidant vitamins (see page 46) and may prevent or reduce the severity of the common cold. The recommended daily intake is 60 milligrams, and consuming more than 1000 milligrams a day can be of no real benefit unless your body has a greater-than-average need for vitamin C, for example if you smoke (see page 51). Vitamin C is a water-soluble vitamin and the body cannot store excess amounts. Therefore, if you consume more than 1000 milligrams a day your body will simply excrete it. I sometimes find that people who take excess vitamin C suffer from sensitive and irritable stomachs and mouth ulcers (vitamin C is, after all, ascorbic acid). So instead of taking a pill at breakfast time it would be much better to eat a couple of kiwi fruits, squeeze an orange, or make a fruit shake (see page 342).

The main sources of vitamin C in the diet are fresh fruit and vegetables; if you eat five portions of fruit and vegetables every day your body's requirements will easily be met. An average bowl of strawberries contains about 70–120 milligrams of vitamin C; a kiwi fruit or a helping of steamed broccoli contains about 50 milligrams; and a large orange contains 70 milligrams.

- Besides broccoli, other vegetables rich in vitamin C are: spinach, curly kale, Brussels sprouts, spring greens, cabbage, cauliflower, red, green and yellow peppers, watercress, potatoes (especially new potatoes in their skins), green peas and mangetout.
- Fruits high in vitamin C, besides oranges, strawberries and kiwis, include: grapefruit and other citrus fruits, blackcurrants, rosehips, guava, mango, papaya, lychees, raspberries, nectarines and peaches.

One of the reasons why so many people choose to take a vitamin C supplement is because they fear that there will be very little of the vitamin left by the time they eat fruits and vegetables that may have endured long journeys – oranges from South Africa, lemons from Spain – and possibly spent weeks in cold storage.

While vitamin C content does diminish with time, I still believe that if we shop regularly and conscientiously, following natural seasons as much as possible, we should be able to glean sufficient vitamin C from our diet without resorting to a supplement.

The way in which you prepare food also affects its vitamin C content. There is very little difference in the vitamin C content of raw and lightly cooked foods; problems occur if you put vegetables on to boil and forget about them, as by the time you eat them all the vitamin C will have dissolved in the water. Keep the cooking time down to a minimum: stir-fry, steam, or boil just until *al dente*, in other words they retain plenty of texture when you bite into them.

Surprisingly, there can be quite a lot of vitamin C in frozen and tinned fruits and vegetables. This comes as a great relief to parents who find shopping for fresh vegetables and fruits daily an impossible task. The time that elapses between the food being picked and frozen or tinned is often a lot shorter than the time it takes for so-called 'fresh' foods to get from field to shop or market stall. So stocking up your cupboards and freezer is a good way of ensuring you and your family can eat healthily with little fuss.

Some food producers add vitamin C to foods which have been heavily processed. This is why you will find ascorbic acid on the labels of some foods. I support the addition of vitamins to foods, where it is appropriate to replace whatever has been lost, but clearly, fresh nutritious produce is the best option.

VITAMIN D

Vitamin D (also known as calciferol) works in conjunction with the mineral calcium (see page 42); both are essential for healthy bones and teeth. Although vitamin D is found in a few foods, it is chiefly made by the skin in the presence of sunlight. This is one of the reasons why you should try to get out in the fresh air every day, if possible. This is particularly important for young children who are in their active growth spurt, but also for people suffering from osteoporosis or who are generally frail.

Patients who have to spend a lot of time resting in bed can quite easily suffer from a poor vitamin D status; for them, it is important to look to foods rich in vitamin D. These include:

• oily fish such as tuna, mackerel, sardines; cod liver oil; liver; eggs; butter and margarine, cheese, milk, yoghurt.

Vegans should be aware that manufactured products sometimes contain animal-derived vitamin D. You can obtain a list of animal-free products from The Vegetarian Society (address on page 352).

VITAMIN E

Vitamin E is needed to help develop and maintain strong cells, especially in the blood. It is one of the group of antioxidant vitamins (see page 46) which have been shown to decrease the risk of heart disease and some cancers. Many people feel, especially my male patients who are worried about the prospect of a heart attack, that they need to take an antioxidant tablet containing vitamin E, but this is unnecessary. The suggested safe intake of 3–4 milligrams a day is easily obtained from a well-balanced diet that includes vitamin E rich foods such as:

• avocados, blackberries, mangoes, tomatoes, sweet potatoes, spinach, watercress; nuts and seeds; wheatgerm and wholegrain cereal; soft margarine and vegetable oils such as sunflower, safflower, corn and olive.

VITAMIN K

The role of this vitamin is mainly that of helping the blood clot to the naturally healthy degree, and maintaining strong bones. Many hospitals routinely give vitamin K (by injection or by mouth) to new-born babies, as the young body does not have an adequate quantity.

It is found in small quantities in most vegetables and wholegrain cereals, but we mainly produce it in our guts, with the aid of healthy bacteria. These bacteria also produce substances that help to prevent cancer and heart disease.

Various drugs such as antibiotics and antifungals tend to kill these bacteria, but you can replenish your stores by eating live yoghurt containing acidophilus and bifidus. People with irritable bowel and other digestive problems should be aware that live yoghurt has been known to cause adverse reactions in some sensitive guts. Discuss the issue with your doctor or dietitian.

Processes such as colonic irrigation can easily destroy the balance of healthy bacteria in the gut; if you need this, perhaps because of severe constipation, it should be done no more often than every two to three months, and always under strict medical guidance.

CALCIUM

Calcium is essential for strong, healthy bones and teeth. Lack of calcium has been linked with the development of osteoporosis, a condition that causes brittle bones. Although this usually affects post-menopausal women, everyone will benefit from a diet that meets their calcium requirement throughout childhood and into adulthood.

The primary source of calcium in the diet is dairy produce. The daily requirement is around 550 milligrams a day for children up to the age of eleven, 1,000 milligrams a day for teenagers and pregnant women, 800 milligrams a day for other adults. To put this into perspective, 250 ml/½ pint of cows' milk or 150 g/ 5 oz of yoghurt contains 300 milligrams of calcium.

You can easily obtain sufficient calcium if you incorporate some milk and other dairy products in drinks and everyday cooking. A glass of milk or a warm milky drink at the end of the day is an excellent way to get children to meet their requirement, and can help them to sleep. You can use milk's soporific properties yourself (although it is not the best way to tackle indigestion; see page 158 for advice). All milk, from skimmed to rich Jersey milk, including goats' and sheep's milk, is high in calcium; so are most types of cheese and cream, but some of these are also high in fat, so watch the quantities. Yoghurt is also a good source; ideally it should be 'live', containing acidophilous and bifidus, as this has other health benefits (see page 47).

If you can't eat dairy products for any reason, other food sources include:
• green leafy vegetables such as spinach, curly kale, watercress, broccoli; okra; tofu; pulses; dried figs and apricots; oysters, canned fish with soft, edible bones (sardines, salmon, pilchards and mackerel); sesame seeds and tahini (sesame seed paste, used to make hummus); almonds, Brazils, hazelnuts. There are also calcium-enriched soya milks and cheeses, which are worth exploring. Breads and flour, especially white flour, is sometimes enriched with calcium.

However, you need to eat a lot more of these foods, other than white bread, because they contain 'salts', chemical substances that bind the calcium and reduce the amount that can be absorbed into your blood. It is doubtful that the majority of people would be able to meet their daily requirement of calcium from non-dairy sources alone. In this situation, therefore, you should seek professional advice about meeting the shortfall with a supplement. There are many different calcium supplements on the market and it is important to check with your doctor or dietitian before you choose one because several medical conditions, including kidney problems, can be aggravated by supplements. If you are taking a supplement, you should try to ensure that your calcium intake is around 1000 milligrams a day, rather than the 800 milligrams recommended above. The reason for the difference is that the body does not absorb as much from a supplement. You should still eat as many calcium-rich foods as possible.

It is important to look beyond the calcium level in your supplement or diet, as the amount your body absorbs can also be affected by factors such as vitamin D and vitamin C intake, smoking and caffeine.

Don't forget that dairy foods provide not only calcium but also vitamins B12 and B2 (see page 38). If you feel you need to make up a shortfall in B vitamins, yeast extract (Marmite) can be used in savoury dishes such as lentil bakes as well as a snack on bread. However, yeast extract is rather high in salt and hence sodium. Sodium can adversely affect your body's ability to maintain strong healthy bones, so it is best to keep the quantity down and make sure you eat plenty of calcium-rich foods.

IRON

Iron is needed for healthy blood and muscles; lack of iron leads to a common form of anaemia (see page 275). Your body's daily requirement for iron varies between 8 and 15 milligrams a day; most women need 12–15 milligrams, men need slightly less, since they don't suffer from menstrual-related iron losses. Some men who have health problems which predispose them to an increased risk of bleeding, such as ulcers or piles, should make sure that their diet is generally high in iron, so that their body is better prepared for the loss of iron, should it occur. Equally if you are recovering from a loss of blood you should boost your iron intake. Children need increasing amounts of iron as they grow, as they are producing more and more healthy cells.

Pregnant women need more iron, to supply cells to the womb, placenta and the developing baby. The baby will very rarely suffer from lack of iron, as it takes the iron from the mother's body. So if you don't have good stores of iron before you become pregnant you may suffer from lack of iron by the time you get to the end of the pregnancy.

At birth, babies need only a small amount of iron as they have laid down stores that will last them for three to four months; one of the primary functions of weaning children is to bring more iron into their diet.

There are two main types of iron in food: haem iron, from lean red meat and offal; and non-haem iron, derived from some plants, grains and nuts. Unfortunately the vegetable sources of iron also contain 'salts' (oxalates and phytates) – substances that obstruct the absorption of iron, meaning that your body cannot use the iron from these sources as effectively. You therefore need to eat a lot more of them to obtain sufficient iron. Egg yolks and oily fish are quite rich in iron, but they too contain substances that prevent the body from absorbing it efficiently. The body can absorb between 20 and 40 per cent of the iron from meat, but only 5–20 per cent of the iron available from vegetable sources. If we eat a mixed diet including vegetables, fruits, meat and fish we are thought to absorb approximately 15–20 per cent of the iron in our food.

In addition to iron, the body needs both vitamin C and folic acid in order to absorb and utilize the iron. Try to include some good sources of these nutrients (see pages 39 and 40) in the same meal as your source of iron. It's a good idea to get into the habit of having a glass of freshly squeezed orange or tomato juice before a meal or a piece of fresh fruit afterwards.

Another step you can take to increase the amount of iron and other nutrients that are available to your body is to make sure that there is nothing in your diet to hinder their absorption. Two of the leading offenders are tannin and caffeine – found in tea, coffee, chocolate and cola-based drinks. If you must drink these, do so between meals – don't round a meal off with a cup of tea or coffee.

Some people with digestive problems such as chronic constipation, irritable bowel or Crohn's disease can have slightly disrupted iron absorption. If you have any bowel problem you should ask your dietitian or doctor for advice.

- The primary source of iron is lean red meat, game, liver and kidney. Pregnant women should avoid offal, as it contains too much vitamin A (see page 37).
- Other iron providers include: eggs (avoid giving egg whites before the age of one year; cooked egg yolks – which are in any case the source of iron – may be given once your baby is established on a mixed diet at the age of eight or nine months); spinach, curly kale, watercress, broccoli, Savoy cabbage and other dark green leafy vegetables; lentils, beans (including baked beans) and peas; oily fish such as tuna, mackerel and sardines; oysters; dried fruits (especially figs, raisins, apricots and prunes); canned blackcurrants; wholegrain cereals and wholemeal bread; black treacle; nuts; liquorice and plain chocolate.

MAGNESIUM

This mineral has a variety of functions in the body, including the release of energy, building strong bones, teeth and muscles, and regulating body temperature. It also helps the body absorb and metabolize various other vitamins and minerals such as calcium and vitamin C. Magnesium deficiency can cause anxiety, irritability, high blood pressure and in extreme cases, heart attacks. Good sources of magnesium include:

- wholegrain cereal products such as wholemeal and granary bread, wholewheat pasta, brown rice; nuts and seeds; pulses; green leafy vegetables, okra, peas, sweetcorn, courgettes, parsnips; milk, yoghurt; lean meat; dried figs, apricots, raisins; bananas.

POTASSIUM

This mineral works with sodium to regulate the body's water balance, heart rhythm, nerve impulses and muscle function. Potassium and sodium levels within the body behave rather like a pair of scales. When the potassium level increases the sodium level decreases and vice versa. It is generally a good idea to make sure that your potassium intake is substantial, because most of us consume too much sodium in the form of salt. An increase in the sodium level can cause the body to retain fluid, which may result in puffy eyes, swollen ankles and a generally bloated feeling. A low potassium intake can ultimately cause high blood pressure or your heart to beat erratically, a condition known as arrhythmias. Some medication can cause the body to lose excessive amounts of potassium, for example loop diuretics and antihypertensive drugs. This may be a problem for elderly people, as they frequently have to take numerous tablets. In this instance it is especially important to boost the potassium intake. Glasses of freshly squeezed orange juice, banana sandwiches, and small bowls of dried fruits to nibble on are all good ways to increase potassium intake. While elderly people may need a potassium supplement, this should only be taken under the guidance of their doctor. Good sources of potassium include:

• potatoes, bananas and other fresh fruit, orange juice, dried apricots, prunes.

ZINC

Zinc has many functions in the body, including the maintenance of a healthy immune system. Deficiency may result in lack of appetite, skin problems, slow healing of wounds, and sexual problems ranging from low libido to sterility and birth defects. Zinc deficiency is most common in women who have been taking the contraceptive pill, as the pill inhibits the absorption of zinc and causes the body to excrete more. Everyone, whether male or female, young or old, should try to include some zinc in their daily eating plan, and it is particularly important if you have just come off the pill or you are run down or unwell in any way.

As with other minerals and vitamins, many people think that they can improve their health by boosting their diet with a zinc supplement. This is not the case: over and above the recommended daily allowance of 15 milligrams, zinc supplements can actually make your body more susceptible to bacterial infections. This is important to bear in mind if you have a blood test to screen for vitamin and mineral deficiencies. You may be told you're zinc deficient, but this could be because in certain circumstances the body purposely lowers your blood zinc level so that you don't get a secondary infection. There are cases for zinc supplements, but they need individual advice. The majority of people simply need to include the following zinc sources in a well balanced diet:

• shellfish such as oysters, crab, mussels, lobster; canned sardines; turkey, duck, goose; lean meats such as beef, lamb, gammon, pork, venison; liver and kidneys; Parmesan and other hard or crumbly cheeses such as Cheddar, Stilton, Cheshire; eggs; wholegrain breads and brown rice.

Additional sources for vegetarians are:

• nuts and seeds (including peanut butter and tahini); wheatgerm and wholegrain cereals; pulses (dried peas, beans and lentils); fresh peas, watercress, spinach, asparagus; dried apricots, figs, raisins; passion fruit.

SELENIUM

Selenium is needed in tiny, but regular amounts, for maintaining a healthy liver, and as an antioxidant (see below). It is found in many foods, such as fruits and vegetables, but the selenium content of foods varies depending on the soil in which they are grown; some parts of the world are known to be deficient, and its inhabitants are advised to take supplements. In other countries, such as Britain, modern farming practices have reduced the amount of selenium found in the produce, which has led some interested parties to advocate a supplement.

Based on current research there is no call for this, as even the reduced levels of selenium are adequate for our nutritional needs.

• Selenium is also found in Brazil nuts, cashew nuts, sunflower seeds, whole-wheat bread, milk, hard and crumbly cheeses, eggs, chicken, lean meat and offal, fish and shellfish.

OTHER MINERALS

Other nutrients are vital to the body, but in such small amounts that they will almost certainly be provided by the food we eat. Some are dangerous in high doses, either in themselves, or because they block the actions of other minerals or vitamins. They include phosphorous, copper, manganese, boron, molybdenum, chromium and iodine.

Antioxidants

In recent years there has been a lot of exciting research into antioxidants, and their health-giving, disease-preventing properties. Antioxidants are a group of substances that includes vitamins C and E, along with beta-carotene, which the body converts into vitamin A, and the minerals selenium and zinc. Antioxidants are believed to reduce your likelihood of developing cancer and heart disease, as well as other diseases of ageing, such as arthritis and cataracts. They do this in several ways: by boosting the immune system, producing anti-cancer substances, preventing blood fats from oxidizing and depositing in the blood vessels (see the chapter on High blood cholesterol), and through their 'antioxidant' activity. Our bodies need oxygen, but the process of oxidation can be harmful, because it results in the unstable molecules known as free radicals. These molecules interact with those that make up our body's cells, causing damage that can lead to cancers and other 'diseases of modern living'. The reason we give them this name is that, while the process of oxidation has always gone on, our bodies are now producing far more free radicals as a result of stress, environmental pollution – including cigarette smoke and car exhaust fumes – and exposure to too much ultra-violet light from the sun.

Despite this apparently gloomy picture, there is no need to grab a supplement. The body responds far better to an all-round antioxidant-rich diet that includes plenty of the foods listed below vitamins A, C and E. This is the main reason we are so often urged to make sure we eat at least five portions of fruit and vegetables every day. Fruits and vegetables also contain another type of antioxidant, called bioflavonoids. These are particularly concentrated in the peel, skin or outer layers of plants. Citrus fruits such as oranges, tangerines, clementines, grapefruit, lemons and limes are good sources of bioflavonoids.

Bacteria

Bacteria are by no means all bad. The healthy gut contains colonies of bacteria that serve a number of functions. As I have already mentioned, these bacteria are the principle producers of vitamin K. They also produce a certain amount of energy. Most interestingly, they seem to produce substances that may be beneficial in preventing many diseases, including heart disease and cancer, and generally improving our immune system.

With this in mind I suggest that we should include some bacteria in our daily diet. This is particularly important when you have been taking antibiotics, as antibiotics kill the good bacteria that live in the gut and expose it to an over-growth of 'bad' bacteria, which can cause irritable bowels, thrush and fatigue. Diets rich in fatty and sugary foods can also adversely change the balance of gut bacteria. In addition, the good bacteria are frequently bombarded by pesticides and additives in foods.

The two gut bacteria which appear to be the front runners are acidophilus and bifidus. Taking in regular quantities of these bacteria helps to replenish stocks and redress the balance. Bowel symptoms frequently disappear as soon as you do this.

You can take acidophilus and bifidus in various forms, but I think they are most easily and effectively absorbed from natural yoghurt. Look out for the 'live' or 'bio' yoghurts containing these substances. A good daily dosage would be 20 milligrams, which provides around 20 million live organisms. This quantity can usually be found in a small pot of yoghurt. Alternatively you could ask your dietitian to suggest another source.

A word of warning; people who have a sensitive immune system or gut, including those with irritable bowel syndrome, Crohn's disease or arthritis, should seek advice from their doctor before taking these bacteria, as they are potentially irritating to the gut in certain cases.

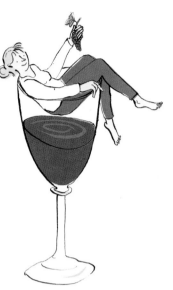

Habits – good and bad

Alcohol

It has become apparent from recent research that not only does alcohol taste good, it also does you good. However, it's not just a question of the more you drink the healthier you will be. In the UK, the Health Education Authority recommends that women drink no more than 21 units of alcohol a week, men no more 28 units – a unit being a glass of wine or half-pint of beer. It is also advisable to have one or two alcohol-free days a week.

Some people either cannot or should not drink alcohol. If you are taking certain medication, you may be told that it will not respond in the presence of alcohol. People with hepatitis or raised liver enzymes, detected in blood tests carried out by a doctor, may be advised to go without alcohol for three months or longer. Some people simply feel bad when they drink alcohol – it just doesn't suit them. They feel hung over after a single glass or develop allergic reactions such as urticaria (nettle rash) or migraine. Young children have very sensitive hearts, lungs, livers and brains, which can be seriously affected by alcohol. If they accidentally drink alcohol they should never be left to sleep it off, but should be taken to casualty immediately for treatment. For teenagers, I think the French have the right idea when they introduce wine in diluted form; it teaches young people the correct use of alcohol, as a pleasant adjunct to a sociable meal.

BENEFITS

The most well-documented benefit of alcohol is the effect of antioxidants on our blood fats. Of all alcoholic drinks, red wine contains the most antioxidants. In simple terms, antioxidants have a protective effect on our overall health. As our body uses oxygen, it creates by-products known as free radicals (free radicals are also produced as a result of stress, too much sun, and environmental pollution, including cigarette smoke). While a few free radicals are necessary to the body, too many will cause damage to cell walls, which can result in heart disease, certain cancers, arthritis, cataracts and ageing of the skin. Antioxidants (which include vitamins A, C and E, minerals such as selenium and zinc, and other compounds, such as the anthocyanin and tannin found in red wine) can 'fight' the free radicals and prevent cellular damage.

Other antioxidant compounds are being researched; some are found in all wine, others are present in far greater amounts in specific wines. Flavonoids found in grape skins, for example, may offer some protection against cancer – the effect will be less powerful in Beaujolais Nouveau, which is relatively low in flavonoids and tannin because the grape skins remain in contact with the juice for a very short time. Other antioxidant compounds include resveratrol,

quercetin, catechin and rutin, which have been demonstrated to help prevent
cancer of the digestive tract. These seem to be higher in red wines grown in
cooler, damper climates, and those made with the Pinot Noir or Pinotage grape.
Resveratrol can also reduce the risk of thrombosis and atherosclerosis.

Apart from the antioxidant effects, regular moderate drinking of any sort
of alcohol can reduce stress and blood pressure and can therefore reduce the
likelihood of heart disease. Moderate drinking has also been shown to increase
the proportion of HDL in the blood (HDL is the 'good' form of cholesterol,
which escorts 'bad' LDL cholesterol back to the liver where it can be recycled
or destroyed) and therefore reduces the incidence of heart disease (see page 256).

Beers, like wines, vary in their health benefits: dark brown beers contain
more flavonoids than light beers, but not as many as wine.

THE DOWNSIDE

If taken in excess, alcohol has many health-hindering effects. Too much alcohol
of any sort can cause cardiomyopathy (disease of the heart muscle), cirrhosis of
the liver and an increase in the 'bad' blood fats – triglycerides and LDL. Too
much alcohol can also adversely affect bone marrow, and the blood's ability to
clot and heal. It can also be psychologically addictive.

Too much alcohol can also affect your sex life. While a tipple can release
stress and remove inhibitions, it tends to make you very tired, and too much
affects men by anaesthetising the nerves in the penis; in women it can decrease
their ability to orgasm. If men consume alcohol to excess over a long period it
can lead to testicular atrophy, shrinkage of the penis and an increase in breast
size. Too much alcohol not only causes a beer belly, it can decrease the level of
testosterone in the body, and increase the level of oestrogen (in men!), both of
which decrease libido and the production of sperm.

People metabolize and tolerate alcohol differently: some can drink copious
amounts before feeling the effects, while others sway after a single glass. One
of the major factors that influences how your body responds to alcohol is food.
Drinking on an empty stomach causes the alcohol to whizz through the stomach
into the duodenum (the first part of the small intestine) where the absorption
is rapid, so the effect of the alcohol is greatly increased. Food helps to keep the
alcohol in the stomach, and slows down its absorption.

Alcohol also increases your appetite by lowering your blood sugar level.
Alcohol prevents sugar that is normally stored in the liver from being used by
the body. This interrupts the body's natural blood sugar control cycle, and means
that your blood sugar level drops soon after you drink alcohol. The result is that
you feel hungry. While this can be advantageous for people with poor appetites,
for the majority of people it causes them to lose control over what they are
eating and how much they need to eat before they feel full. It also causes weight
gain because it provides calories without supplying any useful nutrients (apart
from the antioxidants in red wine). Drinking on an empty stomach can cause

Ginger tea punch

This iced ginger punch is very refreshing and perfect for unsettled tummies.

Makes 12 glasses

900 ml/1½ pints boiling water
8 Assam tea bags
2 teaspoons caster sugar
4 tablespoons peeled and grated fresh ginger
1 litre/1¾ pints sparkling mineral water
20 ice cubes

Pour the boiling water into a large jug and stir in the tea bags, sugar and ginger. Leave to infuse for 8 minutes, then take out the tea bags.

Leave the tea to cool, then cover and chill in the refrigerator for 1–2 hours. Strain the tea through a coffee filter, or a sieve lined with kitchen paper, into a serving jug or punch bowl. Stir in the mineral water, and serve in long glasses with ice cubes.

energy levels to crash, leaving you feeling shattered. If you are aware that your energy levels tend to fluctuate you should definitely take your drink with food, as this helps to cushion the effects of the alcohol.

HANGOVER CURES

Contrary to popular belief, strong black coffee is about the worst thing you can consume as it dehydrates the body even further. Both caffeine and alcohol stimulate the kidneys to produce more diuretic hormones. Drink as much water as you can throughout the day.

The best morning-after cure is to eat some breakfast consisting of carbohydrate foods such as cereal or toast, along with a glass of fresh fruit juice and an analgesic if necessary. If you can't face eating, mix a teaspoon of honey into a glass of fresh juice to help bring your blood sugar up to an acceptable level.

Prevention is better than cure: drinking water before you go to bed is one way to reduce a hangover. Eating something small, even if it's just a piece of fruit or bread, before you go out also helps.

Coffee and tea

Throughout the book, you will find me warning against excessive tea and coffee drinking. It is not that I am totally against these drinks, rather that the way many people drink them leaves a lot to be desired. Often, it is out of sheer force of habit. How many people do you know who can't start the day without two or three cups of tea or coffee? Or who accept cups of coffee or tea without thinking in business meetings or on social occasions? These people are not enjoying aromatic coffee or refreshing tea, whereas if they limited themselves to two or three cups a day they would be able to look forward to and appreciate the experience.

Problems arise because the caffeine in coffee and tea (and in cola drinks) is mildly addictive, the more you drink the more you want. If you have more than two or three cups of caffeine-containing drink a day, the caffeine in your body becomes excessive and inhibits the absorption of vitamins and minerals, leaving you, at best, sapped of energy, at worst, suffering from a deficiency of vital nutrients.

Good coffee can be enjoyed within a healthy lifestyle. You just need to make sure that you choose a good coffee and don't drink too much, or you risk upsetting the balance of vitamin and mineral absorption.

DECAFFEINATED COFFEE

Patients sometimes ask whether they should drink decaffeinated coffee, since it is excess caffeine that is bad for you? The problem here is that the majority of decaffeinated coffee is made using a chemical solvent to remove the caffeine. Not only does this not taste so good, but these chemicals are potentially carcinogenic.

Consumer outcry has led many coffee companies to seek alternative decaffeination techniques, and they have developed the water method and the carbon

Think good

dioxide method. Both are currently more expensive – but produce fine-tasting coffee. Look out for them in speciality coffee shops; the decaffeinated coffee you find in supermarkets is most likely to be a solvent type, unless it is labelled water method or carbon dioxide (CO_2) method. Decaffeinated tea is subject to the same techniques.

Refresh your thirst with water or herbal tea. There are so many delicious herbal teas in the shops, you should be able to find some that you really like. See page 343 for more caffeine-free drinks.

Smoking

Sadly smoking is still sometimes portrayed as glamorous or 'cool'. There is nothing cool about cancer, asthma, red eyes and wrinkles. Smoking has been shown to be a risk factor in sudden infant deaths, asthma, heart disease and many sorts of cancers. Even if you decide to ignore these facts, you should bear in mind that smoking also drains the body of many essential vitamins and minerals. This affects not only smokers themselves but everyone in contact with smoky environments.

A smoke filled body is less efficient at absorbing and retaining nutrients than a smoke free body. The major nutrient to be hit is vitamin C. The more you smoke, the more vitamin C you lose from your tissues and blood. The damage smoke inflicts on your cells causes your body to need more vitamin C to counter-act this damage. You don't need me to point out that smokers are more likely to smoke a cigarette between meals than to eat a piece of fruit, so it is relatively easy to deprive your body of the vitamin C it so desperately needs. Smokers lose out on the beneficial effects of vitamin C because they need more, but eat less, absorb less and excrete more.

Since vitamin C is one of the major antioxidants (see page 46) which has been linked to the prevention of cancer, cigarette smokers are at a much greater risk of developing cancer as a result of poor antioxidant intake and damage to the cells inflicted by the smoke. The main organs to be exposed to an increased risk of cancer are the lungs, stomach, mouth, breast and cervix.

In order to try to counteract the disturbance in vitamin C metabolism, a smoker's requirement for vitamin C increases to approximately 2000 mg a day. See page 40 for the vitamin C rich foods. However, it would be almost impossible to get this amount from food alone – you will need to take a vitamin C supplement.

If you cannot give up, which of course would be the greatest favour you could do yourself and everyone around you, you must make sure that you eat plenty of fresh vegetables and fruits every day as part of a generally healthy diet, to help minimize the damage.

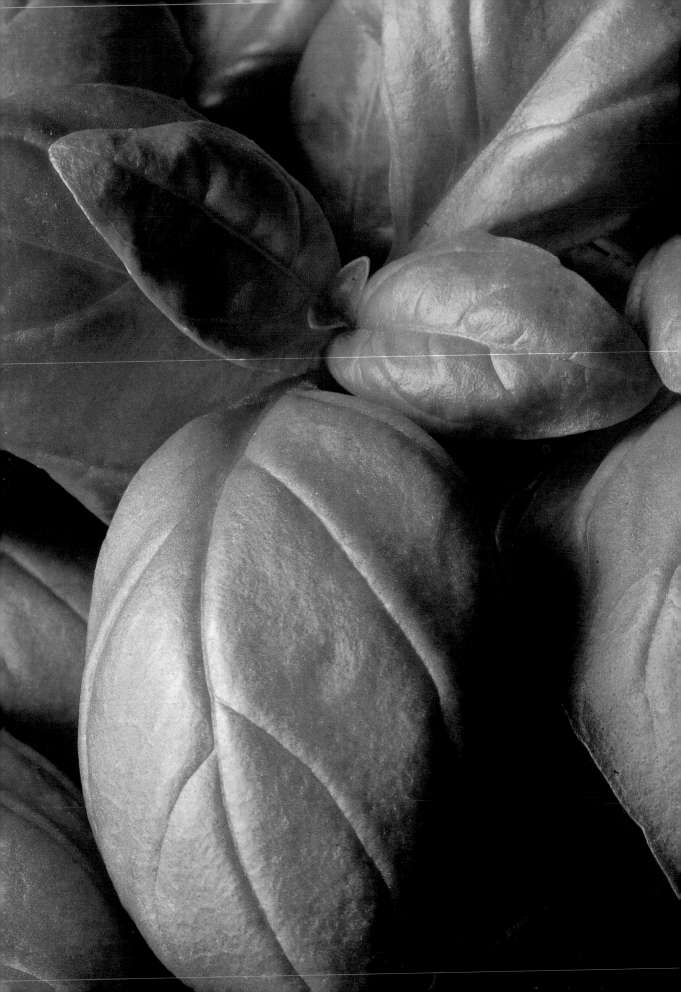

Discovering real food

In choosing real, fresh, unadulterated food over processed and ready-made meals you will be doing your body a huge favour. Not only are the nutrients in real food 'packaged' in the way that nature intended, but also the body will not have to deal with additives that it was not designed to digest.

Fruit and vegetables

Food always tastes better in season. This is particularly true when it comes to fruits and vegetables. Nutritionally there is a huge advantage to choosing fruits and vegetables according to their local season, because the majority of vitamins and minerals fade with time, so the sooner you can eat them after they have been harvested, the higher the nutritional value.

Unfortunately it is often very difficult to notice when things are in season; these days the shops, markets and supermarkets are full of all kinds of items, throughout the year. Buyers scour the world for climates that can produce the fruits and vegetables when our climate can't. The problem is further complicated by the fact that some fruits and vegetables can be stored for a very long time (up to eight months!) before they appear on our shelves as 'fresh'. Until there is legislation to force growers and vendors to tell us when they were picked, our search for genuinely fresh food will remain problematic.

However, there are a few rules of thumb to help you. Seasons in the northern hemisphere are the mirror image of those in the southern hemisphere. For example, apples grown in Britain traditionally crop in autumn (September to October); South African apples crop in their autumn, in May to July. So if you are buying apples in July, choose a southern hemisphere apple such as a South African or New Zealand apple, rather than a British or French.

Developments in glasshouse horticulture have extended local growing seasons, and some fruits and vegetables are now available through the majority of the year. While this produce has the advantage of less distance to travel, it rarely tastes as good and tends to be more expensive than fruit and vegetables grown in healthy soil and sunlight in their natural season.

Herbs

These days the selection of fresh herbs available in the shops is fantastic. Supermarkets sell herbs growing in pots, which stay fresh longer than packs of cut herbs, but if you can grow your own herbs this is the best scenario, as you can pick what you need and they couldn't be any fresher. Fresh herbs have a range of wonderful flavours, some subtle, some vibrant; if you are looking to replace salt, butter and cream in your diet, herbs add variety to all kinds of dishes.

Dried herbs have their uses, but remember that they do not last for ever; they fade with time, heat and light, so buy just a small amount and keep them in dark, airtight jars in a cool place.

Shellfish

Shellfish are divided into two groups: crustaceans, such as crabs, lobsters, prawns and shrimps, which have jointed shells; and molluscs, such as mussels, oysters and scallops, which have hinged shells.

Fresh seafood has a reputation as an aphrodisiac: this is partly due to the suggestive appearance or method of eating some shellfish, but they are also rich in zinc, one of the main minerals involved in sustaining a healthy libido. Zinc also helps to maintain a strong immune system, so seafood is one of the healthiest of foods, besides being low in fat.

Unfortunately some people cannot enjoy seafood because their body produces an 'allergic' reaction. Many of my patients are puzzled as to why it happens with some shellfish and not others, or why they can sometimes eat a particular type of seafood without suffering any ill effects. While some people have a clinical allergy, others react to the presence of toxins that can build up as the shellfish feeds on other tiny sea creatures (this reaction depends on the conditions and food availability in the water in which the shellfish lived). I strongly recommend that you never eat molluscs you've harvested yourself, as water conditions are very unreliable, and the shellfish are likely to be riddled with toxins. Another reaction is to preservatives such as benzoic acid that are used to treat some shellfish, especially those vacuum-packed in controlled atmosphere packaging. I suggest you check the labels carefully. I think that it is best to wait until your child is two years old before you give them shellfish, as this can help prevent their body from adversely reacting. This can be a particular problem for hyperactive children.

Not every town has an independent fishmonger, but supermarkets often have a fish counter; the best way to be sure you are getting the freshest shellfish is to build up a good relationship with the fishmonger. He or she will be able to advise you on which seafood is fresh and how to prepare it. Remember that harvests fluctuate and so should availability. If they always sell the same shellfish it is likely to be frozen – some varieties lose their succulent tenderness and delicate flavour to become rubbery and bland when frozen. You should never refreeze seafood.

Fish

Fish cooks quickly, so it is a good choice for an evening meal when you are in a hurry. It is a good source of protein: white fish are low in fat, and the fat found in oily fish has been shown to be effective at protecting us against heart disease.

White fish are often divided between flat fish – such as brill, Dover sole, halibut, lemon sole, plaice, skate and turbot – and round fish, which include cod, coley, grey mullet, hake, haddock, John Dory, monkfish, sea bass and sea bream. Oily fish include herring, mackerel, tuna, pilchards, sardines, anchovies, red mullet, salmon, freshwater and sea trout, sprats and whitebait.

The drawback to fresh fish is that it needs to be bought on the day it is to be eaten, which is not always a viable option. When buying fresh fish, look for:
• bright, rounded eyes (dull, sunken eyes are a bad sign)
• red gills (not greyish)
• firm flesh
• a sea-fresh smell (it is the 'fishy' smell of past-its-best fish that puts many people off fish)

Frozen fish is an option; although usually inferior in taste, they can be quite acceptable in casseroles and soups. When you cook with frozen fish, you should not then refreeze the dish, as there is a risk of food poisoning. Fish fingers and other shaped products are often made up of scraps, so they are not very healthy to begin with and are frequently oozing with additives and preservatives.

CANNED FISH

Canned fish such as salmon, sardines, pilchards and anchovies, which have soft, edible bones, are rich sources of calcium and are good to keep in the store cupboard for simple supper dishes.

Poultry

Since factory farming became widespread in the 1960s, what was once a delicious treat has become an everyday meat with little of its former flavour. First chicken, but now duck, turkey and quail are all being reared intensively, with the result that their meat is often bland, spongy-textured and fatty. If we want a tasty chicken we have to be prepared to pay up to double the price.

The best-tasting and most nutritious poultry comes from birds that are well looked after – they're given space to exercise and make nests, natural light, natural feed and allowed a natural life as far as possible. Unfortunately, all too often our poultry is reared in factories: overcrowded, windowless sheds which contravene the basic recommendations of animal welfare. A high-protein diet is designed to put on maximum weight in minimum time, and in cramped conditions the spread of disease and infection can pose serious problems. This means that antibiotics and other preventive drugs may be routinely fed to the birds; these drugs produce adverse reactions in some people.

Unless poultry is clearly labelled 'free range' you should assume that the bird has been reared in less than ideal conditions. There is some concern regarding the fact that some birds labelled free range are not allowed to roam out of the barn and, while not kept in cages, do not have a great deal of space. This may be more strictly regulated in the future, but in the meantime I would encourage you to buy organic free range chicken.

Organic birds are fed mainly on grain, which contributes to their flavour. Organic chicken also tastes better because it is more mature. A ready-to-eat organic bird has to be at least 82 days old, whereas a barn-reared bird only has to be 42 days old. (There is no legal requirement for the age of a free range chicken.) You have to be prepared to pay up to 100 per cent more for an organic, free range chicken, but it is well worth it.

Many parents will still be tempted to buy chicken or turkey burgers and other poultry foods for their children. I warn them that they will usually be buying recycled (or re-formed) inferior meat that has been dyed, processed and flavoured to make it look like real poultry. Such products seem a great deal cheaper than free range organic poultry, but if you think about what you are paying for in terms of meat and fillers such as breadcrumbs and starches they represent poor value.

Turkey, duck and quail remain more of an occasional treat – all the more reason to make sure you are buying the best.

Game

The term game is applied to wild animals and birds that are hunted and eaten. It includes grouse, partridge, pheasant, mallard, hare, rabbit and venison to name but a few. In many countries, there is a close season for certain species, when hunting them is forbidden. Others, such as rabbits and pigeons, are not protected by law and are usually available fresh throughout the year. Game farming is on the increase, and we can now buy farmed wild boar, venison, rabbit and quail. Although many types of game are commercially frozen and therefore available all year round, the flavour is at its best in freshly killed and well-hung game, which is available in autumn and winter. Game is generally low in fat, rich in protein and minerals such as iron and zinc.

Before game is ready for cooking, it must be hung in order to tenderize the flesh and develop the flavour. Hanging time depends on the weather and on individual taste. Game birds are hung by their beaks, unplucked and undrawn, in a cool airy place and are traditionally considered ready when the tail feathers can be pulled out easily. Furred game is hung by the feet for one or two weeks.

For roasting and grilling, game birds should be young; the beak and feet should not be stiff, the plumage or fur soft, and the breast plump. Older birds are best casseroled. These days, many of us buy our game prepared and ready for cooking, which takes away a lot of the hassle, but makes it difficult to know the age of the birds. The best thing is to find a reputable butcher who knows the origins of what he is selling.

Lamb

Choosing good lamb is relatively simple. Lambs cannot be factory farmed, and the only issue tends to be the grass they graze on. Organic sheep are bred on pasture that has been certified free of chemicals, but pasture is not normally

Think good

sprayed, so most lamb is free of chemical residues. Lamb is a rich source of B vitamins, iron and other important minerals.

The time of year affects the appearance of the meat. Good-quality winter lamb is dark red, with creamy, marbled fat. Spring lamb is slightly lighter (dark pink) in colour, with white fat. Some cuts are naturally leaner, such as the fillet and lean chops, but cuts such as knuckle can make delicious casseroles, and if you make them a day ahead and leave them to cool the fat will solidify on the surface and can be lifted off.

Beef

In Argentina, North America and Australia, most beef comes from animals raised exclusively for meat; in Europe at least 60 to 70 per cent comes from herds that produce both milk and meat, although the finest beef comes from dedicated beef breeds such as Aberdeen Angus.

The best beef comes from young animals about eighteen months old, but even this must be matured or 'hung' for ten to twenty days at low temperatures, to tenderize the meat and to improve its flavour and keeping qualities. However, since each carcass takes up quite a lot of (expensive) refrigerated hanging space, this is one area where producers may be tempted to save time and money.

On properly hung beef, the lean meat should be a deep plum-red in colour and slightly moist. It should have a good outer covering of fat, creamy to pale yellow and of firm texture. Very bright red meat denotes that the beef has not been hung sufficiently and is therefore not very tender or tasty. Very dark red, sinewy beef indicates that the meat comes from an animal which is not of prime quality and is likely to be a little tough. Such cuts are suitable for slow cooking, provided they are well flecked with fat.

Since the health scares of the 1990s, butchers must label beef with the country of origin. If they are proud of their meat, they will probably supply further information about the region or farm it came from, the breed, and how it was reared. Be aware that producers often use label terms such as 'heritage' and 'traditional', but there is no legal definition of these terms.

As most farmers try to maximize profits by producing meat quickly and cheaply, one method was the use of growth-promoting hormones. These have been banned by the EU since 1989, but are still permitted in other countries. Unscrupulous farmers have found that certain drugs, normally used to treat disease, will promote rapid muscle growth and minimal body fat when fed to healthy cattle. Drug residues have been found in meat products.

Another bone of contention is what the cattle actually eat. The image of a cow grazing on green pasture is sometimes far from the truth; dairy cows are often kept inside and cattle feed can legally contain unnatural extras such as dried skimmed milk powder, dried blood, ground fish and dried poultry manure (chicken litter and carcasses of intensively farmed poultry). You may be aware that since the link between mad cow disease (BSE) and its human form,

Creutzfeld Jakob disease (CJD) has been established, it is no longer legal to feed cows recycled wastes from pigs, sheep or other cattle, but animal protein from poultry is still allowed. Unless you buy beef which is labelled as coming from a beef herd, you can assume it is from a dairy herd.

Your best bet is to choose organic beef, approved by the Soil Association. Farmers who maintain organic standards use natural food, no growth-promoting drugs, and have animal welfare very much in mind.

Good-quality beef will be more expensive, but will taste better and you will not be exposing your body to all sorts of potential health risks. As with other foods, you get what you pay for.

Having said that, while grilling steaks are expensive because only a given number can be cut from one animal, that still leaves a lot of meat which is just as tasty and nutritious, but which needs longer cooking in order for it to tenderize (the fat marbled through the meat melts and bastes the meat as it cooks). The cheaper cuts such as brisket, chuck and shin are ideal for casseroles, curries and hot pots. Many of these dishes are even more tender if made a day ahead, and this is excellent for anyone who needs to watch their saturated fat intake, because once the casserole is cooked, you can let it cool, then lift off the solidified fat.

Pork, ham and bacon

Pork and bacon, like poultry, suffered greatly from the rise of factory farming in the 1950s and 1960s. The tastiest and healthiest pork comes from pigs that are kept outside and allowed the freedom to live as natural a life as possible. Organic pork is definitely a good option.

Lean pork is highly nutritious; it contains more thiamin (vitamin B1) – which prevents fatigue – than any other meat, along with other B vitamins and minerals such as zinc. The best pork should be pink, smooth and firm to the touch; freshly cut surfaces should look slightly moist and there should not be excessive fat. The fat should be firm and clear, milky white. Avoid cuts with soft, grey and oily fat. The skin, or rind, should be thin, pliable, smooth and free of hairs; in older pigs the skin tends to coarsen and thicken. For crackling, make sure that the butcher scores the rind carefully so that the cuts are close together and penetrate the rind, otherwise the heat will not reach to the meat.

In order to enjoy the meat of the pig all year round, our ancestors devised many delicious ways to preserve pork by salting, smoking and air-drying, as bacon, gammon, hams and sausages. Somewhat unfortunately, they also discovered that nitrates and nitrites help to preserve meat; these preservatives, though traditional, are not helpful to our health, so we should limit our intake of bacon, sausages and salami. Ham should be less of a problem – with the proviso that what you buy resembles the thigh of the pig. If it is cut off the bone before your very eyes, it will be a far purer product than ham that has been formed into boneless blocks so they are easy for the retailer to slice. In any case, ham should never be shiny and watery, just matt and slightly moist.

Cheap sausages and meat products are likely to contain poor-quality, recycled meat (MRM), as well as cereal fillers. As with most food you get what you pay for – in this case, not much meat! In addition, they will be packed with additives such as flavour enhancers, which can adversely affect your body in various ways.

Dairy products

Western societies traditionally rely on milk, cheese, yoghurt, cream and butter as major food sources. However, in many parts of the world dairy products are not eaten in any form, so vegans and people who cannot tolerate lactose (milk sugar) should be assured that they are not essential, although I think they are by far the best way to take in calcium and a range of other vitamins and minerals. Some regions use mainly sheep's, goats' and buffalo milk, but here I shall concentrate on cows' milk products.

MILK

Commercial pressure to produce vast yields of milk can lead dairy farmers to feed the cows concentrated, high-protein pellets derived from grains, fish meal, soya beans and animal waste; far removed from the cow's natural diet of pasture. This can upset the cow's gut and cause excessively swollen udders, both of which lay the animal open to infection; the farmer then has to use antibiotics. Despite strict screening procedures, there have been cases of the antibiotics breaking through the testing protocols and entering into our diet. Cows' milk is also a very sensitive indicator of environmental pollution. If the cows are farmed in polluted areas, the pollutants can easily pass into our milk.

To avoid such problems, the simple message is that organic milk reduces your exposure to toxins, antibiotics and other undesirable components. Organic herds are generally smaller and the good health of the cow is maintained by high standards of welfare, including natural feeding.

Most milk is pasteurized, then sold as full fat (whole), semi-skimmed and skimmed. All contain practically identical amounts of calcium and other nutrients. Full fat milk contains between 3 and 5 per cent fat, semi-skimmed contains 1.5–1.8 per cent fat and skimmed milk contains 0.1–0.3 per cent fat. Many people are under the impression that full fat milk is very high in fat and therefore unhealthy. This is really not the case, although if you do need to reduce your saturated fat intake, switching to semi-skimmed is an easy way of doing this. Young children need to have whole milk up until the age of three years as they need its beneficial fats. It is usually inadvisable to give a child under the age of one large amounts of cows, milk; small amounts in cooking are fine, but glasses of milk can cause problems in the immature gut.

BUTTER

Butter is made by churning cream; the fat solidifies to form butter. Salted butter can have up to two per cent salt added. People sometimes ask me whether it is healthier to eat unsalted butter, but it really makes very little difference unless you have severe high blood pressure or kidney problems, when you are advised to change to unsalted butter. Unsalted butter tastes better in some dishes, whereas salted butter can enhance others.

For the best taste and to avoid the possibility of chemical residues, it is worth spending a little extra for good quality-butter. Organic butter is excellent, as are some of the butters from small on-farm dairies. Some French butters are protected by AOC (Appellation d'Origine Contrôlée) status; the provenance of the milk is strictly controlled.

YOGHURT

Yoghurt has a reputation as a healthy product, but with so many different styles, this can be misleading.

In simple terms yoghurt is milk, either whole or skimmed, that has been heated and soured by the addition of lactic cultures, such as Lactobacillus bulgaricus, Streptococcus thermophilus, or bifidus and acidophilus, which are most beneficial to the gut. Set yoghurt has had the cultures added to it in the pot. Yoghurt can be made from cows', sheep's and goats' milk, and from soya milk.

Fromage frais and quark are not yoghurt, but fresh cheeses made by curdling milk with enzymes, which means that they don't contain the beneficial lactic bacteria I recommend people include in their diet.

The fat content of yoghurt ranges from 0.1 per cent to about 10 per cent in some thick, Greek-style strained yoghurts. So plain, natural yoghurt can be a healthy alternative to cream in soup or with your dessert, as the fat content of even single cream is around 20 per cent. However, I have serious reservations about fruit-flavoured yoghurts. Firstly, they often contain no fruit, just flavourings and colourings. Secondly, along with the fruit flavours, there is often a large amount of added sugar. Thirdly, just to complete the cocktail of additives, 'reduced fat' yoghurts, whether fruit flavoured or plain, are often thickened with modified starches. Parents of hyperactive children who have problems with additives should be aware that many yoghurt-based desserts are certainly not a healthy or helpful option.

Instead, choose a plain yoghurt, preferably organic, and add your own chopped, puréed or stewed fruit. Yoghurt is also good as a savoury sauce or dip; add chopped cucumber and mint, or see page 312 for more suggestions.

CHEESE

Names like Brie, Parmesan and Cheddar refer to so many different qualities of cheese that it is hard to recognize a good cheese. Farmhouse and handmade cheeses are usually worth buying, as are labels which use the French term AOC (Appellation d'Origine Contrôlée). Specialist cheese shops generally stock good-quality cheese, often from small producers who cannot meet the high yields the supermarkets demand. They will usually let you taste a few cheeses.

Think good

Although cheese is usually high in saturated fat, it is well worth splashing out on a good one so that your taste buds will be happy with only a small amount! Using mature cheese in sauces along with a small amount of mustard to enhance the flavour means you will need less cheese. Avoid 'low fat' and 'diet' cheeses; they are usually tasteless.

The finest cheeses are made with raw (unpasteurized) milk; these tend to have a better flavour and overall character. Hard, unpasteurized cheeses are the best choice for pregnant women, as the natural organisms in the cheese will have fought off the bacteria that cause food poisoning (listeriosis). If you are pregnant you need to avoid all soft cheeses, whether pasteurized or not, including those with white rinds and blue veins.

Here are some guidelines to bear in mind when buying cheese:

- Cheeses should be appropriately wrapped and not wrinkling or drying at the edges.
- Hard cheese should look smooth, not with large dry cracks. Soft cheeses should look moist, not withered.
- If you get the chance to taste the cheese, it should smell inviting. Anything without a smell is probably a cheap cheese. Strong-smelling cheeses shouldn't be rancid or smell of ammonia.
- The cheese should taste good – not bland, soapy or metallic.

Processed cheeses and cheese spreads can contain many additives and preservatives. Mild goats' milk cheeses or Brie and Camembert types have a similar creamy, cheesy flavour, and it is much better to start your children on these rather than the processed cheeses, as they will receive health-giving calcium and other beneficial nutrients, and less health-hindering additives and preservatives.

Eggs

A fresh egg provides you with a cheap, good source of lean protein and lots of vitamins and minerals, all in one little unit. I would not suggest you eat them every day, however – we need a varied diet.

Choosing an egg which is fresh and tastes like an egg is becoming increasingly difficult. Many eggs are either pale, tasteless and insipid or their yolks are bright orange, the chickens having been fed artificial colourings. There have been cases of children developing allergies not to the eggs themselves, but the additives in the chicken feed. We really cannot expect hens kept under the appalling stress of battery farms to produce decent eggs, but whether you are concerned with animal welfare or the taste of real food, you should always buy free-range eggs, organic if possible.

Pregnant women, elderly people and those already suffering from illness should avoid raw egg products, as these carry a greater risk of food poisoning. Fit, healthy individuals can to some extent cope with a bout of food poisoning, but for these vulnerable groups it can be particularly hazardous.

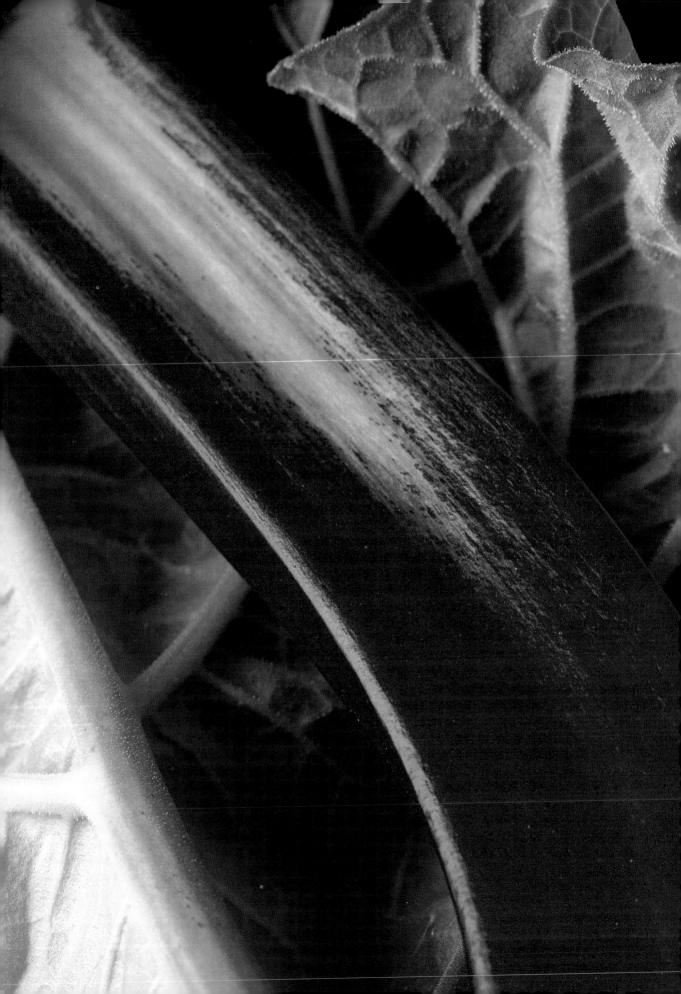

Organic food

I am an ardent supporter of organic food; it is real food, and it tastes like it.

The main reason for choosing organic produce is that artificial pesticides, fertilizers, antibiotics and livestock feed additives are prohibited in its production. This means that organic food contains fewer chemical residues which, if allowed to build up in our bodies, can cause free radical damage (see page 46) and diseases such as cancer and heart disease. In the shorter term, the body complains by developing irritable bowel, colic or hyperactivity. (Sadly, it is almost impossible to find food that is completely chemical free because the atmosphere and ground water are already heavily polluted.) The fact that your system is not constantly bombarded with pesticides and chemicals means your body will generally become more efficient.

Since organic producers generally do not force-grow fruit and vegetables by filling them with water, your body will glean more nutrients per mouthful. This is one of the main reasons why organic food tastes better than perfect-looking, forced food (like those waterlogged tomatoes sitting in neat rows in your super-market), where you are getting, and paying for, a mouthful of water.

I think this is also one of the reasons why people think healthy eating is time-consuming and a little boring. If you buy non-organic fruit and vegetables, you will need to devote more time to making them taste good. Fruit will be a duty rather than a delicious snack. If food tasted as it was meant to, we would all enjoy the fresh, natural tastes.

Thankfully, more and more organic suppliers of all kinds of food and drink are popping up around the country. There are also co-operative companies who deliver nationwide, it's just a question of incorporating ordering into your schedule. I recommend that you contact the Soil Association (see page 352) for lists of suppliers.

At the moment organic food is a little more expensive, but the price will come down if there is greater demand. Bear in mind when you tot up the cost of buying organic that the intense flavours mean you need to do less to the food to get it tasting good. You lose less water from organic meat, so poultry doesn't collapse and joints of meat don't shrink as much once they are cooked.

Some people wonder whether the produce is genuinely organic or just a marketing ploy. The most reliable way of checking is to look for a certification mark from a registered organic producer. They are subject to an annual inspection to ensure that they meet the very strict organic standards laid down under European legislation. You can also look for the names of The Soil Association or the Organic Farmers and Growers Ltd (OF&G); these bodies will only endorse organic food which is produced to the EU standard 2092/91.

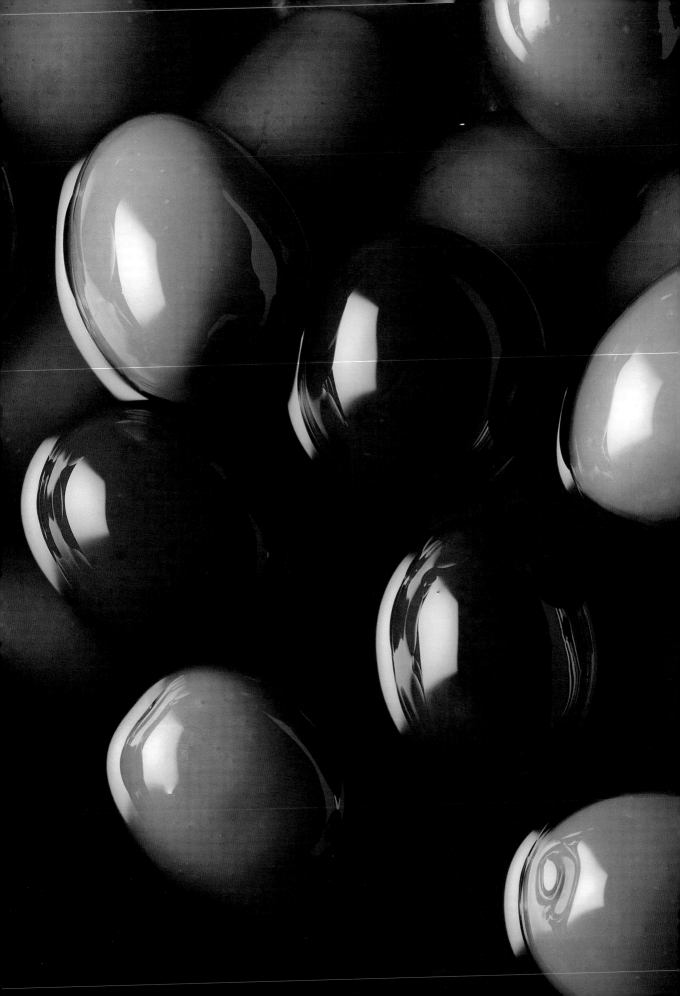

Stocking your larder and fridge

Many people find shopping either boring or daunting, as they wander around the supermarket staring at row after row, label after label. With a little organization, shopping should be a pleasure; you can automatically stock up on routine items and concentrate on choosing the things you'd really like to eat. Some supermarkets now deliver bulky items such as washing powder and loo paper, so find out if this is possible in your region. In some areas you can order food off the Internet. With foods such as cheese and meat, I recommend you find a specialist shop or an approved organic supplier who can deliver to your door, as you will be able to discuss the foods and find out what is best and in season.

To make shopping as easy as possible I have popped down a few ideas for a well-stocked kitchen.

Larder
Wholegrain bread, pitta bread, crackers, oatcakes
Breakfast cereal, oat flakes
Pulses (dried and canned – lentils, chickpeas, kidney beans, baked beans)
Flour
Sugar (demerara, caster, icing, soft brown)
Golden syrup
Dried pasta, couscous, rice (basmati, risotto, wholegrain, wild)
Oils (extra-virgin olive, sunflower, groundnut, walnut, sesame)
Vinegar (white wine, cider, balsamic, raspberry)
Mustard, chutney
Pesto and olive pastes
Capers, olives
Onions, garlic
Potatoes (try different varieties, for baking, mashing and boiling)
Fruit (apples, oranges, lemons, limes, grapes, bananas)
Dried fruits (apricots, figs, raisins, dates), coconut flakes, banana chips

Nuts (almonds, cashews, hazelnuts, pecans, walnuts) and seeds (sunflower, sesame)
Organic peanut butter, jam, marmalade, honey
Dried wild mushrooms (porcini or ceps)
Dried herbs (bay leaves, marjoram, oregano, thyme)
Spices (cinnamon, ginger, nutmeg, saffron, curry powder, garam masala, cumin seeds, coriander, cloves, paprika, chilli powder)
Natural vanilla essence, vanilla pod
Canned tomatoes, tomato purée, sun-dried tomatoes (in oil or dried)
Canned artichoke hearts
Canned fish (sardines, salmon, dolphin-friendly tuna)
Soy sauce or tamari
Elderflower cordial, orange blossom water
Free range organic eggs

Fridge
Avocados, organic carrots, red, yellow and green peppers, tomatoes
Fresh herbs
Fresh ginger
Seasonal soft fruits (mangoes, peaches) for juices and shakes
Unsweetened fruit juices
Mineral water
Butter
Milk/soya milk, crème fraîche, natural yoghurt
Cheeses
Charcuterie (Parma ham, salami)
Smoked fish (salmon, trout, kippers)
Lean minced meat, steaks or lean chops
Lean bacon, good-quality sausages
Fresh roasted or uncooked chicken

Healthy snacks

Many men, women and children find their bodies are not comfortable with just three meals a day, and need a mid-morning and mid-afternoon snack. Tempting as it is to grab a chocolate bar or a bag of crisps, because that's what everyone else has, these will not help your body feel good. If you know you need regular snacks, take the opportunity to introduce some more health-giving foods; I've listed a few ideas below.

FRESH FRUIT

You don't need me to tell you that these are perfect snack food. Rather than just munching an apple, why not slice your apple and eat it with a few cubes of cheese? Grapes and pears are also good with cheese. Oranges can be messy to eat at work, so prepare a simple fruit salad with, for example, sliced oranges, dried figs or black grapes and kiwi fruit.

Poached fruit, apple purée or a compote of seasonal fresh or dried fruits can be served on its own or with yoghurt. See also Raspberry fool, page 338.

DRIED FRUITS

Apricots, figs, prunes and raisins are rich in minerals such as magnesium, calcium, potassium and iron, and are high in fibre. Their only drawback as a snack is that they are quite high in sugar, so I suggest you eat no more than two or three, with a glass of water; this will help the fibre swell and stimulate the fullness centre of your brain (see page 015). In any case it's not a good idea to eat large amounts of dried fruits, as they can cause indigestion and wind.

Try to get fruits that don't use sulphur dioxide (E220) as a preservative. Sulphur dioxide preserves the colour, so unsulphured fruits can look less vivid, but sulphating agents can cause food sensitivities in some people.

FRUIT SHAKES

The mixture of fresh fruits and perhaps some yoghurt or milk gives your body an amazing healthy energy boost. Many fruit shakes can be made in advance and taken to work or college in a small flask. Look at the recipe suggestions on page 342.

WHOLEGRAIN CAKES AND BISCUITS

Many cake and biscuit recipes can be adapted to incorporate wholemeal flour and/or oats. Using these higher fibre ingredients slows down the absorption of sugar into the body, thus preventing energy swings. Fibre also helps your body produce substances that can reduce the risk of heart disease and certain types of

Think good

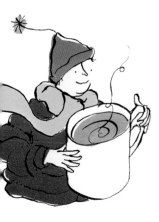

cancer. Try fruit and malt loaf or flapjacks made with apple purée or chopped dried fruit (see page 331 for recipes).

MUFFINS
Buy wholewheat muffins or make oat muffins (see page 328) and top with sliced banana.

OATCAKES
Top with a slice of salami, lean ham, roast chicken, or maybe some sliced tomatoes with a few olives, or sliced cucumber and chopped fresh dill.

HOMEMADE SOUP
A bowl of soup is ideal in the middle of the afternoon if you are at home or have a flask to take to work. It's also a great way to stave off hunger pangs as soon as you get home. Children enjoy sprinkling croûtons or roasted sunflower seeds on top.

Homemade soups contain fewer additives, preservatives, salt and other potentially health-hindering ingredients than ready-made ones, and they are so easy to make. What's more, you can choose your own combination of vegetables and fruits, such as roasted pumpkin or parsnip and lemon. See pages 306–309 for more ideas.

Soup-making is most definitely worth the small amount of effort. If you make a large pot of soup, you can freeze it in portions and then thaw it out as you need it. Base it on a simple stock: get into the habit of using the bones and leftover vegetables from your chickens and Sunday roasts to make your own stock. Failing this, use bought stock or stock cubes. A good investment is a hand-held blender, which can be used in the pan in which you've simmered the vegetables, hence saving on the washing up. A blender also makes your soup more versatile: it can turn a chunky minestrone into a smooth vegetable soup.

RAW VEGETABLES
Cherry tomatoes, sticks of carrots, celery and cucumber can be served with hummus or a simple dip of yoghurt mixed with spring onions and grated cucumber. This is a very good snack for people who have given up smoking.

GRILLED VEGETABLES
If you are roasting vegetables for your evening meal, make extra and take them to work in a plastic container. Remember that you only need to use a small amount of olive oil. Mushrooms, peppers, asparagus, courgettes and aubergines are delicious at room temperature.

How do we know what goes into our food?

Shopping for food should be something you enjoy, but it can easily become a nightmare. Concerns over food safety, unnecessary additives and preservatives, sugar, salt and fat levels mean that people often feel they have to spend hours examining food labels. In theory, the fact that manufacturers have made the effort to tell you what is in their foods should instil confidence, but we have a long way to go before we get to the truth behind the labels.

How fresh is 'fresh'?

The words 'natural' and 'fresh' are two of the most abused words in the English language when it comes to food. There is no legal definition of either.

Words like 'natural' and 'traditional' are often deliberately misleading. When you buy food with no information about how it was grown, or that is not labelled organic, you should assume that it was grown with the aid of chemicals – in other words it is not 'natural'.

Food can sit in a dock for days before it appears as 'fresh' in the shops. Unfortunately, once fruit or vegetables have been harvested they rapidly begin to lose certain vitamins and minerals. The longer food is left before you eat it, the fewer nutrients remain. Frozen vegetables can have a higher vitamin and mineral content than fresh ones, because there are very strict legislative guide-lines governing their production; they have to be frozen within a set period of time after they have been picked. I would like to see 'picked on' dates on fresh foods, so we have at least some idea of freshness and subsequent nutrient value.

Loopholes in labelling

Nearly all foods which come within the scope of either UK or EU food labelling regulations must carry a list of ingredients. There are a few exceptions, including fresh fruits, vegetables which are not prepared and cut into pieces, butter, most cheeses, and foods which consist of a single ingredient.

The British Heart Foundation estimates that 70,000 people in the UK die prematurely every year because of misleading labels which hide the real amounts of salts, fats and sugars in food products. At the moment the nutritional panel need not state the quantity of each ingredient. It only has to list the ingredients in descending order of weight, the first-named ingredient making up the largest part of the product. Without a quantity figure, you cannot judge how healthy the food is. Is a dessert that has butter as the fourth ingredient after apples, flour and sugar, healthier than a pasta dish that lists butter third? Ideally, the total quantity of each ingredient used in a product would be listed, together with the amount in a typical portion, rather than in 100 grams as is usually the case.

Cook things so you can
tell what they are.
Good plain food ain't
committed no crime
an' don't need no disguise.
Fancified cooks is the
criminals.
Mary Lasswell (1905–94)

Worryingly, you cannot always believe what food manufacturers say on their labels. In the UK, the Consumers' Association tested 70 products and only ten per cent contained the exact quantities stated on the labels. Many were way out, and this is not just the case with small producers. One of Britain's most respected chain stores was 72 per cent out in the measurement of fat in its ice cream. A well-known brand of 'slimming' food's baked beans contained 72 calories per 100 g, when the pack claimed 56.

Don't forget that just because a food has a small amount of sugar or animal fat listed on the label, doesn't mean it is unhealthy. Sugar is an important preservative and fat contains fat-soluble vitamins. Foods containing these ingredients can be healthy if they contain fibre or other nutrients.

HIDDEN SUGAR

The sugar content of foods can be disguised in many ways: fructose, maltose, lactose, dextrose, sucrose and glucose are all sugars, as are honey, concentrated fruit juice and anything described as 'syrup'. Partially hydrolysed starch, or maltodextrin, is halfway between a starch and a sugar. It is often used a bulking agent or filler; the body 'reads' it and processes it as sugar.

The label 'sugar free' may simply mean that a food does not contain sucrose; 'no added sugar' means that it is naturally sweet. All sweet foods should be treated with some degree of caution. Any form of sugar, while not harmful in itself, contributes to tooth decay, and can cause obesity and aggravate behaviour problems in hyperactive children. I would not recommend replacing sugar with artificial sweeteners, as this only encourages a 'sweet tooth' in both children and adults.

SALT

You may think that you can tell when a food is high in salt, simply by trusting your taste buds, but there is a lot of hidden salt in foods we generally consider sweet or bland, such as desserts and bread; cornflakes have a higher proportion of salt than Atlantic seawater! Foods labelled 'low fat', 'low sugar' and 'diabetic' may contain huge amounts of salt to make up for the flavours lost in processing the products.

Salt (sodium chloride) is often listed as sodium on labels. People for whom excess salt can cause problems include those with high blood pressure, fluid retention, diabetes, atherosclerosis (furring of the arteries) or kidney problems.

ADDITIVES AND E NUMBERS

All categories of additives must be listed in the ingredients. In all cases other than flavourings the additive must be described by its generic name, for example acidity regulator, and either its specific name, such as sodium citrate, or its E number (E331). Don't make the mistake of thinking that if a food is free of E numbers it must be safe. Instead you should be questioning whether a list of chemicals sounds like real food. Some additives are necessary to preserve food, but most are not.

Manufacturers do not need to list the ingredients used to flavour the food, nor ingredients that have already been processed before they are added to the food, such as the red colouring in raspberry preserves. People who may be allergic to a particular additive may be exposed to it without realizing.

ALCOHOLIC DRINKS – WHAT THE LABELS DON'T TELL YOU

While low-alcohol and non-alcoholic ciders and beers with less than 1.2 per cent alcohol by volume have to list their ingredients, there is no legal requirement for the labels on full-strength beer, cider, wine or other alcoholic drinks to tell you anything about the ingredients, except for the alcohol content.

Preservatives (see page 76) such as benzoates and sulphites are used in many wines; these can cause allergic reactions in some people, or may just make you feel lousy or hung over.

How healthy is the 'healthy option'?

The quest for health and fitness leaves many people wide open to the food producers' claims. Manufacturers play with consumer ignorance by using expressions such as 'lite', 'natural', 'healthy', 'fresh' and 'nutritious' to tempt you into buying their food.

Alarmingly, 'freshly squeezed' fruit juice may contain more sugar, in the form of fructose, than a canned artificial drink. The fruit juice is also likely to contain preservatives, which can cause problems for some people. In theory, freshly squeezed juice has the health advantage over canned drinks because of its vitamin C and folic acid content, but until it is marked with the date that the fruit was picked, we cannot know whether it will actually contain significant amounts of these vitamins.

'SLIMLINE' FOODS

People wonder why they do not remain fit and lose weight when they fill their shopping baskets with diet, slimline, low sugar, reduced fat products. But did you know that

• low fat foods can contain as much as 40 per cent fat?
• low fat foods may contain huge amounts of sugar?
• low sugar foods may contain more fat than the standard version of the food?

Even when you allow for the above facts, you may decide that a low fat product still has to be healthier. I seem to spend hours explaining that just because a fat spread is labelled lite or low fat, it doesn't mean you can use lashings of it. While a spread with 60 per cent fat (not exactly 'lite'!) is lower in fat than butter and traditional margarine (with 80 per cent fat), these fat spreads may also contain hydrogenated fats or oils, which raise 'bad' cholesterol in the blood, reduce 'good' cholesterol and expose your body to a greater risk of developing heart disease, premature ageing and cancer.

Many women have such cravings for chocolate that they buy low fat chocolate bars. They are not doing their bodies any favours: the product they are eating is a vegetable oil-based confectionery item, full of additives, preservatives and artificial sweeteners – more like vegolate than chocolate! The flavour is inferior by such a wide margin that the taste buds switch off and the whole eating experience is a waste of time. They would be much better off enjoying a small amount of real, fine, high-cocoa chocolate and incorporating it into a healthy eating plan, either as a treat after meals or melted as a dip or sauce for fruits such as strawberries, bananas or pears.

Real ice cream, made from milk, vanilla, eggs, sugar and cream, is rich in calcium and other vitamins and minerals. Yes, it is high in fat, but who eats ice cream every day? As a treat, it can be part of a balanced diet, and will be both better for you and more satisfying than the frozen desserts and low fat 'ice creams' with their additives, bulking agents, and (usually) astronomically high sugar content; in no way can these be described as healthy.

ADDED VITAMINS AND MINERALS

The more foods are processed, the lower the vitamin and mineral content. For this reason many food manufacturers add vitamin and mineral mixes to foods at the end of processing, to ensure that we receive some goodness. It would be much better if we could get the vitamins and minerals from the food's natural reserves, as they are much more readily absorbed by our bodies.

Added vitamins or minerals don't automatically make a product healthy. There may be other ingredients in the food which prevent the body from absorbing the 'health-giving' nutrient. For instance breakfast cereals with added vitamins and minerals frequently have a high fibre content. Fibre can inhibit the absorption of nutrients and there may be little benefit to be had from choosing a cereal with added vitamins and minerals.

SURELY OUR DIETS NEED FORTIFYING?

Some experts feel that we need to supplement our everyday foods with vitamins and minerals because many people will not otherwise receive the required amounts of nutrients. They say that people who live on cereals, ready-made meals and fast food are not going to start cooking healthy foods. Why not? Instead of fortifying foods (and boosting food manufacturers' profits) I believe we should be trying to educate and inspire people with ideas and the confidence to prepare meals using cheap, simple ingredients.

Cereals with a little folic acid or iron, but with high levels of sugar, salt and additives, can have an unhealthy overall effect. Some manufacturers are trying to improve this situation by liaising with government bodies to find the best ways to incorporate vital nutrients such as folic acid into breakfast cereals. However, it is important to understand that fortified foods should also be healthy foods, and the consumer should not be lulled into a false sense of security; when you buy a vitamin-enriched food you should still look to more natural foods as your main source of vitamins and minerals.

In the majority of cases we don't need to supplement our diets with fortified foods or vitamin pills. However, there are situations where fortified foods can be helpful. For example, if you can't tolerate dairy products, soya milk fortified with calcium is a good alternative.

'HEALTH' DRINKS

The health drink market is growing daily. You only need to visit a health food store, gym or trendy bar to find a selection of power, sports, herbal, revitalizing, memory-boosting concoctions. Unfortunately there is little legislation to help you decide whether the drink is healthy and delivers its promise. Frequently the buzz you get from these drinks comes from sugar or caffeine – it has nothing to do with herbs, ginseng, amino acids or natural fruit derivatives.

FUNCTIONAL FOODS

'Functional' foods are products that claim a specific medical or physiological benefit because of an added ingredient. In some cases the products are just junk food with some functional ingredient added. Manufacturers even produce drinks with added 'beneficial' oils, which has led to teenagers in Japan buying cans of cola with essential fatty acids, to improve learning ability. Breads with added fish oils are meant to give the impression that they help reduce the risk of heart disease. The real facts are that they are white loaves with little fibre, copious amounts of salt and only a small amount of omega 6 and 3 fatty acids – certainly not enough to bring about any beneficial change in your body. The salt and low fibre characteristics far outweigh the potential effect of the beneficial oils.

Fibre is generally a healthy thing to boost in your diet, but as with most other nutrients 'balance' is the key word. Some people with irritable bowel choose fibre-filled drinks believing that their symptoms will improve, but in the setting of a sugary drink, the bowel reacts adversely.

As with nutritional supplements, it is possible to overdose on functional foods. This is easily done if you start the day with an enriched breakfast cereal or toast made from fortified bread and top up with sports drinks with added vitamins. This can lead to your body being exposed to excessively high doses of some vitamins and minerals. You may think that a few of these products can't do any harm, but I have seen people who desperately want to improve their health and consume these products in vast quantities.

If you are still not convinced, tot up the cost. Functional foods are generally more expensive than normal foods. People on limited budgets should not be misled into buying these so-called wonder foods, then not having enough money to buy the foods that make up a healthy, balanced diet.

Irradiated food

Its supporters hail irradiation as a wonderful new way to keep food fresher for longer. But to many people the word irradiation is linked with cancer and they feel scared at the prospect of their food being exposed to it.

Ionizing radiation was discovered in 1896 and its practical use of killing micro-organisms in food was first pursued in 1921. The process uses electromagnetic radiation to produce an effect in food which is very similar to pasteurization, cooking and other forms of preserving. The rays reduce the level of bacteria and prevent spoilage; they can also delay ripening in fruits and vegetables. This makes irradiation a very attractive prospect for supermarkets; it greatly increases shelf life and, in theory, reduces the risk of food-borne illnesses. Opponents point out that irradiated food may look fresh, but in fact could be old and have lost many of its vitamins.

Many committees, including the World Health Organization and the US Food and Drug Administration, continue to investigate the safety of irradiated food. They seem to be concluding that irradiation, if correctly applied, is safe. Consumers need, firstly, to be convinced and secondly, but equally importantly, to be informed of when a food has been irradiated. Labelling should be quite clear, so you have a choice as to whether you eat irradiated food.

There are, as with most food labelling legislation, loopholes which need to be closed before the consumer is able to make an informed choice. At the moment, while European Union law requires that whole irradiated foods for sale must be labelled, if an irradiated ingredient makes up less than 25 per cent of the whole food, such as meat in a vegetable and meat pie, the food need not be labelled as irradiated. In the UK, irradiation is only being used on herbs and spices, which may be ingredients in the food we buy. Imported food is not as tightly controlled as home-produced foods, so it is possible that other irradiated food will get into our cupboards without our knowledge. Another amazing loophole is that while UK law states that all catering outlets declare irradiated food, schools are exempt, so our children may be eating irradiated food!

Genetically engineered food

Genes within food can be modified to improve a particular quality of a food, a peach can be made more juicy, a strain of wheat can be made more resistant to frost or pests. Both these scenarios sound attractive, as it means we receive a superior product. However, no one knows what the long term effects will be of introducing them into the food chain, or whether there will be side effects for the consumer. If a vegetarian knew that the peach they were eating contained some of the genes of a fish, I think they would spit it out!

Why do we have to aim for the perfect food? Supermarket tomatoes may be perfectly round and uniformly red, but ninety nine times out of a hundred you can close your eyes and you would fail to notice whether you're eating a tomato or a piece of watermelon. Let's stop putting appearance before our health.

What the labels tell us

Additives usually appear after the food ingredients, grouped under their category headings (flavouring, preservative, antioxidant, emulsifier, stabilizer or colour) and itemized by their code number, full chemical name, or both. Flavourings, however, do not have to be itemized. Code numbers that are preceded by the letter E show that the additive has been approved for use in all European Union countries. Additives whose code has no E have been approved only in the United Kingdom.

New additives are all tested very thoroughly, although there are rarely tests on humans – rats, mice, bacteria and human cells cultured in a test tube are the main subjects used for testing. There has also been some concern about how accurately tests are carried out. A commercial laboratory in America, which was responsible for over 30 per cent of the world's safety testing, was found to have been fabricating its data for many years. Although the laboratory was closed down, many of the additives that were passed as safe on the basis of its tests are still in use.

Antioxidants (E300 to E321) An additive that delays or prevents food from turning rancid or changing in taste, smell and appearance. Those most likely to cause health problems are BHA and BHT (E320 and E321).

Calorie A measure of the energy value of food, correctly called kilocalories (kcal). The metric equivalent, the kilojoule (kj) is equal to about 4.2 kilocalories.

Carbohydrate The primary source of our energy, consisting of sugars and starches found in plant matter, especially fruits, root vegetables and cereals (edible grains).

Colourings (E100 to E180) An additive that imparts a characteristic or appetizing colour to foods, or intensifies the colour. About half the permitted colours are extracts from natural sources, the rest are man-made. There is a new trend towards colours produced by fungal cells or plant cells in culture – these too can be labelled 'natural', even though we would not consider eating the items from which they are derived.

Such colours are being sought as a replacement for the synthetic colours known as azo dyes, which have caused much concern. Apart from their potentially carcinogenic effect, many of the azo dyes have been reported as causing sensitivity reactions, especially in children. Azo dyes include colours such as tartrazine, sunset yellow and amaranth. Eighteen of these artificial colours are permitted in Britain; of these, eleven are banned in the United States, and six are not approved by the EU, because they are suspected of being carcinogens.

Two of the 'natural' colours – caramel (E150) and vegetable carbon black

Think good

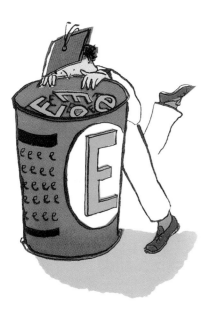

(E153) – are also potential carcinogens (some forms of caramel appear to be safe but not others. Carbon black is banned in the United States.

Dextrose A form of sugar found in animal and plant tissue and derived artificially from starch.

Emulsifiers, stabilizers and thickeners (E322 to 495) Additives that affect the texture of foods; they help distribute particles evenly in liquids and prevent mixtures such as oil and water from separating into layers; they are used in mayonnaise, salad dressings, ice cream, frozen yoghurts and margarines. Several of those permitted in Britain are not approved by the EU – these include 430, 433 and 435.

Energy see **Calorie**

Enriched Some of the nutrients lost during processing have been put back into the food.

Fat A concentrated source of energy. Labels may list saturated fats (mainly from animals) and monounsaturated and polyunsaturated fats (usually from plant sources).

Flavour enhancers (E620 to E635) An additive that modifies the taste or smell of a food without imparting a flavour of its own. The most important of these is monosodium glutamate, or MSG (E621), and its relatives, E620–623. Eating large amounts of MSG may produce a set of symptoms known as 'Chinese restaurant syndrome'. The symptoms described for this condition vary considerably: 'tightness, pain and tingling in the front of the chest, radiating to the arms, often associated with palpitations and faintness' according to one authority, but 'flushing, sweating, loss of co-ordination, headache and hypo-tension (low blood pressure)' according to another. Some studies have failed to confirm the existence of a reaction, but it has been suggested that the source from which the MSG is manufactured is relevant. There are reports of MSG triggering attacks in some asthmatics.

Flavourings There are over 2,000 flavourings; many are herbs and spices, but many are man-made. Unlike other additives, these do not have to be itemized on food labels, they do not have E-numbers, and manufacturers can currently use the word 'flavouring' without specifying what it contains.

Many were tested for safety a long time ago, so the results are questionable. However, they are used in extremely small quantities, and are assumed to be non-harmful for this reason. Although this may be true for the majority, there are doubts over some flavourings, particularly a group known as the allyl alcohols, which are potential toxins. Anyone eating large amounts of sweets, crisps and soft drinks would get a higher than average dose and therefore a greater risk of exposure to any adverse reaction.

Fortified Extra nutrients that were not originally present in a certain food have been added to it during processing. For example, breakfast cereals are often fortified with vitamins and minerals. Just because a food is fortified doesn't mean it's healthy: high sugar and high fat products are often fortified.

Fructose A form of sugar found in fruit and honey, which is often used as a food preservative and flavour enhancer. It contains just as many calories as other forms of sugar.

Glucose A form of sugar found in fruit and starches.

Kcal, Kcalorie, kj, Kjoule and Kilojoule see **Calorie**

Lactose A form of sugar found in milk.

Maltose A form of sugar found in malt and cereals.

Meat products Foods described as consisting of 'meat products' often contain a large amount of fat. For example, beef sausages only need to have 50 per cent meat content, half of which can be fat.

Preservatives (E200 to E283) An additive that helps prevent deterioration of the food product until its 'sell by' or 'best before' date. Preservatives slow the development of bacteria and other micro-organisms that would make food go off and cause food poisoning. Those most dangerous to health are the nitrates and nitrites (E249–E252), which have been used for hundreds of years to make bacon, ham, sausages and salami – they are potentially carcinogenic. Because of the long tradition of use, and the fact that the characteristic flavour of bacon cannot be produced in any other way, these preservatives are difficult to outlaw.

One group of preservatives, the benzoates (E210–E219) sometimes seem to cause sensitivity problems in people who are also sensitive to aspirin and/or tartrazine (E102), a yellow colouring. Sulphur dioxide and sulphites (E220–E227) can trigger asthmatic attacks because they have an irritant effect on the airways.

Protein A nutrient needed for repair and growth of body tissue. Found in meats, fish, dairy products, nuts, seeds, grains, pulses and some vegetables.

RDA The Recommended Daily Amount (or Recommended Dietary Allowance) an adult should consume to prevent any type of deficiency developing, as specified by the government. Labels show the percentage of vitamins and minerals found in a typical serving, or in 100 grams of the product, compared to the RDA.

Some manufacturers refer to Dietary Reference Values, which try to take account of the fact that people have different needs, for example during pregnancy or illness. The figures may be different in other countries, perhaps to take account of national eating habits, and may be updated as new evidence appears.

Stabilizer see **Emulsifiers**

Starch see **Carbohydrate**

Sugar free The product does not contain sucrose, but may contain other sweeteners such as concentrated fruit juice or honey. 'No added sugar' simply means the product is already sweet enough.

Sweeteners Artificial sweeteners have a sweet taste but few, if any, calories.

Food safety

In the past decade, food poisoning seems to have hit the headlines with disturbing frequency. The serious outbreaks and one-off tragedies have had a positive outcome: an increased awareness of the importance of food hygiene, improved labelling regarding shelf-life, and more attention focused on the way our food is produced.

The ironic fact is that as hygiene has improved over time, it is precisely our good health that makes us more prone to serious bouts of food poisoning than our forebears. In the distant past it was quite common for children to suffer from gastro-enteritis, vomiting and diarrhoea, but now if a hundred people go down with the same symptoms there is an outcry. I regularly stress to parents that keeping their child in a 'sterile', artificially clean environment means their exposure to bacteria and viruses is limited, so they are less likely to build up immunity and more prone to succumb to food poisoning as they grow up.

Modern society must accept some responsibility for the outbreaks of E. Coli 0157 poisoning, listeriosis, salmonellosis, and Creutzfeld-Jakob disease (CJD, the human form of 'mad cow disease' or bovine spongiform encephalitis, BSE). We are used to having everything we want in the shops throughout the year and at a very cheap price, which can place some food producers under so much pressure to deliver the goods that they have been tempted to cut corners.

While I am strongly in favour of tightening standards in the food production industry, there is a down side. Certain traditional foods have disappeared because of over-cautious food hygiene legislation. In Britain, only a handful of cheese producers still use unpasteurized milk; all the others have succumbed to pressure from their biggest customers, the supermarkets, to pasteurize. Pasteurization does not make cheese safe to eat; the issues are slightly more complex (see page 79, Listeria).

Modern farming and food manufacturing methods have a lot to answer for, but so do we, the consumers. To the surprise of many people, most cases of food poisoning occur through food and equipment being mishandled at home.

Shelf-life dates

Nearly all foods have to be marked with a date up to which the food can reasonably be expected to 'retain its specific properties, if stored properly'. The time that any food will keep in good condition depends largely on the moisture level within the food and the storage temperature. Where storage temperature is important, food producers will be very cautious about the 'life' they claim for the food. It is important that you understand the significance of the dates, so that you can eat foods at their best and avoid exposing your body to food poisoning organisms. This is vital when you are feeling 'under the weather' or suffering from a medical condition which taxes your immune system, be it an infection such as a cold, or cancer. Strong fit people can normally fight a bout of food poisoning, but elderly people and children don't fare as well, because their bodies are not as well equipped to fight infection. It amazes me that some of my patients don't seem to understand that food poisoning can kill you. The only group of people who tend to take the issue seriously are pregnant women, who realize that it is not only their health, but also their babies' health that is at risk.

The first rule of avoiding food poisoning is to abide by the dates on the label. Certain foods are exempt from date labelling, including foods that are not pre-packed, foods that have a shelf-life of longer than 18 months, eggs, fresh fruits and vegetables (unless they are pre-prepared), frozen foods and ice cream (which carry a star marking), breads and cakes which are intended to be eaten within 24 hours. However, many food manufacturers choose to put a date on the label, to guide either the person selling or buying the food.

- The 'sell by' date is to let the retailer know when to remove food from the shelves. The majority of foods are perfectly safe to eat after the sell by date.
- The 'use by' date provides you with a guide as to when the food is at a low level of contamination. It is usually seen on foods that perish from micro-biological damage relatively easily, in other words they go off quite quickly. They are perfectly safe to eat up to and including the use by date. Although food manufacturers generally err on the side of caution, chiefly because they are not sure how cold your refrigerator or larder is, you shouldn't eat foods after their use by date. Fridges should be kept between 0 and 5°C – it might be a good idea to buy a fridge thermometer.
- 'Best before' dates are found on foods with an expected life of six to twelve weeks. These foods rarely expose you to any food poisoning risk, but this date gives you an idea of when the food tastes at its best.

Food with an expected shelf-life of more than 18 months doesn't have to carry any date. However, the food manufacturer is legally bound to tell you whether there are any special storage conditions you need to adhere to.

Hygiene in the home

In addition to paying attention to food dates and labels there are other steps you can take to reduce the likelihood of developing food poisoning.

- Wash your hands carefully after you have touched any animal or used the lavatory.
- Keep work surfaces clean and wash tea towels regularly.
- Make sure that meat and poultry are cooked appropriately before you eat them. Rare meat is fine for most people, as long as you are certain that the meat is fresh and of superb quality. Poultry, however, should always be well cooked, with no trace of pink.

Think good

- Wash all fruits and vegetables before you eat them.
- Always keep cooked and raw foods separately in the refrigerator, so that the bacteria from raw foods do not infect cooked foods.
- Use separate chopping boards for raw and cooked meat and fish; and another for vegetables and fruits (or mark separate sides of two chopping boards).
- Avoid tins with blown ends as this could, even if only rarely, signify the presence of the bacterium that causes botulism.
- If cooked food is to be kept, it must be cooled as quickly as possible, then, when it is cold, wrapped and refrigerated.
- Always reheat cooked rice until it is piping hot. *Clostridium perfringens* may be found in rice that has been cooked and left in a warmish environment, then not thoroughly reheated. If you eat rice dishes in restaurants, make sure that it is piping hot all the way through, as more cases of food poisoning come from rice than from any other food.

Washing and peeling

It is particularly important to wash fruits and vegetables thoroughly, not only to reduce the risk of food poisoning, but also to remove the pesticides, waxes and other substances used to protect them. If not removed, these substances can lead to free radical damage within the body's cells, which can cause cancer and heart disease (see page 46), and have been linked to other health problems.

I recommend you buy organic food as much as possible, as it is produced without the use of chemical pesticides, fertilizers and other artificial substances; organic produce should be washed to remove dirt.

Some people recommend that you peel fruits for children, as they believe you cannot remove the harmful substances by washing alone. I think children should be perfectly safe eating washed fresh fruits and vegetables and indeed we should be encouraging them to do so, for a number of health reasons. Just make sure you wash produce carefully, especially when you buy from street markets, which are exposed to exhaust fumes.

Avoiding risks

LISTERIA

Listeria monocytogenes is the full name of the bacterium which causes listeriosis, a potentially harmful condition. It produces 'flu like' symptoms, but can cause miscarriage in pregnant women, or can damage the unborn child.
Unfortunately, there is a lot of misunderstanding about listeria bacteria, which are particularly dangerous because they can grow at refrigeration temperatures, unlike most food poisoning organisms. Many people believe that unpasteurized cheeses were to blame for the listeria outbreaks that caused so much concern in 1988–9. In fact, cases were traced to a soft cheese made from pasteurized milk, the Swiss Vacherin du Mont d'Or. The outer moulds of cheeses act to some extent as a protective bandage, keeping bad bacteria from adversely affecting

the inside of the cheese. Cutting away the white rind just before you eat the cheese should remove any potentially harmful bacteria. Softer, moister cheeses, including blue cheeses, are most likely to provide a breeding ground for listeria; soft cheeses without rinds are the most vulnerable. Unpasteurized hard cheeses that have been matured for nine months or more are virtually problem-free for pregnant women.

Other foods that have a greater-than-average risk of listeria infection are pâtés, salad vegetables such as lettuce and prepared salads such as coleslaw and potato salad. Pregnant women should also avoid soft whip ice cream. Ready-made chilled foods should be thoroughly reheated; be especially careful if you are using a microwave oven.

SALMONELLA

Salmonella thrives in foods that are insufficiently heated to kill the bacteria, particularly eggs, poultry and unpasteurized milk. It causes diarrhoea and vomiting, and possibly fever and headache, 12 to 48 hours after eating the infected food, and in rare cases has proved fatal. The very young and elderly, pregnant women and people recovering from an illness, whose immune systems are not working at full strength, are particularly vulnerable and should be treated by a doctor immediately.

To avoid salmonella poisoning, steer clear of foods containing raw and lightly cooked eggs, such as mayonnaise and some sauces and mousses. Egg dishes should be freshly and thoroughly cooked. All poultry and meat should be well cooked. Take extra care at parties, where food is left in warm rooms and the bacteria grow quickly.

TOXOPLASMOSIS

Toxoplasmosis is an infection caused by a parasite; it is not transferred from person to person. It is harmless to most adults, but if caught during pregnancy it can cause miscarriage or damage to the baby in the womb. It can only be diagnosed by a blood test, but sadly the symptoms don't usually appear until two to three weeks after contracting the disease. The symptoms, described as 'mild flu like', may include a slight fever, swollen glands, fatigue or a rash.

The bacterium lives in cats for about three weeks, but cats' faeces can remain infectious for up to eighteen months. Toxoplasmosis can be transmitted through the soil to other animals such as dogs.

In addition to the basic rules of hygiene listed on pages 78–9, the following will help pregnant women avoid toxoplasmosis:
- Avoid eating undercooked or raw meat, such as steak tartare, as these can harbour bacteria. Don't feed raw meat to your cats or dogs as this provides a route for infection. Make sure meat and poultry are well cooked before you eat them.
- Do not allow cat litter near food. Wear rubber gloves to clean up pet mess.

Think good

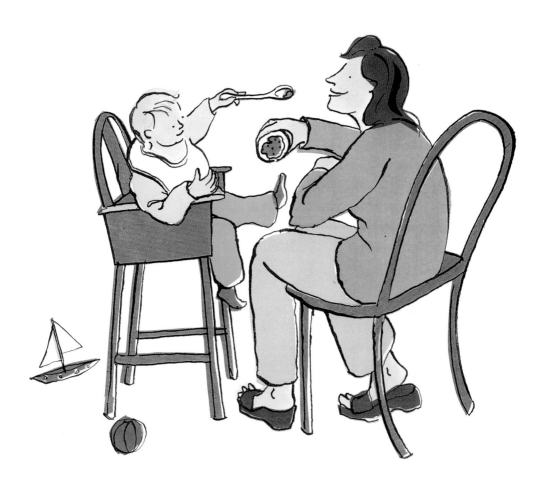

Family health day

If only we had time to be more proactive about our food: to evaluate how we are feeling, what we are eating and how the two can be improved. Eating well requires some organization at the outset. You need to plan how you are going to get good foods into your body with as little effort as possible. The last thing you want is to be stressed out about eating, or to slave over a hot stove only to sit down exhausted and unable to appreciate the experience. It is a good idea to set aside a day to tackle the issues head on. If members of the family ask why they need to change their eating habits, explain that it is to make them stronger and fitter, with clearer skin and loads more energy.

The aim of the family health day is to enjoy the time together, preparing food that is both delicious and nutritious, sorting out kitchen cupboards, throwing away out-of-date food and starting your healthy life on the right foot.

Evaluate your eating and drinking habits

Once you have set the date I suggest that, a week or two before your health day, everyone should fill out a food and symptom diary (see page 85). Take it with you to work or school. Children should try to keep a simple note of the food they eat at lunch and break times and to and from school. Don't forget cups of tea during the day and after-work drinks.

Use the diaries to build up a picture of the food you are putting into your body and the effect your eating habits are having on the way you feel. Remember, too, that food is a valuable preventive medicine: a few simple changes now could save you years of worry and pain in the future.

- Are you managing to eat five portions of fresh fruits and vegetables every day?
- Are you forever grabbing biscuits and cups of tea to keep you going?
- Do you always feel shattered?
- Does indigestion plague you?
- Do you often feel bloated?
- Is your child tetchy and unpredictable in mood; one minute 'hyperactive', the next, slumped in front of the TV, unable to motivate himself?

It's not just what you eat that's important, but also how you eat. Do you eat in front of the TV? Is it possible for you to share your child's eating times? Even if you cannot all eat together, perhaps because the children need to eat before adults are home from work, sitting down and spending a few minutes with them is a valuable activity. If you are eating your main meal later you could have a bowl of soup with them or some fruit. Seeing grown-ups dash around with no time to eat or eating a cake on the run tends to make children rush their food and not appreciate the importance of resting while you eat. Don't get into the habit of finishing their food; if you are not eating with the children, you should not use your body as a waste bin. During the family health day, take the opportunity to sit down together to eat and enjoy your food.

Shopping

Before planning the food you are going to eat during your family health day, think about your shopping habits. Do you rely on 'convenience' meals? Do you frequently turn to pasta because there is nothing else in the cupboards?

- Many of us don't like to stock up on vegetables and fruits because they go off before we manage to eat them. But tomatoes, carrots, peppers, citrus fruits, apples and pears keep well in the refrigerator. Leafy vegetables such as lettuces, spinach and rocket are the least sturdy, so buy them no more than a day ahead. Frozen vegetables such as spinach are useful standbys.
- Would it be a good idea to organize a substantial weekly shop? Many supermarkets will deliver to your home and can be accessed via the Internet. Even if you only use this service for bulky goods such as loo rolls, mineral water and canned beans it can help reduce the stress of lugging shopping around.

- Does your supermarket or local shop sell organic produce? The more organically produced food you can incorporate into your family's diet, the healthier you will all be.
- If members of your family suffer from bloating, look for 'live' or 'bio' yoghurts that contain bifidus and acidophilus cultures. Eat the equivalent of a small pot every day, with fruit or breakfast cereals or as a savoury dip or dressing.
- Does your shopping trolley get filled with the same items every week? It is amazing how many people think their partner or children won't eat certain foods, when in fact they would be happy to try. Don't let meals become so predictable they are eaten just out of habit. Talk about the meals you eat together and introduce a variety of foods.

Plans into action

The aim of the day is to see how you can maximize your physical health and mental well-being. When thinking about your eating habits, remember that food is there to be enjoyed, not to fill you with stress or guilt. There is always something delicious and healthy to be eaten, which should take but a few minutes to prepare, if you are well-organized and in control.

- Discuss beforehand what you are going to eat. Try some new dishes and base the day's meals around vegetables, fruits, lean proteins and starchy carbohydrates.
- Make fruit shakes for breakfast, thick vegetable soups for lunch and plan a special meal full of fresh vegetables in the evening. Have a good stock of fresh fruits in the house for between-meal nibbles.
- If you are having a health day as a couple or with friends, enjoy preparing the food together. If you are on your own, take the time to spoil yourself.
- If you have children, think of things they can do to help with the preparation and serving of the meals. This could be peeling potatoes, washing salad leaves or, if they are very young, just watching and stirring occasionally. Involving children in the preparation of meals helps to teach them how food is made. They are much more likely to eat foods they have 'helped' to cook. Children could help you make biscuits or cakes, such as flapjacks or gingerbread men. These can be part of a healthy diet if they are eaten in moderation, and really appreciated. It is rarely the people who sit down with a drink and a homemade biscuit who have health problems; it is far more likely to be those who eat a bag of sweets in the car and then still want some chocolate when they get home.
- Do some exercise. Staying physically fit is a vital part of a healthy lifestyle. Allow time to go for a long walk or a bicycle ride, and plan how your work and family life can accommodate regular exercise in the future.

Drinking healthily

Make sure that you all drink plenty of water. For optimum health, adults need two to two and a half litres/four to five pints of water every day, five-year-olds one litre/nearly two pints. Results can quickly be seen in a clearer skin and healthy hair. If you are unused to drinking water, begin your health day with two litres of mineral or tap water in the refrigerator and drink it throughout the day, with slices of lemon, orange or lime if you like.

Try to have a day free of caffeine – your body will feel much stronger in the long run. Instead, experiment with herb teas: add about a quarter teaspoon of honey to bring out the flavour. Remember that cola-based drinks contain caffeine; encourage your child to drink sparkling water and freshly squeezed juices, which can be fun to make.

Planning ahead

Besides preparing food for today, get your new healthy lifestyle on the right track by stocking up your refrigerator or freezer so you don't need to turn to ready-made meals and takeaways in the week.

- Make a large cauldron of soup. Freeze some portions to have 'on tap' when you need something warm and nourishing when you get home from work. It is much better to sit down and have a bowl of soup than to pick at crisps and nuts.
- Consider planting some herbs; children can help with this. Having fresh herbs to hand is a godsend when you want to make a simple dish a little more special. Torn basil jazzes up sliced tomatoes, rosemary turns a chicken breast into a tasty meat.
- Make fruit compotes to stock in the refrigerator. These can be mixed with yoghurt or breakfast cereals.
- Make some fruit puddings such as fruit crumbles made with a mixture of fruits – apricot and apple or blackberry and pear – and a wholemeal or oat topping. These can be baked in ramekin dishes as individual portions, which can be frozen and served as an after-work or after-school treat. They are much healthier than chocolate bars or bags of crisps, and because they are full of fibre you will eat less at your next meal (assuming you have drunk plenty of water to help the fibre swell).

After you have enjoyed the day as a family, round off the day with a relaxing healthy meal. If you don't want to cook anything complicated make a main course salad with some chicken or fish, or some hearty vegetable soup with warmed wholemeal bread, green salad or cold meats. Indulge in a special half bottle of wine. Finish the meal with some mint or camomile tea; caffeine at night can cause indigestion and sleep problems.

Keeping a food diary

Throughout this book I stress the importance of a well balanced and varied diet. So often, worrying symptons can be easily explained by an excess of a certain food or drink, or a lack of one of the essential nutrients discussed in the section on Understanding your nutritional needs. A food diary is a useful tool that can inspire you to look afresh at your eating habits.

Record everything you eat and drink for at least seven days. Write things down as soon as possible after eating them, rather than trying to remember them all at the end of the day. Along with the food, make a note of how it is prepared: grilled, fried, raw. If you eat foods from packets or tins and you suspect that there may be an additive which upsets you, you will need to record details of all the ingredients and additives. Remember to include all drinks, from a glass of water to a cup of tea. For young children, ask them to keep a note of what they eat away from the home, ask their teachers and parents of their friends to keep a note of everything they eat and drink; even a sweet or biscuit can be important.

The third column is for quantity; don't worry about exact measurements in ounces or grams, but for instance did you eat a breast of chicken or a slice? This will not only give you an idea of whether you are eating too little or too much, but if you are worried about a food intolerance or allergy you will be able to juggle the quantities of the food you eat – some people can take a small amount of an ingredient, but a large helping will cause a problem.

In the fourth column, record how you feel: do you have indigestion, are you very tired or do you notice that your energy level goes sky high? The more hypochondriacal you are during the time you keep the food diary, the more information you will be able to glean about the way you eat and the way your body feels. It is also worth noting in the fourth column why you are eating or drinking. Are you hungry, stressed or eating for comfort? The answers to these questions will tell you a lot about the emotional aspects of your eating habits.

DATE & TIME	FOOD OR DRINK CONSUMED	QUANTITY	SYMPTOMS
29 Aug 9 am 1.30 pm	coffee, lots of milk granary bread sandwich, egg mayo + cucumber	1 mug 2 slices	shaky fine

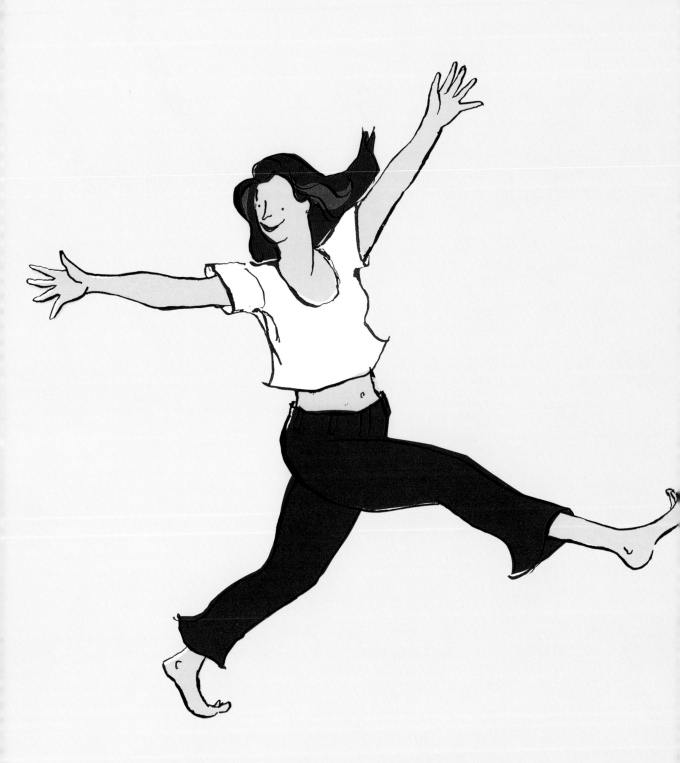

2
look good

Building strong bones

In order to look good, you have to begin with the basics. Although you can't see them, the bones form the basic framework for the body. A strong skeleton is the foundation for a healthy, vital appearance from childhood through to old age.

As a person grows from infancy to adulthood their bones evolve. The bones gradually become harder until the late teens, when the 'long bones', those in the arms and legs, reach their maximum strength and length. Then the process reverses: after the age of twenty, the bones begin to lose their density. For women, this decline in bone mass accelerates when they reach the menopause. Because of this, women are far more likely than men to develop osteoporosis, a weakening of the bones. Sadly, some children and young women develop an infantile or early form of osteoporosis, especially when they suffer from anorexia nervosa. Another cause of bone loss, which applies to men, women and children, is the use of steroid drugs. These are sometimes prescribed for conditions such as severe asthma.

Childhood is the most important time for bone growth. The more bone you have to start with, the greater cushion your body has to fall back on in later years when new bone tissue is no longer deposited. Once you are past your teens, you should continue to pay attention to bone maintenance, making sure that your body has adequate levels of certain essential nutrients. Chief among these is calcium, which needs the support of vitamins D and K, magnesium and several other minerals.

Calcium

The recommended daily intake of calcium is 450 milligrams a day for children up to six years old, increasing to 550 mg until they are eleven, then shooting up to 800 mg a day for girls and 1000 mg a day for boys. The discrepancy between the figure for boys and girls is a medical convention, and I do not think that it is necessary to curb the eating habits of children if you feel they are eating more calcium-rich foods than the daily allowance.

After the age of twenty, the recommended adult intake of calcium is 700–800 mg a day for both men and women. However, when I see patients suffering from brittle bone disease (another name for osteoporosis) I have no hesitation in suggesting a daily intake of 1000 mg a day, to help retain the maximum level of calcium within the bones.

A cup of hot chocolate is an occasional calcium-rich treat for both children and adults. Although large amounts of chocolate can inhibit the body's absorption of calcium, if you use top-quality chocolate, which has a high cocoa bean content, you only need a small amount.

Allow two squares of chocolate to a small cup (about 200 ml) of milk. Put the milk in a saucepan. Break the chocolate into another small saucepan, add a little of the milk and place over a gentle heat until the chocolate softens. Gently heat the remaining milk to just below boiling point, then turn down the heat. Remove the pan containing the chocolate from the heat. Using a whisk, whip the chocolate mixture to a smooth paste. Slowly add the hot milk, stirring constantly. The drink should not be allowed to boil.

Milk and other dairy products are the main providers of calcium in the Western diet. It makes little difference whether you drink skimmed or the richest Jersey milk, low fat or whole milk yoghurt. Goats' milk is slightly lower in calcium than cows' milk, sheep's milk is slightly higher. Hard and semi-soft cheeses (such as Brie) have high levels of calcium; cottage cheese and fromage frais contain similar amounts to yoghurt. To achieve the recommended daily intake a child could have 500 ml (just under a pint) of milk or 300 g (two small pots) of yoghurt or 75 g/3 oz of cheese. To get 750 mg of calcium an adult would need 650 ml (about 1¼ pints) of milk, 400 g/14 oz of yoghurt or 100 g/3½ oz of cheese. Teenagers or people with a low calcium status would need 850 ml (nearly 1½ pints) of milk, 500 g (a large pot) of yoghurt or 125 g/4 oz of cheese. Don't feel you have to force down a pint of milk at one go – it can be used in drinks and cooking throughout the day – and a combination of different products provides a wider range of nutrients than sticking to just one.

If either you or your children are unable to consume dairy products, it may help to consult a dietitian to help you plan a calcium-rich diet. Non-dairy calcium-rich foods include tofu, spinach, sesame seeds, dried apricots and canned fish such as salmon and sardines. See page 42 for more on calcium.

Vitamin D

Vitamin D is required in conjunction with calcium to create and maintain strong bones. It is produced by the body through exposure to sunlight. If you are an active person who regularly goes outside you shouldn't have any problems with your vitamin D status. Children should be encouraged to play outside. As we get older, however, our skin becomes less efficient at metabolizing vitamin D, so it is a good idea to include some vitamin D rich foods in your normal eating plan. The best sources are the oily fish and dairy products (see page 41).

Vitamin K

This is needed to help form strong bones. Vitamin K is mainly produced in the bowel by bacteria, and little is derived from food. Therefore if you have a normal healthy gut, your vitamin K status should be good.

Magnesium, boron, zinc, manganese and copper

All of these minerals are needed for a good bone status. If you eat a well balanced diet and lead a healthy lifestyle, your intake of these nutrients should be adequate. If you are worried that your intake may not be high enough, keep a detailed food diary for a week (see page 85), and compare your diet to the lists below to get a real idea of how well you are doing. If you are still concerned, consult a dietitian before you turn to supplements.

- Dietary sources of magnesium: wholegrain cereal products, such as bread and brown rice; nuts and seeds; dried apricots; green vegetables, such as watercress and spinach (see also page 44).

- Dietary sources of boron: cabbage, peas, lettuce, alfalfa sprouts, apples, pears, plums, prunes, grapes, raisins, dates, nuts.
- Dietary sources of zinc: shellfish, canned sardines; turkey, duck, lean red meats, liver and kidneys; hard or crumbly cheeses such as Parmesan, Cheddar, Stilton, Lancashire; wholegrain breads and brown rice (see also page 45).

There are no particularly rich sources of manganese and copper; they will be provided by a balanced diet.

Exercise

Regular load-bearing exercise throughout life helps to build up both a strong muscular frame and strong bone mass. Everyone should exercise for at least twenty minutes on at least three occasions every week. The exercises that will achieve the best results are those that involve standing or resting your weight on your limbs, for example running, hockey, tennis, brisk or 'power' walking.

Exercise is a habit for life. For children and adolescents it is important because this time of life is when bones are still developing. It is also the time when the seeds of a healthy lifestyle are set. Later in life, exercise helps to reduce the rate of bone loss and reduces the risk of heart disease.

Potential pitfalls

Certain factors inhibit the body's absorption of calcium and other nutrients.
- Caffeine inhibits the absorption of calcium and other vitamins and minerals from the gut and can cause your body to excrete more. You should therefore keep your caffeine intake down to three cups of tea, coffee, cola or other caffeine-containing drinks a day. See page 343 for some delicious alternatives.
- High-fibre foods contain substances that can inhibit the absorption of calcium from the gut. If you follow a well-balanced diet this shouldn't be an issue, but if you are vegan or a strict vegetarian you should try not to overdo the fibre content. Instead of having loads of wholegrain bread and rice, try to include some of the white varieties. In fact, white flour is often fortified with calcium.
- Researchers have found that a high intake of salt can cause the body to excrete more calcium. This is one of the reasons why it is best to keep your salt intake down – look to fresh herbs and spices to help you flavour foods and limit your intake of salty snacks such as crisps and nuts.
- Research shows that there is an increased risk of osteoporosis in people who smoke. Smoking also increases requirements for many vitamins and minerals.
- If young women lose so much weight that they cease to menstruate regularly, they will not produce sufficient oestrogen to protect their bones and build up bone mass while they can. It is healthiest to maintain a body mass index in the range 20–25 (see page 109). Similarly, men who follow extreme restrictive diets can cause their testosterone levels to drop to such a low extent that their bones can lose density, putting them at risk of osteoporosis.

Healthy teeth for life

A bright smile, showing clean, white teeth, is undeniably attractive. By beginning to take care of your children's teeth at an early age, you will set the groundwork for their adult smiles. But no matter what your age, you should never take healthy teeth for granted: a healthy diet and good dental hygiene are vital if you are to avoid that 'down in the mouth' feeling.

Your child's teeth

The first set of baby teeth, commonly called 'milk' teeth, are forming in the gums before birth. Usually children have their full set of milk teeth by the time they are two and a half years old and they keep these until they are six years old, when their adult teeth start to push through.

It is important to care for your child's teeth from day one by not only giving them the best foods to nurture the growth of healthy teeth, but also by teaching them correct oral hygiene. Although the milk teeth are temporary, they protect the developing adult teeth – and good habits are best established early.

Today most dentists advise that parents begin brushing their children's teeth as soon as they appear, using a baby toothbrush and a smear of fluoride tooth-paste; after eighteen months use a children's brush and a pea-sized amount of paste. Try to teach your children not to swallow the toothpaste, but to rinse with water and spit out the excess.

Children should have their first official visit to the dentist when they have their full set of baby teeth (I encourage parents to take their child to the dentist with them on their own visits, because this can help familiarize the child with the dentist's chair and set-up). This early visit will allow the dentist to make a preliminary evaluation of the child's teeth, spotting potential problems early. If the child is treated appropriately from the beginning, they are far less likely to have to undergo many treatments.

Fluoride

Fluoride is a mineral that can reduce tooth decay. It works by creating an environment in the mouth that is hostile to the harmful bacteria that cause tooth decay. It occurs naturally in water in some areas, and in other areas it is added to the water supply as a means of preventing tooth decay. It is useful to know whether the water in your area is fluoridated; be aware that if you and your children drink bottled water, you will not benefit from this fluoridation. Getting the balance right is very important: too little fluoride means that the teeth will not be adequately protected, but too much can lead to a condition known as fluorosis, which causes permanent staining of the teeth. At the first visit to the dentist, additional fluoride treatments, such as drops, may be recommended – but these should be applied only on a dentist's advice.

Food for healthy teeth

As for bones (see previous section), the foods that help you build and maintain strong teeth are those rich in calcium, vitamin D and magnesium. The other crucial factor here is your gums; for these, the most important nutrients are vitamins A, C, the B complex and zinc. In other words, to keep a happy smile and disease-free mouth for as long as possible, a well-balanced diet, with plenty of vegetables and fruit, is as important as regular brushing and dental care.

Sugar – the enemy of teeth

Sugar is the single biggest cause of tooth decay. It is found in many forms, and sometimes in surprising places. In addition to the sugar you buy in bags (sucrose), it is an ingredient in many foods and drinks, both sweet and savoury. On labels, sugar may hide under the following names: sucrose, fructose, glucose, honey, dextrose, maltose, concentrated fruit juice, hydrolysed starch. Artificial sweeteners such as sorbitol, aspartame and saccharin can be just as damaging. The claim 'no added sugar' means that the food was already sweet enough.

Fruit and herbal drinks, including those diluted with water, often contain a lot of sugar (fructose or fruit sugar). In addition, fruit and fruit drinks may contain acid that attacks tooth enamel, clearing the way for the decay-causing bacteria. Rinse your mouth with clear water after a fruit snack or drink.

Cravings for sweet foods are generally established in childhood, when sweets and biscuits are given as gifts and rewards. Try to think of savoury foods and non-food items in the same way. Encourage good habits in your children, but remember that it is never too late to change.

- Choose savoury foods as snacks, for example, a selection of raw vegetables such as celery, carrot and pepper strips, or a piece of cheese with a few grapes.
- Foods that need chewing, such as toast, pitta bread, raw vegetables and fruit, help keep teeth and gums healthy.
- Make eating the occasional sweet a real treat and try to avoid toffees and other sweets that remain in the mouth for a long time.
- Eat sweets soon after meals, then brush the teeth.
- Never dip a dummy in a sugary drink or allow a child to suck on a bottle filled with sweet fruit juice. Babies should not go to bed with a bottle of milk in their mouths, because milk also contains natural sugars.
- Don't eat or drink anything other than water after teeth have been cleaned at night.

Once you have a healthy set of teeth, you should actively preserve them. Eating a healthy diet, flossing, brushing and visiting your dentist regularly are all equally important.

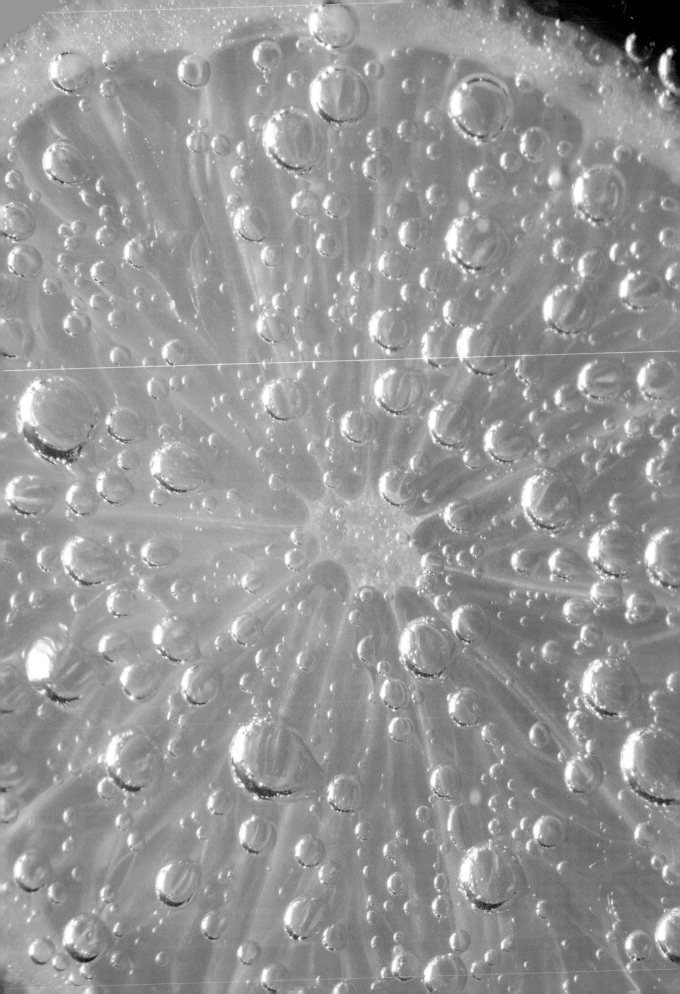

Keeping skin young-looking

The skin is the largest organ of the body. Through its many sensitive nerve endings, it provides us with a phenomenal amount of information about what is going on around us. And although it is highly sensitive, it is also tough enough to protect our inner organs from the stresses and strains of the outside world. It survives years of bombardment with heat and cold, bumps and cuts, environmental pollution and cigarette smoke, and the stress of poor sleeping and eating habits.

The skin consists of millions of living cells that rely on a regular supply of oxygen and nutrients. Adverse changes in the balance of nutrients or your general health quickly start to show in your skin, because skin cells have a very short life span – remarkably, they are replaced every few days. As most people find out after a bad cold or when work has eaten into your leisure and resting time, the appearance of the skin gives a very good indication of your overall health. A clear, glowing, moist skin reflects a healthy body, whereas dull, dry or greasy skin suggests that things are not as they should be within your body.

Unfortunately, your genetic makeup also affects your skin: families pass on the tendency to develop acne, eczema and psoriasis. Some medical practitioners fail to appreciate that while skin problems rarely pose a serious health risk, they can have profound effects on psychological well-being.

Even if you are born with fantastic skin, you still need to look after it. You can't work hard, play hard and cut corners in your eating habits and expect it not to show. Millions of pounds are spent on creams, lotions and tablets designed to tackle spots or dry skin, prevent wrinkles and prolong a youthful appearance. Although cleansing and moisturizing are an essential part of a skin health routine, it is not enough just to tackle the surface. If you are to build and maintain healthy skin, you need to provide it with health-giving foods and eliminate from your life those factors that hinder its function.

Understanding your skin
The skin consists of three layers. The deepest layer is the subcutaneous layer, which contains the main blood vessels, fat, and two types of protein: collagen, which provides the skin with a smooth, firm texture; and elastin, which makes your skin resilient. The middle layer, the

dermis, protects the deeper subcutaneous layer and contains small blood vessels, hair follicles and sweat glands. The dermis also supplies the upper layer, the epidermis, with new skin cells. Over the epidermis is an outer layer of dead skin cells, which swell in response to water. These cells are shed and replenished every day.

Patients frequently ask me why their skin has changed for the worse? The answer could be that they are simply not drinking enough water or getting enough of a particular nutrient, such as vitamin C. It could also be excessive amounts of caffeine or alcohol, or the build-up of chemicals that can come from pesticides and additives in the food we eat and even from nutritional supplements. Poor skin could also be caused by hormonal or emotional problems, which need to be addressed if you are to improve your skin.

The elements of healthy skin

WATER

One of the most common causes of tired, unhealthy, grey-looking skin is dehydration, both on the surface and within your body. The skin helps the body regulate its temperature by allowing heat to escape, in the form of water evaporating from the skin – sweat. Dashing around, living in centrally heated houses and eating a diet high in salts, additives and preservatives all exacerbate the loss of water from the body, and your skin is the first organ to show the signs of water deprivation.

How many of us have dry skin, despite using good moisturizers? Rather than buying yet another cream, I prefer a cheaper and more effective remedy – start boosting your water intake. An adult body needs at least two litres/four pints of water every day.

Water is truly the essence of life. It should ideally be taken as plain water and not as tea, coffee or soft drinks, which often contain caffeine, sugar or both.

It is important to establish the habit of drinking water as early as possible. Many children and teenagers who suffer from skin problems drink very little water, choosing colas, sports drinks, hot chocolate or sweetened juices throughout the day. As soon as they get into the water habit, their skin improves dramatically. Many teenagers are able to stop or reduce antibiotic medication, frequently used to control spots, and young children can reduce their use of creams. To encourage children to drink water, try providing them with a small, colourful water container to carry in their satchel or sports bag. You should also place a jug of water on the table at meal times.

Adults whose liquid intake is mainly of tea, coffee and alcoholic drinks will notice the improvement in their skin when they switch to water. Carry a small mineral water bottle in your handbag or briefcase and get into the habit of having water at your desk. Instead of a tea or coffee break, choose water for a truly refreshing drink that will help you look and feel good.

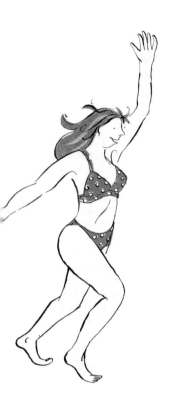

FRUIT AND VEGETABLES

A well balanced diet provides your skin with a regular supply of nutrients and oxygen. Fresh fruits and vegetables contain a huge array of skin-replenishing vitamins and minerals, as well as providing additional water. Children may be reluctant to eat a whole piece of fruit, but it is easy to incorporate fruit into their diet by giving them fruit purée with their breakfast cereal or in pots of yoghurt. Encourage them to take a bunch of grapes or some easy-to-peel satsumas to school instead of a chocolate bar.

Equally it is never too late to bring fruits and vegetables into your diet. Wrinkles will never disappear, but you can reduce the appearance of new lines and improve the texture and general bloom of your skin.

VITAMIN A

Many adults, especially women, take vitamin A supplements in the hope of improving their skin. It is true that doctors sometimes prescribe vitamin A creams for severe skin problems, but these are used under close medical super-vision. It is relatively easy to overdose on vitamin A if you take a supplement, and vitamin A toxicity can cause liver problems; in pregnant women it can lead to birth defects in the baby. I would strongly advise against taking vitamin A supplements. Instead, boost your intake of the fruit and vegetables that contain the vitamin A precursor beta-carotene, including carrots, spinach, watercress, apricots, mangoes and melons. See page 37 for more suggestions.

ZINC

Zinc helps to reduce the inflammatory processes within the body and aids healing, which is why it can help improve skin conditions such as eczema and psoriasis. Zinc-rich foods include seafood, hard and crumbly cheeses, nuts, seeds and pulses (see page 45). If you feel your diet is low in zinc-rich foods, you may wish to take a daily supplement; the dose should not exceed 15 mg, because high zinc levels make your body more susceptible to infections.

Where could I be going wrong?

Contrary to popular belief, bad skin is not generally caused by any one food, unless allergies are involved. However, particular foods can aggravate skin that is already poor and inappropriately nourished.

THE SUGAR MYTH

One of the greatest myths about the skin is that sweets, in particular chocolate, directly cause spots. However, if your diet contains excessive amounts of sweets, it frequently means that it is lacking in health-giving foods. People who snack on a chocolate bar generally do this instead of grabbing an apple or orange. The vitamins within fruits and vegetables, especially vitamin C, are incredibly import-ant for helping to resist the infections that can plague poorly nourished skin.

Also, people tend to eat more chocolate and sweet, quick-fix foods when they are feeling hormonally low, stressed or in need of comfort, all of which suggest that the body, including the skin, is running low on good fuel and helpful hormones. The skin looks bad at this time simply because you are low, not because you have eaten sweets.

CAFFEINE

Caffeine (and also tannins) found in coffee, tea, cola drinks and some of the new 'sports' drinks not only has a dehydrating effect that drains the skin, it also inhibits the absorption of vitamins and minerals from the gut, thus diminishing the potential benefits of healthy eating. Children's bodies are particularly sensitive to the effects of caffeine, but I recommend that even adults drink no more than two to three cups of caffeine-containing drinks a day.

ALCOHOL

Not only does alcohol have a dehydrating effect on the body, but, in excess, it causes the skin to become coarse and to develop thread veins and open pores. You shouldn't develop these symptoms if you stay within the recommended weekly maximum of 28 units for men and 21 for women. A unit means a glass of wine, half a pint of beer or a single measure of spirits.

However, certain additives, preservatives or natural substances such as salicylates or moulds in particular drinks may cause skin reactions. The most common allergic reaction to alcohol is hives (small, itchy red spots under the surface of the skin); intolerance to alcoholic drinks can also worsen psoriasis and eczema. The most common reaction is to salicylates, found primarily in beer. Gin, vodka, whisky and most wines are relatively low in salicylates, but trial and error is the best way to find out what suits you as an individual.

SMOKING

Smoking undoubtedly ages the skin. The nicotine attacks the blood vessels that supply the skin with nutrients and oxygen, as well as those that drain away the skin's waste products. It also affects the body's ability to metabolize vitamin C (see page 51). If you want to have a youthful healthy appearance, give up smoking.

Avoiding wrinkles

The search for everlasting youth drives people to spend hundreds of pounds on creams and even drugs, some of which claim to be able to banish wrinkles and halt the ageing process. While creams can help protect the skin, nourishing the skin takes place on a deeper level.

Within the skin are two types of protein, collagen and elastin. Collagen gives the skin a strong, firm texture, while elastin makes it resilient. If you want to avoid wrinkles, you need to try to preserve these two components in your skin. Wrinkles start appearing as the collagen and elastin fibres start to deteriorate, from around thirty years of age. Excessive exposure to sunlight speeds this process.

DIET AS THE FIRST LINE OF DEFENCE

The food you eat can help in the fight against wrinkles by reducing the effect of free radicals on the skin. Free radicals are unstable molecules that occur naturally in our bodies and are also produced by sunlight, smoke, air pollution and certain foods. They have a damaging effect on cells within the body, including skin cells. It is possible to reduce the damage caused by free radicals in two ways: by making sure that our diet contains foods that limit the effect of free radicals, and by avoiding foods that encourage the production of more free radicals.

A group of nutrients known as antioxidants can protect against free radical damage by 'soaking up' the rogue molecules and limiting the cell damage. A diet rich in antioxidants (beta-carotene, vitamins C and E and selenium) is the best way to protect yourself against wrinkles and a host of more serious health problems. See the chapter on Understanding your nutritional needs.

On the down side, certain foods are thought to increase the number of free radicals produced in the body. Hydrogenated vegetable oil or fat (found in some margarines and in nearly all processed foods, from cakes and biscuits to stock cubes) is one of the major foods suspected.

Chemicals and pesticides present in the wax used to protect fruit and some vegetables have been implicated in the free radical scenario. Fruit and vegetables are also susceptible to air pollution as they grow. You should therefore wash them thoroughly before eating and try to choose organic suppliers whenever possible.

EXERCISE

Exercise helps keep a good blood flow to the skin, ensuring that it is well provided with oxygen and nutrients and cleared of waste products. Regular cardiovascular exercise keeps your skin and the rest of your body fit and younger looking. In addition, facial exercises help preserve good tissue drainage and a good muscular structure. It is important not to let your facial muscles sag from lack of use. Keep smiling!

AVOID YO-YO DIETING

Losing dramatic amounts of weight can cause you to develop saggy skin; conversely gaining large amounts of weight stretches the skin and up pop the unsightly stretch marks. Changing your weight gradually, by a kilo or a couple of pounds a week, allows your skin to shrink or stretch gently, so the elastin and collagen fibres can accommodate the change.

The stretch marks that appear during pregnancy are due to hormonally triggered changes in the protein within the skin. They should disappear after birth, or at least fade significantly. Unfortunately no creams will stop them.

Skin problems

Problem skin can affect all age groups. It causes physical discomfort and embarrassment, but worse still, the psychological scars can remain long after the blemishes have cleared.

Skin conditions, including eczema, acne, psoriasis and even skin cancer, are often triggered by an allergic reaction to a food, a vitamin or mineral deficiency, or an excess of either a substance or an activity. There can also be a strong genetic link: for example, children born into a family with a history of asthma or hay fever are more likely to develop eczema. Although most skin problems are not directly caused by food, many can be helped by the correct food.

Food-related skin allergies need to be investigated with the help of either a dermatologist or dietitian, especially when young children are concerned, because it is potentially risky to start cutting out foods from the diet without a nutritious substitute.

ACNE

Acne vulgaris is one of the most dreaded conditions affecting young people, but even adults suffer, and some only start developing spots in their middle years. Fundamentally acne is the result of the over-production of sebum, which is produced by the oil glands of hair follicles. When the pores become clogged with sebum, blackheads, pimples and large spots erupt on the face, chest and back.

Many people wrongly believe that acne is caused by eating too many fatty and sugary foods, such as chocolate. It is primarily a hormonal problem, which is why it is usually found in adolescents, but it is also true that eating sweet or fatty foods in place of a healthy diet with plenty of fresh vegetables and fruits will aggravate the condition. Acne also tends to be worse during times of stress or emotional upset, which is when we tend to cheer ourselves up with sweets or cut corners in our meal preparation and grab fatty or sugary convenience foods.

A balanced diet, with an emphasis on foods rich in vitamin A and zinc, is helpful in clearing up skin. Boosting your intake of oily fish can help to reduce inflammation (see Psoriasis).

If you are taking antibiotics to control acne, you may suffer from certain side effects, such as thrush and irritable bowel symptoms. This is because antibiotics kill the good bacteria in the gut. A good bacterial balance needs to be established, so I suggest you take a small pot of 'live' yoghurt containing acidophilus and bifidus, every day (see page 47).

PSORIASIS

Psoriasis is an extremely common, chronic skin disorder that can afflict people of all ages. It begins with red, dry patches that become covered with white scales. The worst areas to be affected are the elbows, knees, legs and scalp. It is itchy, and the skin can become so sore that it bleeds; in the worst cases, infections develop.

Although there is no cure for psoriasis, correct nutrition can have a dramatic effect. Results take several weeks to appear, so don't expect an overnight cure.

One of the most effective nutritional therapies for psoriasis uses oily fish, such as herring, mackerel, tuna and salmon. These fish contain substances called omega 3 fatty acids and omega 6 fatty acids, which have been shown to alter the body's biochemistry; in particular they alter the inflammatory reaction that is thought to bring on psoriasis. One portion a day can bring about astounding results, and even three helpings a week can provide substantial relief. What is important is that in order for the omega fatty acids to be effective, your total fat intake, especially of saturated fats, must be low (see page 32 for information about saturated fats).

Dermatologists often recommend exposure to natural sunlight or special sun-lamps as a treatment for psoriasis. Interestingly, if your diet is rich in a substance called psoralen, the sunlight will have a greater effect. Psoralen is found in limes, lemons, lettuce and parsley – all perfect additions to salads.

Stress can aggravate psoriasis, and it helps to make sure that your body does not become 'run down', either as a result of incorrect nutrition or of rapid weight loss or gain.

A reaction to substances found in alcoholic drinks often seems to worsen psoriasis and eczema. Rather than depriving yourself of all wine and beer, it is worth experimenting with different types. One of my patients suspected that his psoriasis was aggravated by his heavy red wine intake at the weekend. The interesting fact was that he nearly always drank Chianti, so we started to explore other wines made from different grapes. And hey presto his psoriasis improved dramatically! This is a good example of why it is important to look at suspected allergies and intolerances in fine detail. It would have been easy, but such a pity, to say no red wine.

ECZEMA

Eczema is one of the most common skin conditions. There are several forms of eczema, all characterized by inflammation of the skin (dermatitis), usually red, itchy and flaky. Constant itching, followed by scratching, can cause the skin surface to break, causing bleeding and weeping. The worst aspect of eczema is when you scratch the skin so much that the skin becomes infected. Eczema is an allergy disorder, belonging to the group of conditions that includes asthma, hay fever, urticaria and irritable bowel syndrome. Often a predisposition to these conditions runs in families. Eczema is known as an atopic condition: this means that the symptoms can arise in any part of the body, not necessarily related to where the triggering irritation is occurring. The trigger may be certain foods, dust, pollen or other external irritants.

A nutritional cure of atopic conditions has two angles of attack: avoiding any food irritants, and helping your immune system to stay calm after it has been exposed to the offending allergen.

One of the most successful areas of nutritional treatment of eczema is exclusion diets – avoiding the food that triggers the reaction. Although not every case of eczema is tied to a food allergy or intolerance, it is always an avenue worth investigating, as it is much better to avoid the trigger than have to placate the symptoms. Exclusion diets can be a useful tool to identify any food intolerance, but unless they are carried out appropriately, they can lead to malnourishment, and many physical and emotional problems. If you have severe eczema you require specialized advice from your doctor or dietitian. People with mild eczema can begin by making their own experiments.

Cows' milk and eggs are common triggers for eczema. Try eliminating one item at a time from your diet, replacing them with nutritionally similar foods (see the chapter on Managing allergies for more on food intolerance).

Other common irritants include chicken, azo dyes (certain yellow, red, brown and black food colourings, used in a wide range of processed foods) and benzoates, found in the greatest quantities in processed foods.

Oily fish may help to reduce the inflammation in the skin (see Psoriasis).

Non dietary treatment includes avoiding biological washing powders and synthetic bedclothes and undergarments. Cotton is the best fibre to use. You could also take steps to keep the amount of dust, house mites and pet mites down to the minimum. If you find that you scratch a lot, keep your fingernails short, to reduce the damage caused by scratching.

SKIN CANCER

One of the most prevalent forms of cancer, skin cancer affects thousands of people every year and the incidence is rising. Women are more likely to develop it than men. If caught early, the majority of skin cancers can be treated very successfully. For this reason, everyone should keep a regular check on skin blemishes, freckles, moles and other bumps to monitor any changes such as increase in size, weeping, soreness or itchiness. Any changes must be checked by your doctor.

The best way to avoid skin cancer is to protect yourself against exposure to the sun. Any skin not covered by clothing must be protected by sunscreen creams or lotions. Sunbeds must be avoided at all costs – for a safe summer glow, try bottled tanning products instead.

Food neither causes nor cures skin cancer, but it can improve your ability both to fight the cancer and respond to therapies. The nutritional aim in treating any form of cancer is to make your immune system strong. See the chapter on cancer for more advice.

Healthy hair and nails

At first sight, hair differs far more than skin. Beyond the natural variation we are born with, we can change its style, length, colour and texture to a greater or lesser extent, yet everyone wants a full head of healthy-looking hair. Hair loss can cause a great deal of distress; sometimes it is a factor of growing older, but it can also be a sign of illness in the body. Diet can play a role in limiting hair loss and in facilitating the growth of healthy new hair.

About your hair
There are roughly 100,000 to 350,000 follicles on the human scalp, but not all of them are productive at any given time. Hair growth is cyclical: on the scalp each follicle is active for around 1,000 days (three years) and then rests for a period of 100 days (three months). This hair cycle varies from individual to individual and is influenced by age, diet and general state of health. The old hair from the last hair cycle may remain in the hair follicle until it is dislodged, for example by brushing, or pushed out by a new hair. Hair length is determined by the length of your growing phase. If you have a short growing phase of around 600 days, at the average rate of 0.33 mm a day your hair will grow to approximately 200 mm/8 inches. With very long growth phases the hair can grow down to the ground!

Hair food
Any 'food' you put on your hair in the form of conditioners can have no more than a cosmetic effect. Whether you buy the most expensive conditioner or make your own using eggs, the principles are twofold: protein clings to the hair shaft and thickens it, while oils lubricate, making the hair look shiny.

Remember that your hair reflects your general state of health; it is therefore important to look to your lifestyle if you want to keep your hair in good condition: eat a well balanced, healthy diet, take regular exercise, get plenty of fresh air and sleep, and don't smoke. To check that your diet is providing a wide variety of nutrients, I suggest you first read the section on Understanding your nutritional needs, then keep a food diary (page 85) for a week or two.

One of the simplest ways to improve the look of your hair (whether it is too dry or too greasy) is to drink more water. After all, it cannot look its best if it is dehydrated. This is not an occasional 'instant' remedy, but a lifelong necessity.

Caffeine has the opposite effect to water – it dehydrates the body. It also inhibits the absorption of vitamins and minerals and increases their excretion. People who are constantly drinking cups of tea, coffee or other caffeine-containing drinks such as cola can drain their body's iron stores to a level that can cause or aggravate hair loss. Choose water and within a couple of months you should notice an improvement in your hair and your general health and vitality.

Understanding hair loss

We all lose some hairs every day. It is important to realize that the amount lost is less significant than a change in your usual pattern. For example if you have been losing forty hairs a day and this increases to eighty, you will notice twice as many hairs when you brush or shampoo. Although eighty is still well within the normal range for hair loss, in this case it represents a 100 per cent increase.

Around 95 per cent of hair loss complaints are caused by just two conditions: increased hair shedding and genetic hair loss. Thyroid disease causes two per cent, alopecia areata (hair loss in patches) two per cent and scarring alopecia less than one per cent.

INCREASED HAIR SHEDDING

Most of the time there is a simple explanation for increased hair shedding. Certain illnesses and drugs, particularly chemotherapy for cancer, anti-coagulants for thrombosis and even the contraceptive pill, may be the cause. If you are not taking any new drugs, you should see your doctor to ensure that there is no underlying physiological cause. Viral illnesses can cause increased hair shedding eight to twelve weeks later. Stress can also cause hair loss, particularly bouts of acute stress, shock or bereavement. Excessive hair loss may be associated with skin conditions such as psoriasis, eczema or seborrhoeic dermatitis. It can also occur in children or young adults with malabsorption problems such as Crohn's disease, or people suffering from eating disorders such as anorexia nervosa. In the latter case the hair loss stops when body weight reaches an acceptable level and nutrient stores are replenished.

When there is no obvious physiological reason for the hair loss, it is most probable that it is caused by a nutrient imbalance. There has been a great deal of research into the role of nutrients in the cause and therefore the treatment of hair loss, but it is only recently that the correlation has been found between hair loss and low iron stores in the body. This is more of a problem for women than for men because of menstruation: every month women lose iron from their bodies and if this is not replaced, in time the body's iron stores become so low that hair loss occurs.

Women suffering from sudden hair loss should see their doctor to have both their serum ferritin and their haemoglobin levels tested. The serum ferritin level measures total iron stores in the body, whereas the haemoglobin level measures the iron in the blood. It is possible to have a low serum ferritin level and yet have a normal haemoglobin level because the body tries to maintain its haemoglobin level, drawing from its iron stores. A low haemoglobin level suggests iron-deficiency anaemia (see page 275), but if you find you have low serum ferritin the nutritional treatment is exactly the same.

- Boost your intake of iron-rich foods such as lean red meat, game and offal, and secondary sources such as eggs (yolks), dark green leafy vegetables and pulses (see page 44).
- Boost your intake of vitamin C (see page 40) and folic acid (see page 39); both are important to help your body absorb the iron from your food.
- Maintain a good balance of proteins. Hair follicles have extremely high requirements for essential amino acids (see page 30). In addition, researchers have found a link between the intake of lysine, one of the essential amino acids, and serum ferritin levels. Poor protein levels compromise the body's ability to build good ferritin stores. Vegetarians and vegans need to be particularly vigilant.
- Biotin deficiency can also cause hair loss. This nutrient is mainly produced by bacteria in your intestine, which could be a problem if antibiotics or other drugs are disturbing the balance of bacteria. It is also found in food; rich sources of biotin are cooked eggs (raw eggs severely inhibit biotin absorption), peanut butter, wholegrain foods (especially oats) and liver.

GENETIC HAIR LOSS

Many men are distressed by their thinning hair, but unfortunately there isn't any simple cure for hair loss due to a gene that has been with them since before they were born. Women can often be treated successfully with a drug therapy based on androgen hormones in combination with oestrogen; consult a doctor or trichologist for advice.

Nails

The skin is the nurturing bed for both nails and hair, so it is important to look after it well. If you suspect that your weak, brittle or blotchy nails are linked to poor skin, turn to page 96. To maintain good, strong healthy nails you should strive to eat a well-balanced diet, drink plenty of water, exercise regularly, avoid stress and generally look after your body by not smoking or drinking too much coffee or excessive amounts of alcohol.

It is rare that a deficiency in any one nutrient can cause poor nails. In fact, overdoses of some vitamins and minerals can lead to ridged, brittle and yellowish nails. In some cases, poor nails can signify health problems such as iron-deficiency anaemia or liver problems. You should definitely point poor nails out to your doctor if you also suffer from symptoms such as severe tiredness, nausea or lack of appetite. Severe calcium deficiency can manifest itself in brittle nails. Brittle nails often respond well to an increased intake of biotin (see above).

Non-nutritional therapies

Regular hand massages help to keep the nails supplied with blood (and therefore oxygen and essential nutrients). Manicures also encourage strong nails.

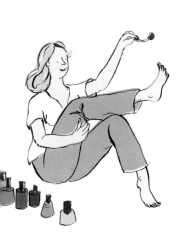

Healthy hair and nails

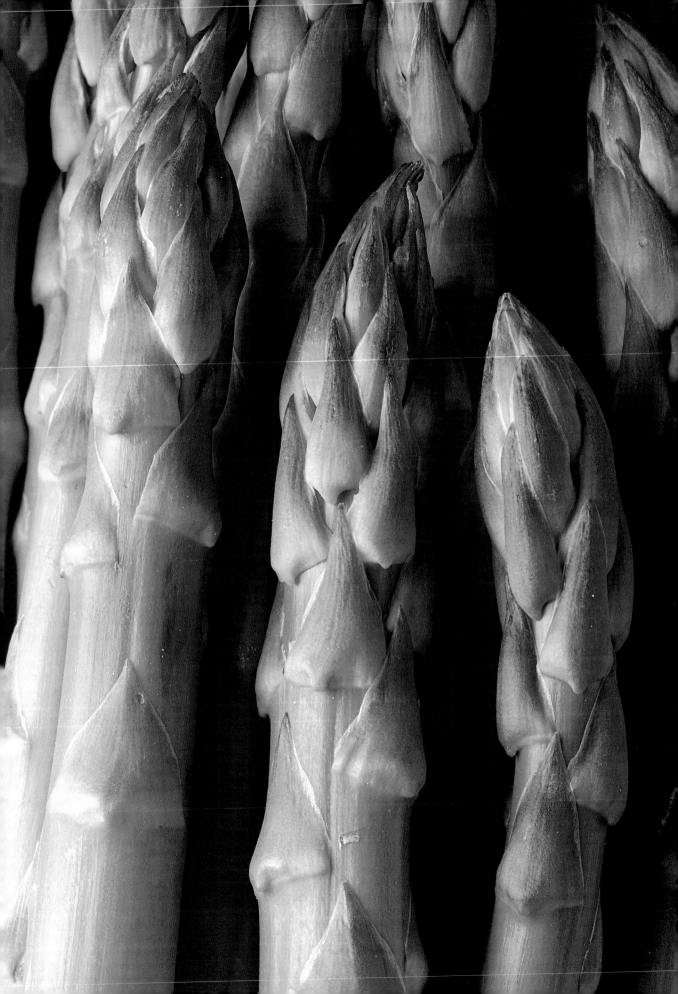

Achieving your ideal weight

Carrying excess weight affects the physical and psychological well-being of many members of society. The incidence of weight-related diseases, such as hypertension, diabetes and heart disease, is on the increase, and adults who grow heavier each year are more likely to enter their twilight years hindered by arthritis and less likely to feel full of 'joie de vivre'. In addition, more and more children are entering adulthood carrying excess body fat that will plague them for the rest of their years. Overweight children are suffering the pain of prematurely worn joints and are even showing the first signs of atherosclerosis (furring of the arteries).

There are a number of reasons why a fat adult or child may store too much fat.

- *Hereditary factors* Obesity does tend to run in families; possibly this is due to lifestyle and eating habits, which we can do a lot about. There is also a genetic element involved, as some children and adults will never be slight and slim, however much they try. It is essential to remember this and to be realistic.
- *Comfort eating* Food can a source of comfort, and therefore unhappy people may eat more than happy ones. If you notice that your child is putting on a lot of weight, try to find out if there is any reason why he or she is unhappy. We all have been known to use food as a bribe or a reward, but to use food as a replacement for love and attention is not healthy, especially as sugary and fatty foods are the ones normally offered in these situations. Instilling children with these inappropriate associations with eating can lead to problems in later life.
- *Lack of exercise* Remember that obesity often results from a simple imbalance of calorie intake versus expenditure.
- *Hormonal reasons* Conditions such as Prada Willi syndrome, where a child never feels full, are very rare and therefore I shall not refer to their specific treatments. You should seek the advice of a professional dietitian or doctor.

The slimming industry

A massive industry has grown up around our concern about our weight. January finds many people buying yet another diet book or starting another season in the gym, hoping and praying that this time the weight will come and stay off, easily. What they all need to realize is that radical diets don't work. To change one's lifestyle drastically, filling the cupboards with low-fat diet products, spending hours in the supermarket studying the calorie and fat levels on the side of packets, depriving oneself of favourite foods, is not only a miserable preoccupation, but it is also only a short-term solution. You may initially get good results, the pounds will in many cases fall off, but in six or twelve months time you will be back to square one, or even fatter than you were before.

Learning to lose excess weight, and most importantly maintaining your new body, is not about restriction in a negative way. It is more about understanding which foods your body needs, how best to deliver the essential nutrients and how to avoid the excesses. This sounds much more of an effort to begin with; to drink a milk shake or take diet pills only takes a few seconds in comparison, but the initial time investment will lead to lasting results.

However tempting it is to take a little tablet to help you lose weight…don't. There are several types of weight-loss drugs: some are based on amphetamines (which interfere with your body's metabolism) or thyroxine (a synthetic or animal-derived hormone) and some fill your stomach up with fibre-like substances. They all have side effects, ranging from extreme mood swings, depression, hyperactivity, stomach cramps, diarrhoea and above all dependency.

Once you start taking these drugs it is extremely hard to lose weight without them. You may lose some weight while you take them, but as soon as you come off them, your weight goes back to its starting point and frequently goes higher. I see hundreds of patients every year who have taken slimming drugs in the past, and who find losing weight without them exceedingly difficult. But when they try the drugs again they need to take more and more to achieve the same results. These drugs are potentially lethal: they can cause heart problems, kidney damage and severe digestive problems. They should never be given to children, unless your paediatrician prescribes them. And of course they don't address the problem of why you are overweight and how you can change your eating habits and general lifestyle to conquer the problem. Slimming pills should be prescribed by doctors only for patients whose obesity is such that their health is endangered, and never for social or cosmetic reasons.

Setting weight loss goals
Your sensible weight loss journey begins with two questions. How much weight do you want to lose? Is this target reasonable and achievable?

It is also worth asking yourself why you want to lose the weight. Is it for yourself or someone else? In the case of children, is it you the parent who wants them to lose the weight, or are you both determined to work together? Without the will to lose weight, it will be a struggle from day one.

This is particularly important with children. It is essential not to pressure them into losing weight, making meal times into battles. This may trigger a pattern of behaviour of eating secretly or using food as a control mechanism. The best scenario is to agree with your child that he or she will benefit from getting into better shape, to make them feel and look stronger and fitter.

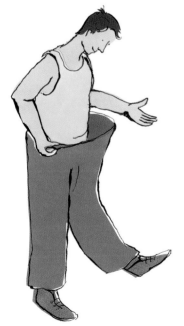

Ideal body weight

Obesity Grade	Body Mass Index	Weight ((kg) to the nearest 1kg)									
	45	101	104	107	110	112	115	118	121	124	127
	44	99	102	104	107	110	113	115	118	121	124
3	43	97	99	102	105	107	110	113	116	118	121
	42	95	97	100	102	105	108	110	113	116	119
	41	92	95	97	100	102	105	108	110	113	116
	40	90	92	95	97	100	102	105	108	110	113
	39	88	90	93	95	97	100	102	105	108	110
	38	86	88	90	93	95	97	100	102	105	107
	37	83	86	88	90	92	95	97	100	102	104
2	36	81	83	85	88	90	92	95	97	99	102
	35	79	81	83	85	87	90	92	94	96	99
	34	77	79	81	83	85	87	89	91	94	96
	33	74	76	78	80	82	85	87	89	91	93
	32	72	74	76	78	80	82	84	86	88	90
	31	70	72	74	75	77	79	81	83	85	88
	30	68	69	71	73	75	77	79	81	83	85
	29	65	67	69	71	72	74	76	78	80	82
1	28	63	65	66	68	70	72	74	75	77	79
	27	61	62	64	66	67	69	71	73	74	76
	26	59	60	62	63	65	67	68	70	72	73
	25	56	58	59	61	62	64	66	67	69	71
	24	54	55	57	58	60	61	63	65	66	68
0	23	52	53	55	56	57	59	60	62	63	65
	22	50	51	52	54	55	56	58	59	61	61
	21	47	49	50	51	52	54	55	57	58	59
	20	45	46	47	49	50	51	53	54	55	56
Under	19	43	44	45	46	47	49	50	51	52	54
weight	18	41	42	43	44	45	46	47	48	50	51
	17	38	39	40	41	42	44	45	46	47	48
Height	m	1.50	1.52	1.54	1.56	1.58	1.60	1.62	1.64	1.66	1.68
Height	ft ins	4.11	5.0	5.0¼	5.1½	5.2¼	5.3	5.3¾	5.4½	5.5½	5.6

Body Mass Index (BMI) = $\frac{\text{Weight in Kilograms}}{(\text{Height in Metres})^2}$

This is an ideal body weight chart which gives you a rough idea of the weight you should be. Remember the most important thing is how you feel in yourself.

Weight ((kg) to the nearest 1kg)													
130	133	136	139	143	146	149	152	156	159	162	166	169	173
127	130	133	136	139	143	146	149	152	156	159	162	166	169
124	127	130	133	133	139	142	146	149	149	155	159	162	165
121	124	127	130	130	136	139	142	145	145	152	155	158	161
119	121	124	127	127	133	136	139	142	142	148	151	154	158
116	118	121	124	127	130	133	135	138	141	144	148	151	154
113	115	118	121	124	126	129	132	135	138	141	144	147	150
110	112	115	118	120	123	126	129	132	134	137	140	143	146
107	110	112	115	117	120	123	125	128	131	134	136	139	142
104	107	109	112	114	117	119	122	125	127	130	133	136	138
101	104	106	108	111	113	116	119	121	124	126	129	132	134
98	101	103	105	108	110	113	115	118	120	123	125	128	131
95	98	100	102	105	107	109	112	114	117	119	122	124	127
93	95	97	99	101	104	106	108	111	113	116	118	120	123
90	92	94	96	98	100	103	105	107	110	112	114	117	119
87	89	91	93	95	97	99	102	104	106	108	111	113	115
84	86	88	90	92	94	96	98	100	103	105	107	109	111
81	83	85	87	89	91	93	95	97	99	101	103	105	108
78	80	82	84	86	88	89	91	93	95	98	100	102	104
75	77	79	81	82	84	86	88	90	92	94	96	98	100
72	74	76	77	79	81	83	85	87	88	90	92	94	96
69	71	73	74	76	78	80	81	83	83	87	89	90	92
67	68	70	71	73	75	76	78	80	80	83	85	87	88
64	65	67	68	70	71	73	75	76	76	79	81	83	85
61	62	64	65	67	68	70	71	73	73	76	77	79	81
58	59	61	62	63	65	66	68	69	69	72	74	75	77
55	56	58	59	60	62	63	64	66	67	69	70	72	73
52	53	55	56	57	58	60	61	62	64	65	66	68	69
49	50	52	53	54	55	56	58	59	60	61	63	64	65
1.70	1.72	1.74	1.76	1.78	1.80	1.82	1.84	1.86	1.88	1.90	1.92	1.94	1.96
5.6¾	5.7¾	5.8½	5.9¼	5.10	5.10¾	5.11¼	6.0½	6.1¼	6.2	6.2¾	6.3¾	6.4½	6.5¼

FRAME

Light Frame	Heavy Frame	
< 15	-	Seriously undernourished
15	19	Underweight
20	25	Acceptable/Desirable
26	30	Slightly overweight
31	40	Seriously overweight
-	40+	Dangerously overweight

Many adults and children associate sweets with rewards. It is important to reward ourselves and our children with non-food activities, such as seeing a movie or playing a favourite game.

With both children and adults, it is essential to find positive motivational points, rather than focusing on issues of vanity. The best motivation is health: if you lose excess weight, you have a decreased risk of heart disease, cancer, joint problems and diabetes. You should also feel more positive and more confident.

How much weight should you lose?

One guideline for healthy weight is the body mass index (see table on page 109). On average your ideal weight gives you a body mass index (BMI) in the range of 20 to 25. A body mass index of 25 to 30, although not in the seriously over-weight category, takes your weight into a range in which raised blood pressure and joint problems may start to occur. A body mass index of 30 and over is the dangerous area. It is really only heavy weight lifters with very high proportions of muscle to fat who can reside in this area without damaging their health.

Having said this, you should bear in mind that tables are constructed from a sample group of people. They do not take into account your individual body and weight history. Some people don't look or feel right within the 20–25 range: men who play a lot of sports have a greater than average muscle mass which means that their optimum weight is higher than the recommended ideal. If you feel comfortable at a certain weight and know that it is within a few pounds of the ideal, your body will not be compromised at your current weight.

Equally, if your weight is within the ideal range, but above the point at which you feel happy with your body, it is all right for you to lose a few pounds. However, a BMI in the region of 18 or 19 is the lowest acceptable: if your weight drops below this, you are increasing the likelihood of nutrient deficiency problems, halting your periods (for women), compromising your bone status and increasing the risk of developing osteoporosis (see page 89). Young women who keep their weight too low are particularly at risk because the first twenty-one years of life are crucial when it comes to building strong bones.

Many fitness centres offer body fat measurements. There are a number of ways in which this can be done: impedance meters calculate your body fat by using small amounts of harmless electromagnetic current; skin fold callipers measure the thickness of fat around various areas of your body; the measure-ments are then used to calculate your percentage body fat. The latest electronic scales can measure percentage body fat quite effectively. Bear in mind that many body fat charts were compiled in the 1970s when ideas on health and nutrition were very different to today. Their recommended body fat measurements are far lower than the ideal range of 19 to 24 per cent for women and 14 to 17 per cent for men. Even the most accurate reading of your percentage body fat will not tell you any more than you already know and can see by standing in front of a mirror.

Charting your progress

The best way to assess your progress is not by getting on the scales. It is far better to consider how you feel in yourself and in your clothes. However, if

Look good

you want to be able to make some more objective comparisons, take some body measurements. Using a tape measure, take the circumference of your arms, upper thighs, waist and chest and make a note of them, along with a starting weight, if you so desire. If you repeat the process monthly, you should notice that the measurements are decreasing.

I often see people who weigh themselves every day. This behaviour is destructive as you frequently end up being reactive: on days when you have lost weight you let the eating habits loosen up a bit, and on days when no weight loss shows on the scales, you become depressed and tempted to cut down even more. Daily weighing tends to show changes in body water. Some days we carry more water than others, so you are reacting to a factor which should be ignored.

In addition, fat is lighter than muscle, so if you are combining a change in eating habits with a healthy increase in exercise, your muscle to fat ratio will improve, but you may become despondent that you are not losing weight as quickly as you want to.

A good guide is to lose only about a kilo/2–3 lb a week. Usually if you lose more weight than this your body is either losing water (as is frequently the case during the first week of a change in diet) or muscle. In either case you should adjust your diet to slow the weight loss to this recommended rate. Controlled, steady weight/fat loss is what we are after. Rapid weight loss has a number of negative effects: it can lead to depression, stress, hormonal imbalances, low libido, decreased fertility and an increased risk of heart attacks and strokes.

How much weight should your child lose?

The easiest and most reliable way to tell whether your child needs to lose weight is to consult their growth charts with your doctor or health clinic.

In terms of monitoring progress, the same rules apply to children and teenagers as to adults; it is much better to use a tape measure to show them how their body is changing for the better, or simply go by how they look and feel in their clothes. Encourage your child to eat a healthy diet to enable their weight to catch up with their height. Guide them into good eating practices, such as eating at the table, eating slowly and concentrating on their food, not watching the television at the same time. They should also be encouraged to be physically active, playing sports, swimming, walking and doing some fun exercise such as dance or tai ch'i. For more information on good eating habits, read the chapter on developing a positive relationship with food (page 13), especially the section devoted to children (page 21).

Control your weight by positive thinking

Changing to a healthier lifestyle means thinking about the food you put into your body. It is not realistic to expect a miraculous overnight change in your weight, or any other aspect of your health.

• Set small achievable targets. Take one step at a time and allow yourself to achieve one goal before you attempt the next. This way you will stay positive, in control and confident.

- Try a family health day. Taking a day to look at how the whole family eats will help you to change your eating and living habits for the better (see page 81).
- Understand your appetite mechanism. If you learn how your body recognizes hunger and fullness (see pages 15–16), you can avoid overeating. This is one of the most valuable lessons you can teach your child.
- Stock your cupboards, refrigerator, drawer at work or school bag with healthy snacks, so that you are not tempted by chocolates and crisps.
- Try to eat regularly. Basing your eating pattern around three meals a day, plus snacks of fruit or vegetables, will stop your body from becoming desperately hungry and prone to grabbing sweet or fatty snacks.
- Take regular exercise to help you burn up some calories, raise your metabolic rate and keep your muscles toned.

Eating for weight loss

At the end of the day, weight loss is based on a simple equation: eat fewer calories than you expend. You can use more calories by increasing the amount of exercise you take, but if you are already – honestly – doing at least 20–30 minutes of exercise, three or four times a week, you should look at how you can reduce your calorie intake. Practically everything you put in your mouth provides calories (units of energy). Foods with a high percentage of water (such as fruit and vegetables) contain fewer calories than those with a high percentage of fat. Gram for gram, carbohydrates and protein provide less than half the calories of fat. By understanding the different food groups and how they react within the body, it will become easier to plan a healthy diet.

Fats

We all need some fat in our diets, to carry important fat-soluble vitamins, to help our bodies produce and regulate hormones, and to provide flavour. However, fats are concentrated sources of calories. One of the best ways to reduce your total calorie intake is to reduce your fat intake.

A common mistake is to think that margarines and oils have fewer calories than butter; they don't. However, many oils and some margarines are a better choice than butter healthwise as they do not produce cholesterol in the blood. Unless you have a cholesterol problem (see the chapter on High blood cholesterol), I think the best way to treat fat is to use one you like the taste of, be it butter or extra-virgin olive oil, but keep the quantity down to the minimum. To cut down your fat intake:

- Leave good food alone. Don't think that every dish needs to be smothered in a creamy or buttery sauce. Choose the best quality fish, meat, poultry or vegetables (ideally organic) and cook them simply. Grill a fillet steak; wrap a trout in foil and bake it in the oven to seal in the flavour.

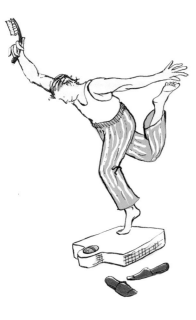

- Chargrilling gives a tasty slant to vegetables, fish and lean meats and they only need a little fat to stop the food from sticking.
- Instead of cream, base sauces on tomatoes (see page 313) or a reduction of wine, perhaps with a little yoghurt.
- Experiment with yoghurt in dishes where you would normally use cream. It can be added to soups, served with vegetables such as baked potatoes, and used in salad dressings (see page 312). Serve it with fresh fruit salad or mix it with fruit compote to make a dessert sauce. Remember not to add yoghurt to boiling liquids – let them cool very slightly – as it can curdle.
- Choose lean dishes. Cut visible fat off meat and the skin off poultry. Resist pastries, fried and battered foods.
- Beware of false promises. Food labels may claim that a food is low-fat, even when fat can be contributing up to 40 per cent of the calories, as long the fat content is lower than it would have been in the original product. 'Fat-free' foods often need something to replace the flavour, and that something is probably a form of sugar.

Sugar

Natural sugars are found in fruits and vegetables. Refined sugars (which include honey and both white and brown sugar) are found in soft drinks (squashes, cordials and canned drinks), cakes, biscuits, jams and other preserves. All sugar has the same number of calories, but refined sugars are the ones to avoid as far as possible, as they provide 'empty' calories, in other words there is no positive nutritional benefit from eating them. Fresh fruit and fruit desserts will satisfy your sweet tooth at the same time as they contribute valuable vitamins and minerals. Fruit also provides fibre, the sensible dieter's number one ally see pages 27–29.

Carbohydrates

The reason why people are often confused when they look at food labels is that sometimes sugar is called carbohydrate. Sugar is one form of carbohydrate, the other is starch. Both provide the same number of calories. As with sugars (see above), starches can be natural or refined. Natural starches are found in wholegrain, wholemeal and wholewheat breakfast cereals, wholemeal flour and bread, wholewheat pasta, brown rice, potatoes, lentils, chickpeas and beans, bananas, parsnips and other root vegetables. These foods are high in fibre and when you eat them they send signals to the brain telling you when you are full. Spoonful for spoonful, they are more satisfying than other kinds of food.

Foods containing refined starch – sugary breakfast cereals, biscuits and cakes, white bread, pasta, white rice – tend to be less satisfying, meaning you want to eat more of them, which is when you can easily put on weight.

A successful, healthy weight loss diet will be based around high-fibre carbohydrate foods. They can only help if they are also low in fat, so don't load them up with butter or other fats, and be sure to keep to low-fat cooking techniques.

Another good reason for choosing these foods is that they don't aggravate hunger and energy levels. They are processed by the body at a slow, steady pace, whereas sugary foods are digested and absorbed into the blood very quickly. Rapid changes in your blood sugar level can cause your body to go into overeat mode. Eating a chocolate bar on the way home from work may give you an energy lift, but its high refined sugar content is dealt with by the body in a way that is followed by a drop in blood sugar level – and soon you will be ravenously hungry again. In this state you are much more likely to eat more than your body really needs in your evening meal. So not only do you consume the 200 or so calories from the chocolate bar, you also consume excess calories in your meal.

The converse happens when you eat a banana late in the afternoon (before you are desperate for a snack). Because the carbohydrate in the banana is a combination of natural sugar and starch, its energy is released into the blood more gently, avoiding the blood sugar crash and subsequent appetite stimulation. Not only will you be able to enjoy your meal more because you won't be rushing through the food in a bid to feel better, but you will also be able to judge the point when you have had enough.

Fibre

For adults, the secret to successful weight loss is fibre. (Young children generally don't need much fibre, even if they are trying to lose weight; their fibre needs will be met through a balanced diet. Too much fibre can interfere with the absorption of vital nutrients, so, for children, it is best to reduce their calorie intake in other ways; see page 23 for some ideas). Fibre within food swells in the stomach in the presence of water, stimulating the stretch receptors that send signals back to the fullness centre of the brain (see page 16). For fibre to work efficiently, adults need to drink at least two litres/four pints of water every day.

The main providers of fibre in our diet are, firstly, cereals (edible grains) such as wheat, corn (maize), oats and rice and foods made from them, preferably wholegrain or wholemeal types, including bread, pasta and breakfast cereals. The other great fibre providers are vegetables (including the dried beans and lentils known as pulses) and fruits (see pages 27–29 for more about fibre).

If you have a problem with wind when you start increasing your fibre intake, I suggest you stagger your intake throughout the day, so that your body gets used to dealing with a small amount of fibre at every meal time. See also page 153.

Fibre can help your body to deal with sweet foods, both by increasing their satisfaction value and helping you feel fuller, and by slowing the absorption of the sugar into the blood and helping to stave off hunger pangs. In simple terms this means that, while a ripe mango is high in sugar, its fibre content and low fat makes it a far better choice of snack than a chocolate bar. Equally, a slice of cake made with wholemeal flour or oats, such as carrot cake or flapjacks, will have the same number of calories as a slice of buttery Madeira cake, but it will make you feel more satisfied and keep the hunger pangs away for longer. Always try to tie some fibre with a sweet food; if you can't resist chocolate, eat only a small amount after a meal that includes plenty of vegetables.

VEGETABLES AND FRUITS

Within a weight loss programme you can never eat too many vegetables. With the exception of potatoes, which are rich in starch and therefore higher in calories, vegetables contain so few calories and so much fibre that you can hardly avoid losing weight – with the usual provisos that they are cooked and served with a minimum of fat, and that you drink plenty of water.

Fruits are slightly different, because they contain fructose, which is a natural sugar. In theory you could fail to lose weight if you exceed five pieces of fruit a day. Be especially careful with ready-to-eat dried fruits. Although they have many nutritional benefits besides being high in fibre, they are high in fructose. So munching a bag of dried apricots can amount to quite a lot of calories.

Soups are a good way of including more vegetables in your diet. A bowl of soup is an excellent lunch-time snack, or after-school/after-work filler to keep you going until your main meal. If you are looking for a 'free' soup, avoid those based on carbohydrate-rich foods, such as pasta or potatoes, but think of all the lovely soups to be made with red, green and orange vegetables, and fresh herbs.

Protein

Protein ensures that your muscles, energy level and immune systems stay strong. However, people in westernized societies generally eat far too much protein. While lean protein is better for you than fatty or sugary foods, if you take in more than you need, the excess will be converted into fat. Most people need a rich source of lean protein at their main meal, in a portion size equivalent to a chicken breast, and a small amount in a second meal (see page 29).

Alcohol and weight loss

Alcohol is very calorific, providing seven calories (kcals) per gram, compared with nine for fats and approximately four for carbohydrates and proteins. It is very easy to consume excess calories by drinking alcohol. In addition, alcohol provides your body with calories without many other useful nutrients (although some wines do contain antioxidants that help to protect our general health; see page 48).

Alcohol also increases your appetite by lowering your blood sugar level, signalling the hunger centre in your brain. A small amount of your favourite wine or other alcoholic drink can complement your food, but save the alcohol until you have a little food inside your stomach to stop your blood sugar level dropping dramatically. Some people find that cutting out alcohol leads to a major calorie reduction.

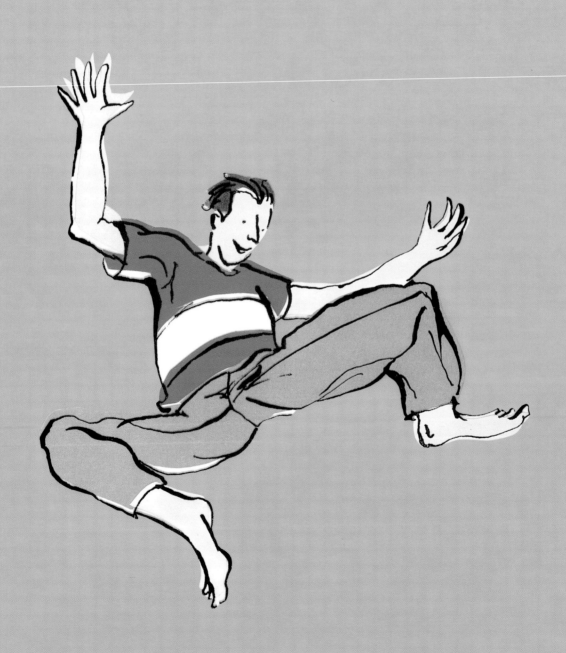

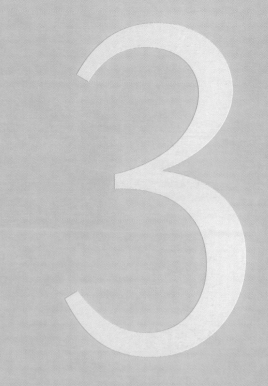

3

feel good

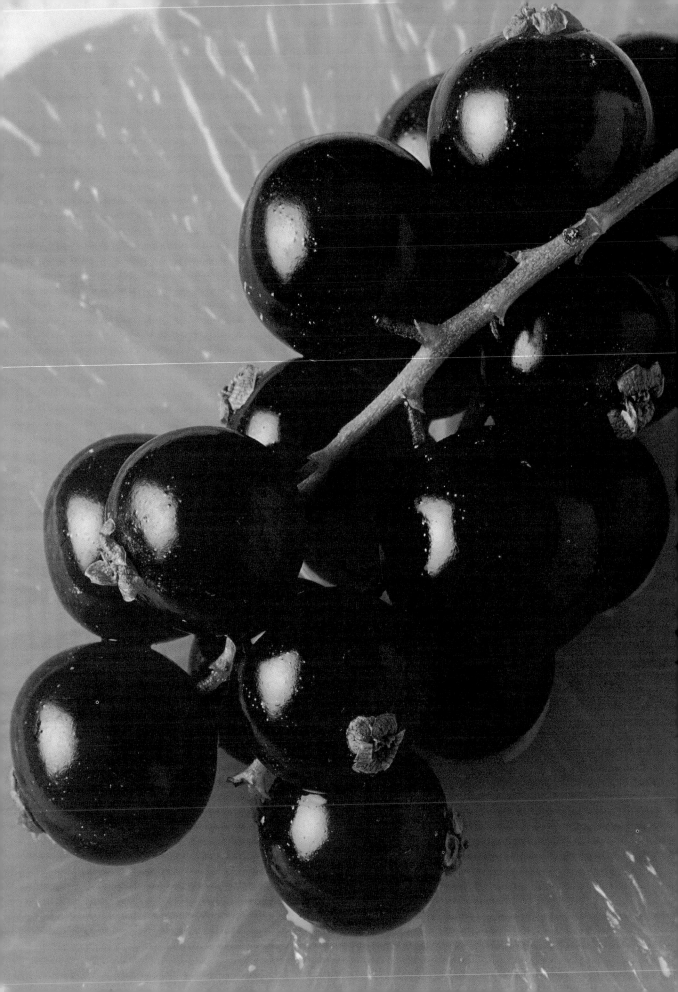

Feeling full of energy

How often do you, and your friends and colleagues, say you feel full of life? It is more often the case that people feel they are pushing their body to the end of the day, then to the end of the week, only to collapse at the weekend or during their holiday.

Much of this is down to what many health experts call 'the disease of modern living'. Environmental pollution affects our body's ability to breathe oxygen and assimilate the nutrients it needs from food; it has to battle with car fumes, cigarette smoke and industrial pollutants in the air, water and soil. The food industry fills our foods with preservatives, additives, fats and sugars which hinder the body's ability to glean the nutrients it needs, and it spends more energy getting rid of the substances it doesn't want. Farming and food purchasing habits have changed so that while we may have perfect-looking foods, nearly all the year round, the nutrient content is not as high as it was in the past.

In addition, we don't take enough time off to recuperate from illnesses – how many people stay at home in bed when they have a cold? The trend is to struggle on. Finally, fewer and fewer people, including children, are actively exercising, which helps to keep the heart pumping blood and oxygen around the body, as well as being a good stress reliever and energy booster. All in all it is no wonder that the majority of people feel tired the majority of the time.

The good news is that there is a lot we can do nutritionally to help our bodies deal with the demands of daily life, to wake up in the morning feeling refreshed and happy to meet the day.

Understanding tiredness

There are varying degrees of fatigue, from normal weariness to debilitating chronic fatigue, which may be caused by post-viral fatigue syndrome, also known as myalgic encephalomyelitis (ME), and glandular fever. If you've been feeling very tired for quite a while and cannot seem to pick yourself up even when you're eating well, you should ask your doctor to investigate. It may be that you are suffering from a virus such as Epstein Barr virus (which causes glandular fever, with episodes of severe fatigue, as well as depression and swollen glands). A blood test can confirm the diagnosis.

Children, especially those brought up in particularly health-conscious households, can suffer from a lack of energy simply because their body isn't receiving enough calories from the foods they eat. Parents who believe that the earlier you start eating healthy food, the better, can be over-zealous about not giving their child too much fat and sugar. While it is good to keep an eye on the amount of these concentrated sources of energy in the diet, the watchword is balance; children need plenty of energy-giving foods as well as cereals, fruits and vegetables.

More and more of my adult patients are complaining of chronic fatigue, with the odd bout of acute tiredness. I have to remind them that the body is not a robot, which can keep on going and going. Despite the tremendous pressures of today's society, we all need to take regular replenishing breaks and find stress-relieving activities. We also need to make sure our body receives the nutrients it needs. If we try to cheat our body by cutting corners, it will eventually falter. As tempting as it is to miss breakfast or keep going until late in the office without eating anything, or expect the body to respond favourably to chocolate bars and endless cups of coffee, these will not bring you health and happiness. Instead, take a little time to organize your life, think about the foods you are eating and how your body reacts and you will reap the benefits.

To help you understand why you are so tired and how you can correct this, I suggest you keep a food, drink and symptom diary (see page 85). After a week or two you will be able to see whether there are any patterns to your tiredness. Is it first thing in the morning – that, 'Oh, I can't get up' feeling – does it appear at four o'clock in the afternoon, or is it sheer exhaustion at the end of the day? Some patients feel as if the plug has been pulled from their body.

The main nutritional causes of fatigue are: lack of the correct nutrients, anaemia, food intolerances, too much caffeine or alcohol, and lack of oxygen in the blood. In addition to these I also see people who are simply not matching their food intake to their natural biorhythm and lifestyle demands. For instance. people who exercise early in the morning without having something to eat first can feel immensely tired late morning. Sports players who expect their body to perform well in a match after work, when they haven't eaten anything for six hours, often run into problems. Women who pick their children up from school often feel exhausted because they haven't realized that their body needs a nourishing snack at three or four o'clock. Simply changing the timings of meals can help your body respond to your lifestyle. Your total daily intake won't change, but you may need to adjust the structure of your meals.

Before looking at ways to boost your energy levels and fight fatigue, I would like to draw your attention to the effect that a certain group of foods can have on the body. Carbohydrate-rich foods such as bread, pasta and potatoes make your body produce sleep-inducing hormones. This affects some people more than others, and of course can be used to your advantage at night, but some of my patients feel sleepy after they have eaten these foods at lunchtime, when they really want to feel energetic in the afternoon. Things improve when they change to eating a meal based on protein, fruits and vegetables. Parents should keep this in mind when they are trying to help their child feel active throughout the day.

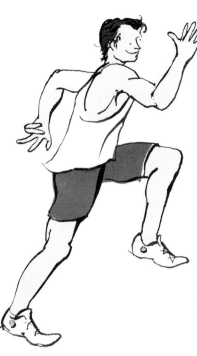

Boosting your energy

If you frequently suffer from tiredness or want to maximize your energy levels, I recommend that you read through the section on Understanding your nutritional needs. Eating well is a fundamental part of equipping your body to feel good and stay well. Include fresh vegetables and fruits, lean proteins, wholegrain foods, dairy products and plenty of water in your daily eating plan. Try to cut out processed, ready-made and high-fat fast foods and cut right down on caffeine, alcohol and nicotine.

LEARN TO BREATHE

A lot of people don't breathe efficiently. Learning to breathe using the whole of your lungs – diaphragmatic breathing – can really help you to feel more energized, as you push more oxygen around your body. Proper breathing techniques can also help you to become more efficient at getting rid of carbon dioxide, the waste product of breathing. Many books on yoga explain this in more detail – or better still take yoga classes, which are suitable for people of all ages and fitness levels.

CORRECT ANY VITAMIN OR MINERAL DEFICIENCIES

If you feel that your diet is already well balanced, but your energy levels are not as they should be, I suggest you ask your doctor to arrange a series of blood tests to find out whether you have any nutrient deficiencies. In the case of a mild deficiency, you can increase your intake of the food sources of the relevant nutrients (see pages 36–47). If you have a serious deficiency you should consult a dietitian for advice regarding supplements.

THINK BEFORE BUYING NUTRITIONAL SUPPLEMENTS

Many multivitamins and other supplements seem to promise increased energy levels, but the true facts are that many of them contain abnormally high levels of certain nutrients, which can upset the natural balance of the body. It's much better to try to get the nutrients you need from a well-balanced diet.

RESIST THE CRAVING FOR VERY SWEET FOODS

One of the commonest mistakes people make when low in energy is to eat something very sweet for a 'boost'. Unfortunately if you take in a snack that contains a lot of easily absorbed sugar (such as glucose or sucrose), the pancreas responds by producing too much insulin (a hormone that 'breaks down' sugar). This leads to a rapid fall in the sugar level, which makes you feel even worse.

The best snacks are those that are rich in natural carbohydrates combined with fibre, such as fresh fruit, a wholewheat or oat biscuit or wholegrain bread with a pure fruit topping. These foods contain some sugar to give you energy, but the presence of fibre means that the rise in your blood sugar level is slow and controlled. See page 66 for some suggestions for healthy snacks.

Fighting fatigue

Now let's look at the main causes of tiredness and how to tackle them.

LACK OF SLEEP

It may sound obvious, but I'm amazed at the number of people who think they can 'burn the candle at both ends', staying up late night after night and then dragging themselves out of bed early the next morning. If you are having trouble sleeping, refer to the chapter on How to sleep soundly.

LACK OF THE CORRECT NUTRIENTS

Every vitamin and mineral plays a vital part in either energy production or hormone metabolism. Therefore virtually all vitamin and mineral deficiencies can manifest themselves as chronic or acute fatigue. If you eat a well-balanced diet and are otherwise healthy it is very unlikely that nutrient deficiency will be the cause of your tiredness. I really only see this in people who either have a disturbed relationship with food, with periods of anorexia or bulimia, or who are on extremely restricted diets because of food preferences, allergies or intolerances (see below).

However, it is quite common to find nutrient-related fatigue in people who decide to become vegetarian or vegan; teenagers are particularly at risk. It is not just a question of living on vegetables and fruits; the body needs protein, carbohydrates and some fats, and you need to be careful about balancing the different food groups so that the body can metabolize the nutrients efficiently. Read the chapter on Understanding your nutritional needs and choose foods from the lists given under each nutrient.

FOOD INTOLERANCES

Time and time again I see people who have been told that their extreme fatigue is due to an allergy. They are sent away with a list of things to avoid, but without realistic alternatives to eat and drink. You cannot just remove something from the diet without acknowledging the body's requirements. For example, if you cut out all sugar and yeast products, or all wheat and gluten, you need to find other foods which will give the equivalent amount of energy and nutrients. It's really not surprising that people feel sapped of energy if they suddenly cut out major sources of carbohydrates such as wholewheat bread and pasta. Look for alternative grains and carbohydrates, such as rice and potatoes.

Some people experience a lot of relief following various exclusion diets, but these must be executed within a good, well-balanced eating plan. This is especially important in children. At first, it takes effort and careful organization to follow an exclusion diet, and this is difficult when you're feeling chronically or acutely tired. I have often found that tiredness is simply due to insufficient energy in the diet rather than an intolerance, so you could try boosting your general nutritional and energy status by following the advice in this chapter.

If you then feel you want to explore the food intolerance issue, see the chapter on Managing allergies for advice.

ANAEMIA

Anaemia is one of the most common causes of extreme tiredness. There are various types of anaemia, but among women and children the most common is iron-deficiency anaemia. Red meat is one of the best sources of iron, but many parents today don't want to give their children red meat and it is quite easy to cause a child to suffer from iron-deficiency anaemia. It is also common in the elderly, people who suffer from digestive disorders such as Crohn's disease, coeliac disease and duodenal ulcers. People taking certain anti-inflammatory drugs can also be prone to iron-deficiency anaemia.

The chapter on Anaemia has advice on this and other forms of anaemia. In mild cases it can be easily corrected with rest and a diet rich in iron, vitamin C and other nutrients, but in more severe cases or in cases where you cannot eat enough of the appropriate foods, you may need to take an iron supplement; ask your doctor for advice.

TOO MUCH CAFFEINE

Caffeine overdose is one of the most common causes of chronic and acute fatigue. I can understand why people drink caffeine-containing coffee, tea and cola-based drinks; they can give a kick start in the morning or stimulate falling energy levels in the middle of the afternoon, but caffeine has several detrimental effects on energy levels.

After the initial stimulation, the energy boost is short lived. Caffeine upsets the hormone levels in your body, in particular insulin and glucagon, which regulate blood sugar; this causes your energy level to crash. When your energy crashes it is tempting to have another caffeine fix to pick you up again. This starts a negative energy cycle: the more you have, the more you need to get the desired effect. Before you know it, you're drinking three or four cups rather than one. Your body doesn't respond well to artificial stimulants. Disturbing your natural energy systems means that your body is never able to find a healthy balance.

Secondly, caffeine inhibits the absorption of vitamins and minerals from the gut, which means that the body cannot use them efficiently. Caffeine also makes your body excrete more of these nutrients, so you also lose out in that respect.

If often seems particularly difficult for patients who work in an office environment, when I suggest they cut down their caffeine consumption. However, many offices these days have chilled water available for meetings, and it's easy to take herbal, fruit or ginger tea bags to work, or a little bottle of elderflower cordial to replace canned drinks. Some decaffeinated versions are worth trying (see page 50).

As a breakfast energy booster, indulge yourself with a delicious homemade fruit shake: try orange, mango and banana.

Some people can enjoy a small amount of caffeine if the rest of their diet is healthy. I suggest that you initially try to go without caffeine for a couple of weeks to help your body clear itself. Once you are feeling stronger, you can reintroduce one or two cups of really good coffee or tea a day, ideally with a high-fibre biscuit or cake such as a slice of fruity malt loaf to help regulate your blood sugar levels. Having said this, the majority of people I see feel so brilliant when their body is free of caffeine that they don't want to go back to it.

Note: If you remove caffeine from your diet, you may find that you suffer from headaches and low energy levels for a couple of days. This happens because your body has become reliant on the caffeine and you need to go through a 'cold-turkey' phase before you can start to feel truly healthy.

ALCOHOL

Alcohol was once thought of as a tonic, but it is now well known that, after the slight pepping up effect of the first glass, alcohol does nothing to lift energy levels and at worst it can grossly exaggerate tiredness. Alcohol suppresses your energy levels most noticeably if you drink on an empty stomach – so the aperitif or after-work drink can be particularly hazardous. Most of us know how it feels on a Friday night when you are tired after a long week – you feel you need a drink, but after one glass you are ready for bed. For many people, drinking alcohol at lunchtime during the week destroys the whole afternoon.

The reason for these scenarios is that alcohol affects the ability of the liver to release energy. Excess sugar is stored in the liver as glycogen. In normal circumstances the liver breaks down glycogen to produce glucose and ultimately energy, when it is needed. Alcohol blocks this response, causing your blood sugar level to drop, which means you feel physically tired. Having a little something to eat, such as fruit, a sandwich or a couple of wholegrain biscuits, before you have a drink, can help reduce this effect by keeping the alcohol within the stomach, where absorption is slower.

You might conclude that since alcohol can send you to sleep it is a good thing to take if you feel desperately tired and need more sleep. Unfortunately, this is not the case: because of its effects in your body, alcohol interferes with your sleep patterns and reduces the amount of beneficial sleep. You may sleep for longer after a few drinks, but you will still feel exhausted the following morning. Herbal tea or warm milk would be much better drinks to help you sleep.

Alcohol is also a diuretic, which causes the body to excrete more vitamins and minerals, especially water-soluble vitamins such as vitamin C. Excess alcohol also disturbs the liver's ability to metabolize fat-soluble vitamins – all in all your vitamin and mineral levels can be compromised.

I recommend that anyone suffering from chronic fatigue should stay away from alcohol until they feel stronger. Instead, choose natural non-alcoholic drinks such as sparkling mineral water or elderflower cordial, ginger beer or lemon and lime fizz (see page 343). Just remember how much fresher you'll feel.

Feel good

CRASH DIETS

Crash dieting and starving yourself can cause you to feel very sleepy. Again, this is because you are interfering with your body's ability to regulate its own energy levels. Sensible, controlled weight loss keeps you in tune with your body (see the chapter on Achieving your ideal weight).

LACK OF OXYGEN IN THE MUSCLES

The most common cause of lack of oxygen in the muscles is smoking. When you fill your lungs with smoke, you diminish the volume of oxygen you can obtain from a single breath. Smoking can therefore cause you to suffer from lack of energy simply because your muscles (including the heart and digestive organs) cannot function properly.

Another problem with smoking is that the satisfaction that accompanies putting a cigarette in your mouth tends to suppress the appetite. So you tend to miss meals or grab an alcoholic drink or a cup of coffee instead; all of which exacerbate fatigue. Being a smoker minimizes the potential benefits of eating well, so do try to give it up, or at least cut down.

MEDICATION

A number of medications can make you feel very tired. These include antibiotics, antihypertensive drugs such as beta-blockers, antidepressants, anti-epileptic medication and the cytotoxic drugs used in the treatment of cancer. In addition, many of these don't mix well with alcohol; your doctor will advise you.

Other drugs can keep you awake, depriving you of your required amount of sleep and leaving you chronically fatigued. For one young patient taking Azothiaprim to help combat Crohn's disease, taking the drug a couple of hours earlier in the day meant he could get to sleep more easily. If you suspect it may be your medication making you feel fatigued, do discuss this with your doctor, who may be able to advise you or prescribe an alternative.

HORMONE LEVELS

Some women find that they feel sleepy just before they get their period. This is a natural response set up by our reproductive hormones. For more information, see the chapter on Learning to live with periods.

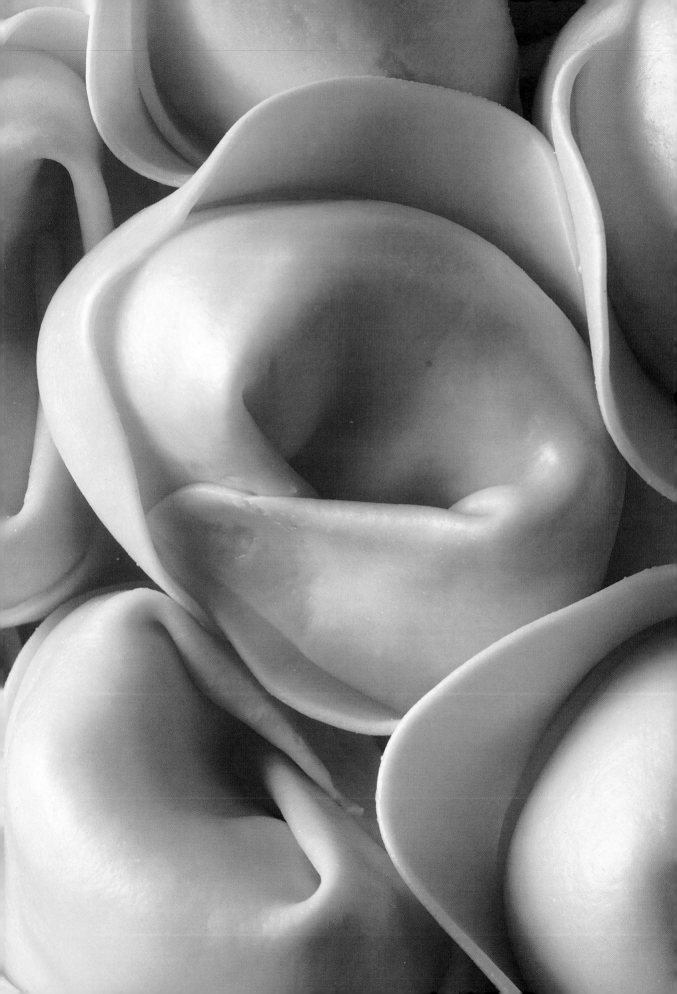

How to sleep soundly

Exactly why we need sleep is not fully understood, but it may be that our brain is rebuilding its stores of chemicals and hormones that are used during the day. Sleep definitely provides a chance to rest and repair all areas of the body. Physiologically, it is interesting that we all need different amounts of sleep: many famous and successful people claim to need only four hours sleep a night, whereas others feel ghastly if they have less than eight hours. Too much sleep can cause headaches and migraines, while too little leaves even the best of us feeling low in energy, ratty and below par.

As we get older our sleep pattern alters; we take longer to get off to sleep and wake more often during the night. We also generally need less sleep. Young children often take little catnaps throughout the day. Many adults retain this ability to catch forty winks, but others either feel that they never get enough sleep or don't feel refreshed when they wake.

There are two types of sleep: slow-wave, orthodox sleep, which is of paramount importance to allow our body to replenish itself, and dream-sleep, otherwise known as rapid eye movement (REM). During the night we alternate between both types. The different types of sleep account for why we feel refreshed after some nights' sleep and not others.

The connection between caffeine and sleep is well known: caffeine can keep you awake at night. But many of my patients are astounded to learn that there are many other links between what and how we eat and drink and our ability to sleep soundly. One of the most dramatic examples of how foods can affect both mind and body is seen in hyperactive children. Sometimes only a minute quantity of an unwanted substance needs to pass their lips before they become uncontrollable. If you think about the amount of food we put into our bodies every day, whether we are a child or an adult, we can begin to appreciate the potential effects. Get the nutrients right and the body can slumber efficiently. But if you continually bombard it with chemicals and incorrect foods the body will complain.

Sleeping pills

I strongly suggest you look to food before turning to sleeping pills. Not only are you filling your body with chemicals, but you are in danger of becoming dependent, so that you need to take stronger and stronger doses, and become desperately anxious if the pills are not available.

The majority of sleeping drugs alter your natural sleep pattern, which is why they should only be taken on a short-term basis. If you have been taking drugs to help you sleep, such as Diazepam or Mogadon, when you come off them you will probably experience a temporary increase in sleeplessness. However, once the body adjusts to not having them you should sleep soundly. If you are concerned about any aspect of the medication you're taking, discuss this with your doctor.

Exploring the natural alternatives to sleeping pills can not only be useful for adults, but can be a life saver for parents with young children who seem unable to sleep properly. By following the advice below you will ensure that you are doing everything you can to help your body.

A good night's sleep

Whether your problem is an inability to fall asleep, frequently waking up during the night, or feeling in the morning that you haven't had a really good sleep, there are several nutritional and lifestyle factors that can improve your ability to sleep well.

THINK CARBOHYDRATES

There is a close link between carbohydrate-rich foods – such as pasta, potatoes and bread – and sleep. A bowl of pasta can act as a perfect natural sleeping pill. The reason lies in the fact that the digestive system is a collection of glands and muscles. Like other muscles, it needs a plentiful supply of oxygen and the appropriate hormones to enable it to work properly. After you have eaten, Mother Nature produces hormones in your body that cause you to feel sleepy so that you are unable to move around and divert the oxygen away from the stomach to your limbs. Carbohydrate-rich foods stimulate the body to secrete copious amounts of these hormones.

You can use this to your advantage by making sure your evening meal is rich in carbohydrates; choose dishes such as lasagne or risotto, or an accompaniment of spaghetti or mashed potatoes.

AVOID STIMULANT FOODS AND DRINKS

Although most people are aware that caffeine can keep you awake, not everyone realizes that it's not just the after-dinner coffee that's the culprit. Caffeine is mainly found in coffee and tea, but it is also present in chocolate, cola drinks and some of the so-called health/vitality/energizing drinks. So hot chocolate before bedtime is not as soporific as it appears. Also, if you have a number of these drinks during the day, it can take your body several hours to clear them from your system.

Sugar is another stimulant, causing a rush of energy shortly after you've taken it, whether in the form of a high-sugar malted bedtime drink, fruit squash, sugary snacks such as chocolate, biscuits or toffee popcorn, or a sweet dessert

Remember the Peter Rabbit stories? Camomile tea induces soporific thoughts and is a delightful way to end the day. If you can't find the flower heads to make your own infusion, many health food stores and supermarkets sell camomile tea bags.

after a late meal. Children's bodies are generally more sensitive to sugar swings, but even adults need to be aware of how easy it is to disturb the pattern of sleep. I am not saying that you need to cut out these things all together, simply look at how and when you eat them.

Try to leave at least a couple of hours between the time you eat your dessert and your bedtime. Another option is to make sure your dessert contains some fibre, in the form of fresh or dried fruit or wholemeal flour for example, to cushion the sugar swings. If you are in the habit of having a snack before you go to bed, choose a high-fibre snack such as an apple flapjack, an oat muffin or a wholemeal roll. See page 66 for other high-fibre snacks.

Instead of hot chocolate, a mug of hot milk or a glass of cold milk will help you sleep easier.

KEEP A FOOD DIARY

Note when your sleep is particularly disturbed and look at the foods and drinks you consumed on the previous day. With this information, after a week or two you may be able to isolate certain foods that make you restless. Common culprits include spicy or fatty foods, as these can sit heavily in the stomach, and foods and drinks high in artificial additives and preservatives.

You may also find that your restless nights coincide with a little indigestion or bloating. This may be as a result of a food intolerance. I suggest you read the chapter on Managing allergies.

WATCH YOUR ALCOHOL INTAKE

While a little drink can help you relax, and a larger amount can make you feel tired, excessive amounts of alcohol disturb your natural sleep patterns and dehydrate you, thereby decreasing the quality of your sleep. You may sleep for longer, but you will wake up with a headache or feeling sluggish, and your energy levels and sense of well-being will be at rock bottom.

Occasionally people find that a particular drink aggravates their tendency to feel headachy and down. This may be because of an individual grape variety or because the drink contains pesticide residues or naturally occurring substances such as salicylates. Keeping a food dairy and then temporarily eliminating the drink that seems to cause the trouble should help you decide whether you need to look for an alternative beverage.

Otherwise, just keep the quantity down and don't drink every night, out of habit.

AVOID TAKING SUPPLEMENTS AT NIGHT

Several vitamin and mineral supplements have a slight stimulating effect. Taking them in the morning should help prevent this.

You may also find that certain medications, for example sugary cough mixtures and antidepressants such as Prozac and Seroxat, can disrupt your sleep pattern.

MAKE SURE YOUR ROOM IS VENTILATED AND AT A COMFORTABLE TEMPERATURE

Excessive heat can cause disturbed sleep; in centrally heated houses bedrooms are often too hot. Cooling your room down and choosing bedlinen made of natural fibres such as cotton may help you to sleep better.

Sleeping arrangements are of paramount importance with babies. Placing them in a secure position should help both you and your child to sleep soundly. Current advice is to:

- Place babies on their backs to sleep
- Make sure they are not too hot
- Make sure babies' heads are not covered
- Refrain from smoking in the house

REDUCE STRESS

Lack of exercise and excessive stress can cause your sleep patterns to be disturbed. Take measures to relieve stress before you try to sleep: listening to music or reading a book or magazine may help.

Encourage your child to be as active as possible during the day, as this will enable them to become physically tired and free of stress. You may question whether children suffer from stress, but don't forget that they are under as much pressure as the rest of us in the modern world, and schools are increasingly competitive places. One of the ways that children exhibit stress can be insomnia. Look to the underlying cause as well as doing everything you can foodwise to help them.

HERBAL REMEDIES

Consider using herbs and flowers, either as tea such as camomile or as drops of aromatherapy oils, either in your late night bath or on the pillow or on the upper edge of the sheets. Good oils to consider include lavender and basil. This is a useful tip if you have restless children.

TRY NOT TO OVERSLEEP

Having too much sleep can make you feel at odds with yourself, unable to get your body going; even worse, you may wake up with a headache or migraine. Many of my patients are amazed to learn that oversleeping can cause headaches and migraines. This is because it causes the release of a hormone called serotonin. Although serotonin is associated with feeling happy, it is not a question of the more serotonin, the happier you feel; it is more important to maintain appropriate levels within your body. The serotonin released when you oversleep is subsequently processed by the kidneys. Sensitive blood vessels within the head dilate rapidly, pressing on surrounding nerves and causing pain. This is why some people wake up with a stinking headache, having slept for many hours and despite not having drunk any alcohol.

Always feeling sleepy?

This problem is discussed in more detail in the previous chapter. The answer, briefly, is to look to your lifestyle. Changing to a regular meal pattern which includes lots of fresh organic food and water, little or no caffeine, alcohol in moderation, and regular exercise, can work wonders. You will sleep more soundly at night and feel awake when you want to, with none of the in-between muzziness and lethargy.

Children who seem to exist on healthy foods – lots of fruits, vegetables and fibre – but very little else, can suffer from lethargy simply because their body is not getting enough energy-giving foods. Look at the chapter on Understanding your nutritional needs.

Those of you who are feeling psychologically low or depressed may find that always wanting to sleep is one of your main symptoms. I suggest you read the chapter on Depression. Children who are unhappy often have this problem. Try to get to the bottom of the problem: are they being bullied at school or having problems with friends? Don't just feed them sweets and treats to comfort them, as these will not help their bodies.

Snoring

On a final note, snoring can disrupt slumber. Excess weight and excess alcohol aggravate snoring. Cut down on alcohol or read the chapter on Achieving your ideal weight to help reduce the problem.

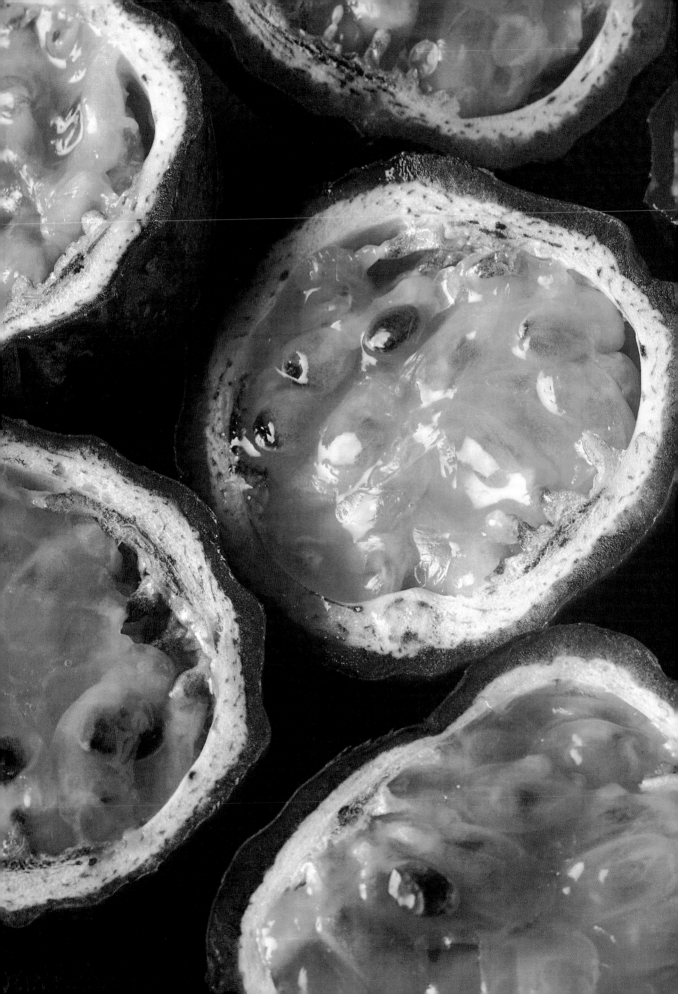

Building a strong immune system

A strong immune system will help your body to ward off infections such as colds and cold sores, gut infections and cystitis. Your natural immunity may be lowered as a result of viruses, stress or other illnesses, or simply when you are chronically tired. With our hectic schedules it's tempting to battle on, but if you don't take your body seriously, problems won't disappear. It's well worth building up your immune system so that it is ready to fight infections, help you recover as quickly as possible, and above all, stay well. Throughout this chapter I refer primarily to the common cold, but the advice applies equally to many other infections. First, here are some general guidelines:

- Eat a well balanced diet, including fresh fruits, vegetables and pulses, wholegrains, lean protein, dairy products and water. See the chapter on Understanding your nutritional needs for details.

- Avoid eating foods that are well past their 'use by' dates. Store and cook foods according to food safety recommendations (see page 77). It astounds me that people can eat food that is just going off; I know they don't want to waste it, but if they stopped to think that they are potentially introducing toxic bacteria into their body, severely challenging their immune system, they wouldn't count the cost in a few pence.

- Get enough sleep – ideally seven to eight hours a night. Sleep requirements vary and it's not just quantity of sleep that counts. If you manage to get to bed early you are more likely to have the most therapeutic type of sleep.

- Try to reduce the amount of stress in your life. Stress adversely affects the immune system, so it is important to allow yourself regular de-stressing times. For you, this could mean reading a good book or having a massage. Think of your body as an engine which needs regular servicing, as well as the correct fuel. The benefits of boosting your nutritional status are greatly reduced if you are stressed or emotionally run down.

- Take regular exercise. Exercise helps to keep a healthy supply of oxygen in the body, which maintains a strong immune system. Outdoor exercise provides an opportunity for your lungs to breathe fresh air, rather than the stale air in offices and centrally heated buildings. Harmful bacteria don't thrive in fresh air, so outdoor exercise 'cleans out' your airways and helps keep you healthy.

- Stop smoking, as this damages your lungs and reduces your ability to fight infections.
- Avoid contact with people who have colds and infections. If a friend has a cold, encourage them to stay at home. Infections wouldn't spread if we all did this. If you have a cold, keep it to yourself.
- Take time to recover from any illness. You are much more likely to pick up further infections if you are 'below par'.

Foods to help prevent the common cold

The common cold plagues us all at some time during the year. It can be caused by one of more than 200 viruses, the symptoms and severity of which vary from one individual to another. Sometimes the virus simply gives you a congested or runny nose and a sore throat. Other viruses affect the lungs, causing bronchitis, or the larynx, giving you laryngitis. It is important to take action as soon as you feel you are getting a cold. If you let it go on untreated, you could develop a secondary bacterial infection which may attack the ears, lungs or throat. Once bacteria become involved, antibiotics may be necessary to clear up the infection.

Essentially there is no cure for the common cold, you just need to manage and alleviate the symptoms and give your body the rest it needs to concentrate its efforts on fighting the infections. There are two issues to address with the common cold: how to stop yourself from catching it and how to get rid of it.

Nutritionally, the plan is to make sure that you have a strong immune system to withstand any viral or bacterial attacks. Many people believe that large doses of vitamin C can prevent or cure the common cold. Although vitamin C does have a profound effect on the immune system, there are other nutrients to consider. Beta-carotene, vitamin E, the B vitamins, selenium, zinc, magnesium and iron each play an important role. Remember that you need to maintain a balance of vitamins and minerals: too much of a single nutrient can hinder the absorption and beneficial effects of other nutrients. This was demonstrated in a study of the effects of beta-carotene and lung cancer in the United States in 1996. Too much beta-carotene seemed to knock the other vitamins and minerals off their 'therapeutic stations'. It is better to get a good, balanced, vitamin and mineral intake from foods rather than supplements.

VITAMIN C

This vitamin has the potential to prevent and also reduce the severity of the common cold. Some people believe that 1000 mg of vitamin C taken every day can prevent a cold. Others, including Nobel prize-winning scientist Linus Pauling, suggest that we take up to 5000 mg a day. I don't feel that it is worthwhile to take such large doses, as vitamin C is a water-soluble vitamin, so the body excretes the excess.

Large doses can irritate the gut and many people find it impossible to take more than 1000 mg a day without suffering from side effects such as indigestion and bloating. I have also seen some people with mouth ulcers caused by taking too much vitamin C (also known as ascorbic acid). The mouth is an alkaline area. If you chew lots of vitamin C tablets the alkaline balance is disturbed and ulcers can develop. However, this usually only occurs with doses in excess of 3000 mg a day.

Rather than buying a supplement, I suggest that you eat plenty of foods rich in vitamin C: fresh citrus fruits (oranges, grapefruits, lemons, limes, clementines and mandarins), kiwi fruits, strawberries, blackcurrants, and dark green leafy vegetables such as spinach, Savoy cabbage and broccoli. Potatoes cooked in their skins, such as baked or boiled new potatoes are another good source.

Vitamin C begins to be lost from fruit and vegetables as soon as they are picked, and many people question how much vitamin C is present in foods by the time we get around to eating them. Tests have shown that, while a freshly picked orange contains about 150 mg of vitamin C, the oranges in supermarkets vary between 115 mg and a mere trace. Obviously, the fresher vegetables and fruits you can buy the better. Don't leave fruit in the fruit bowl for days. Fresh fruit shakes (see page 342) or freshly squeezed orange juice can provide a substantial amount of vitamin C. Eating fruits and vegetables in season will help you glean the maximum amount of this vitamin, and remember that frozen vegetables can have more vitamin C than fresh ones.

Since vitamin C is water-soluble, you will lose a lot if you boil or soak vegetables for a long time. Keep cooking time down to a minimum, and try steaming, stir-frying or baking vegetables, rather than boiling them until soggy.

If you eat five portions of fresh fruits and vegetables every day, your vitamin C intake should be high enough to prevent a cold. However, if you can't manage this, or feel you need an extra boost, I suggest you take a supplement of between 1000 and 1500 mg a day. Take it as three 500 mg tablets throughout the day, with food and a glass of water, to avoid any potential irritant effect. It's no good taking vitamin supplements with caffeine-containing drinks such as coffee, tea or cola, as the caffeine and tannins inhibit the absorption of nutrients.

ZINC

Zinc plays a fundamental role in maintaining a healthy immune system. If you are deficient in zinc you are much more likely both to catch a cold and to suffer for longer. You should therefore ensure that your zinc status is good, by including rich sources of zinc in your everyday eating plan. The best dietary sources of zinc are shellfish (especially oysters), lean meat such as lamb, beef and turkey, wholegrain products, and nuts and seeds (see page 45 for further sources). If you eat a well balanced diet, your zinc intake should be sufficient to prevent colds, but if you feel you want to take a supplement I suggest you take 15 mg a day. It is very important that you don't take more than this. Bear in mind that when you have a viral cold, the body automatically lowers its blood zinc levels, as high zinc levels can make you more prone to bacterial infections.

MAGNESIUM

Magnesium has also been linked with developing a strong immune system. I do not recommend that you take a supplement, but rather make sure that your diet includes magnesium-rich foods, especially green leafy vegetables. Other rich sources include nuts and seeds (including hummus, made from sesame seeds), pulses, wholegrain products.

What to do if you get a cold or other infection

- Rest and keep warm.
- Don't exercise vigorously. Gentle walking in the fresh air can help keep you healthy, but you should not exercise or play strenuous games, as this can damage the muscles and aggravate your symptoms. Encourage your child to play gently and not to go running about.
- Ask your doctor or pharmacist for advice about medication to relieve your symptoms. You may need a decongestant, throat syrup, aspirin or paracetamol to reduce fever, but be careful not to take too many different drugs, as there is sometimes a danger of overdose. My grandmother's honey and lemon drink relieves sore throats (see margin); you don't always need chemical mixtures.
- Try to keep to a well balanced diet. If you don't feel like eating much, I suggest you read pages 230–231 for ideas on stimulating your appetite. It may be that you need a day of plain food such as potato soup (see page 308) or pasta. Fruit shakes and vegetable soups can be useful in keeping up your intake of vitamins and minerals.
- When your senses of smell and taste are badly affected, stimulate them with strong tasting or mildly spicy foods. Think of tangy sheep's milk cheeses, lemons and limes, ginger and lemon grass, or even curries.
- Drink at least two and a half litres/four to five pints of water a day. If you have a high temperature, you should drink more than this, as you will lose water through sweating. You could have it cold or hot, with honey and lemon.
- Some people find a warm alcoholic drink, the traditional hot toddy, can give a lot of relief to cold symptoms. If you are taking antibiotics, check with your doctor that it is appropriate for you to take alcohol. Remember that a tot is fine, but excess alcohol can adversely affect your immune system.

Antibiotics

There is a great deal of concern over the suggestion that overuse of antibiotics can lead to resistance. So far, there is no evidence to support this, as long as the antibiotics are administered appropriately: if the right antibiotic is taken and the course of medication is completed. Remember that antibiotics can cure only bacterial infections. Taking an antibiotic for a viral infection such as a cold is useless, all it will do is cause side effects such as nausea, and expose your gut to possible fungal infections.

Many people go to extremes when it comes to antibiotics. Either they reach for the antibiotics at the first sign of an infection, without giving their body a chance to fight it naturally with weapons such as good nutrition and rest, or they refuse antibiotics and expect their body to be able to fight bacterial infections alone. There are dangers with both attitudes.

If you take antibiotics without having had a bacterial culture grown, from a swab of your throat, or a sputum or stool sample, you may take the wrong antibiotic. While a broad spectrum antibiotic such as Amoxyl may kill some of the bacteria around the infection, you may develop a 'hard core' of bacteria which will then need to be 'zapped' with a specific antibiotic. Using broad spectrum antibiotics or the wrong antibiotic can lead to serious complications, as you can believe you are treating the bug, but in fact the infection is spreading, which may necessitate emergency treatment.

The alternative approach, refusing to take antibiotics when there is a clearly diagnosed bacterial infection, can expose you to secondary and serious complications. Food can do a lot to help fight infections, both viral and bacterial, but antibiotics are necessary on occasions. Bacterial infections such as meningitis can kill; antibiotics if used correctly save lives.

It is also very important that once you start a course of antibiotics, you complete the course and don't stop the moment you start feeling better. Although you may feel better there may still be some bacteria around which need killing. If you need another course of antibiotics, the antibiotic level in your body builds up with each successive course and resistance to the antibiotic is much more likely to occur. Therefore the antibiotic may not be as effective on a future occasion. If you do not experience any relief, consult your doctor, as he or she may be able to change to a more suitable dose or type.

Nutritionally, overuse of inappropriate antibiotics can lead to vitamin and mineral deficiencies, partly as a result of a change in their absorption from the gut, partly from other side effects. Certain antibiotics can make you feel slightly nauseous, which can put you off your food at a time when your body desperately needs nutrients to fight infections. Secondly, antibiotics can adversely affect the flora inside your gut. The balance of good and bad flora can change and many people develop yeast and bacterial infections in the lower bowel, mouth or vagina. These infections can manifest themselves as thrush and cystitis. Some people may also develop diarrhoea or constipation. Even if you are taking antibiotics, make sure you are eating well, taking into consideration symptoms such as diarrhoea and nausea. Try to eat a small pot of live yoghurt containing bifidus and acidophilus every day. This will help keep your gut flora healthy. You could eat it plain, top it with fruit, or use it in cooking.

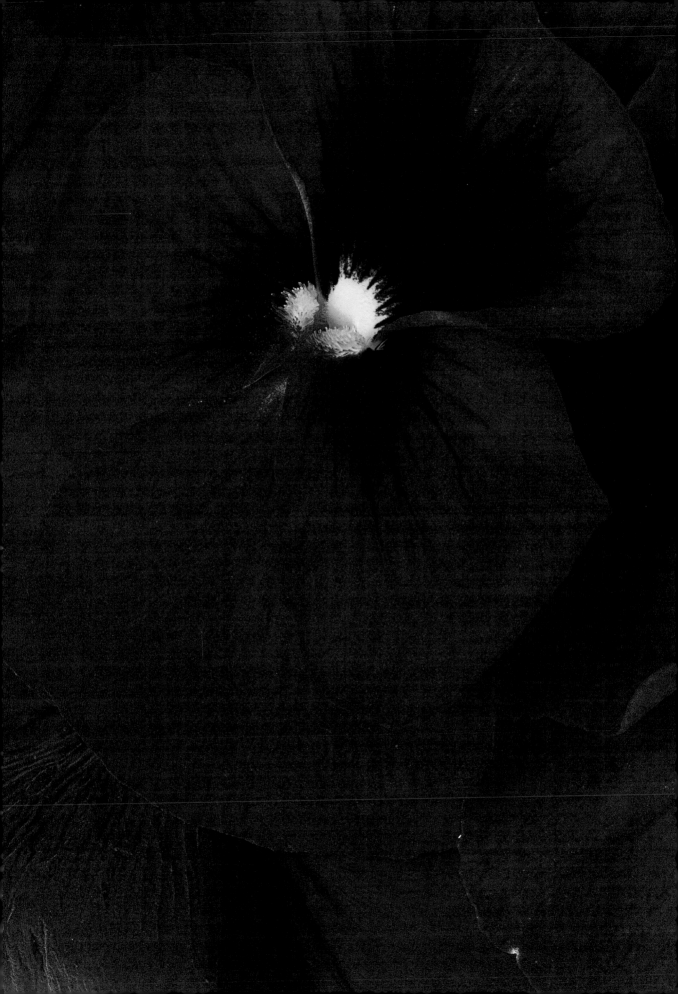

Dealing with depression

Although occasional sadness is part of the human condition – everyone has days feeling gloomy, children sulk off to school, their eyes brimming with tears – true depression ranges from rational sadness and grief to an abnormal state of complete disability. Unless one has actually suffered from depression or been in close contact with someone who has, it is hard to appreciate that the whole body can be overwhelmed by hopelessness, negativity and suicidal thoughts. Clinical depression can include disturbed eating; the sufferer may stop eating – and anorexia nervosa may set in – or overeat, which may lead to obesity or bulimia nervosa. Other symptoms include disturbed sleep patterns, digestive complaints and loss of concentration.

While food on its own cannot cure or prevent clinical depression, a great deal can be done to improve your mood. Changing your eating habits can lift you out of a low period and in more severe cases food can be used in conjunction with psychotherapy and medication.

How food affects your mood
Within your brain, chemicals known as neurotransmitters help pass messages from one nerve cell to another. There are two such substances that seem specifically to affect mood: serotonin and noradrenaline, two types of endorphins. The body makes these endorphins by breaking down the food we eat, and therefore we can, to a certain degree, raise the level of these substances in the brain by eating specific foods.

Unfortunately, it is not simply a question of the more of certain foods you eat the happier you become. Scientifically, food has been shown to have a significant effect on raising the mood only if the level of serotonin or noradrenaline is low before you eat. So what it can do is help to reverse a negative feeling which has been induced by a low endorphin level. In some people endorphin levels are lower during the darker winter months, which is why they feel gloomy until the sun starts shining. Medication can also temporarily lower the levels of serotonin and noradrenaline, which is why you sometimes feel low while you are taking a course of antibiotics, for example. So if we know that levels of these neurotransmitters are low, we can learn how to boost them.

Besides physical effects, there is also the psychological effect of 'comfort food' to consider. Many of our food preferences are laid down in childhood and as adults we can, when we feel down, revive good feelings by choosing certain foods that remind us of moments in our youth. Often these are sugary foods that are given as treats and rewards.

Sources of serotonin and noradrenaline

These endorphins are derived mainly from sugary and other carbohydrate-rich foods, which is why some people feel happier after they have eaten sweets or chocolate, cakes, biscuits, white bread, white rice, jams, honey and sugary soft drinks. It also explains why many people crave them when they are feeling down, especially in the winter months. Syrupy puddings and chocolate bars hold more appeal than a piece of fresh fruit.

Unfortunately, there is a drawback. The sugar from these foods is rapidly absorbed into the blood, which causes an initial boost in serotonin levels in the brain. However, another result of a sudden rise in blood sugar level is the rapid production of insulin. Insulin is a hormone that helps the body use sugar. If there is a sudden rise in blood sugar level, the insulin acts quickly to take the sugar out of the blood into the cells, causing a slump in both the sugar and endorphin levels. The slump leaves you feeling even lower than you were before. The temptation is to eat another sugary snack to give yourself another boost, but this will cause your body to run out of its own natural energy; you'll find yourself needing more and more of these foods to feel remotely happy.

Major swings in endorphin levels can trigger gloom and depression, but in some people, most noticeably hyperactive children, they can cause moods to become totally unmanageable, with tantrum frenzies and hysterical tears; otherwise responsible adults can become violent and then morose.

Luckily the majority of us don't find our bodies react in this extreme way. For most people, eating a small amount of sugary foods can make them feel temporarily brighter. The best way to experience the highs, without the lows, is to make sure that you either have a meal as soon as possible after you eat the sugary food or choose to get your sugar 'fix' from a more slowly absorbed carbohydrate. Good examples include a piece of flapjack, a slice of wholegrain bread or a wholemeal scone, a bowl of fruit crumble with an oaty or wholemeal topping, fresh, dried or stewed fruit. The presence of fibre along with the sugar in these foods helps to lift a low, but not too fast. You are therefore more likely to stay happy for longer.

Even these higher fibre sweet foods can upset some people, especially those with digestive disorders. In this case, remember that it's not just sweet foods that can produce serotonin and noradrenaline; they are also made from tryptophan and L-phenylalanine, two amino acids present in protein foods, such as meat, fish, chicken and eggs. It has been suggested that people with low intakes of these amino acids are more likely to feel down, or even suicidal. This means that strict vegetarians, vegans, and people on crash weight loss diets are all at risk. 'Dieters' may feel low not only because they are depriving themselves of the foods they love, but also because they might be avoiding protein foods.

As with sweet foods, it's not just a question of increasing your consumption of these foods in search of a mood lift. Your brain can only use a certain amount at a time. Vegans and vegetarians should eat a variety of pulses, grains, nuts and other non-animal sources of protein. Keeping a food diary (see page 85) is a good way of monitoring your intake and ensuring that your endorphin levels are high enough to prevent your mood dropping.

Vitamin and mineral deficiencies

Depression is a common symptom of vitamin and mineral deficiencies. A lack of vitamins B12 and C, or of minerals such as iron, potassium and zinc, can cause you to feel low or aggravate depression. There is also a tendency for depressed people to feel uninterested in food, so they don't eat and hence become deficient in various nutrients. On top of this, some antidepressants change your metabolism and cause your body to become deficient in certain minerals and vitamins. People who have gone through periods of not eating properly, feeling unwell, or taking medication that can put you off your food are all at risk. Equally, if you have been bombarding your body with alcohol, coffee, tea or cola, your body can become depleted of nutrients. The best way to confirm whether you lack essential vitamins and minerals is to arrange some blood tests through your doctor. Don't just assume that you are deficient and start taking supplements, as you may not be heading down the right path.

Vitamin deficiencies don't just happen overnight, but if you have neglected your diet for a long time, you may be lacking in vitamins B and C. See pages 38–40 for good sources of these vitamins.

Iron deficiency anaemia can cause you to feel generally run down, if not actually depressed. If you suspect this is your problem, see your doctor and read the chapter on Anaemia.

Potassium deficiency sometimes arises after a period of vomiting or diarrhoea. Various medications, such as diuretics and antihypertensive drugs, can also cause the body to lose excessive amounts of potassium. The best way to replenish your body is to eat foods rich in potassium such as fresh vegetables and fruit (see page 45), but if you can't face food, sip some orange or tomato juice.

Never take a potassium supplement unless prescribed by your GP, as they are potentially very dangerous.

How drinks affect your mood

The positive side is that if you are feeling low a glass of wine with your food can make the whole eating experience much more enjoyable. Alcohol can even rekindle lost appetites. But excessive amounts of alcohol, especially if drunk on an empty stomach, can lead to a hangover, which is never very cheering. Drinking on an empty stomach also causes your blood sugar level to drop, which can lead to a lowering of serotonin levels and hence a 'blue' mood. If taken over a long period of time, excessive alcohol can cause chronic depression.

People taking antidepressants generally have to avoid alcohol, as the two substances interact badly in the body. If in doubt discuss alcohol with your GP.

It's not just alcohol that can interfere with your mood. One of the greatest mood inhibitors is caffeine. Caffeine, found in coffee, tea, cola and chocolate, increases the excretion of vitamins and minerals from the gut and inhibits their absorption. If taken in excess it can lay you open to a vitamin or mineral deficiency. It can also cause you to become hyper-agitated and even 'out of control'. Try to keep your intake down to a maximum of two or three drinks a day. People who cut caffeine out of their diet completely usually start to feel brighter and happier. Just remember that the initial detoxification of caffeine from your body can cause headaches and a withdrawal low.

Exercise

Exercise can be an empowering activity; in a situation when you feel hopeless and helpless, going out and exercising can improve your mood in many ways.

Lack of fresh air is a great depressant, so taking some outdoor exercise can make you feel happier. Exercise as a physiological process helps your brain to produce mood-lifting endorphins such as serotonin. Getting into contact with other people can give you a new perspective on problems, and exercise can distract you from comfort overeating. Exercising gives you an opportunity to burn up some calories if you're worried about excess weight gain, which can be a problem if you are taking antidepressants.

Using food to pick yourself up

It is all too easy to get into a vicious circle: when you feel depressed you are less likely to feel like eating, which, as explained above, makes you feel even more depressed. You may not feel capable of going out shopping for foods rich in vitamins, minerals and other essential nutrients, or of cooking even the simplest meal. In an extreme scenario, I would suggest you take a general vitamin and mineral supplement, just to boost your nutrient status to a level that will make you feel stronger. However, do try to eat small amounts of nutritious food – fruit, salads, wholemeal bread, eggs – as a little is better than none.

- Consider a family health day. (see page 81). Devoting a whole day to your eating habits, tackling the problems of shopping and finding the foods you know you should eat, can do wonders for your mood. Some people like to take the opportunity to cleanse themselves of all the junk food they have been eating. I would support this desire. Don't feel guilty for spending time on yourself; just think how much better you'll feel at the end of the day.
- Look at the nutritional content of your meals. A well balanced and varied diet (see pages 25–47) will give your body the nutrients it needs.
- Choose foods you can prepare easily, even if this doesn't involve more than cutting some cheese and serving it with warm wholegrain bread and a selection of fruits. If you can think about the presentation and sensory aspects

of the food, your body will glean a lot more from the experience than from a meal of dreary colour, texture and shape.

- If you need a short burst of 'happiness', you could have a sugary 'treat' or a piece of lovely fresh bread. However, you must remember that a mood crash will follow unless you eat some fibre with them, or shortly afterwards. Fresh, poached or dried fruit, flapjacks and cakes made with wholemeal flour are good mood boosters.

Antidepressant medication

However much food can lift your mood, some people need the extra helping hand of medication. There are many different types of antidepressants, with various side effects.

A common side effect, particularly with Largactil, is an increase in hunger and an inability to recognize when you are full. Largactil blocks the action of a neurotransmitter (brain chemical) called dopamine. Dopamine generally decreases your feelings of hunger, therefore if you take a drug that interferes with this process, you permanently feel hungry. For some people this can be an advantage, as it can help you eat more of the foods your body needs. However, for the majority of figure-conscious people, especially if they are not aware of this side effect, it is easy to find their weight escalating upwards. The best way to counteract this is to ensure that your meals are as healthy as possible and that you pay attention to the issues of satiety (see page 15).

Some people find that their antidepressant medication causes them to develop sugar cravings. Try to resist sugary snacks, as rapid changes in blood sugar levels will make your mood worse, not better. Instead, treat yourself to a juicy ripe peach, some grapes or a slice of pineapple.

Other antidepressants, such as Prozac, can cause you to feel either nauseous or permanently full, or can take away your appetite. Remember that your body needs a range of nutrients to function efficiently and try to eat nutritious snacks and meals whenever possible. Keeping a food diary (page 85) can help you to get a grip on the situation and enable you to adjust your eating patterns if necessary.

Lithium tends to be used in severe cases of depression. Nutritionally, people taking lithium often experience an increase in appetite and also in thirst and fluid retention. Whatever you do, do not restrict your fluid intake; this can be dangerous as it can disturb the body's sodium level, which in turn can affect your serum lithium level. Serum lithium levels should be closely monitored, so if you're tempted to change your eating or drinking habits you must discuss the issues with your doctor and dietitian. See page 198 for advice on reducing fluid retention.

One of the most crucial aspects of treating depression and low feelings is to talk to people – don't suffer in silence. Food can only go so far; professionals are around to help you further.

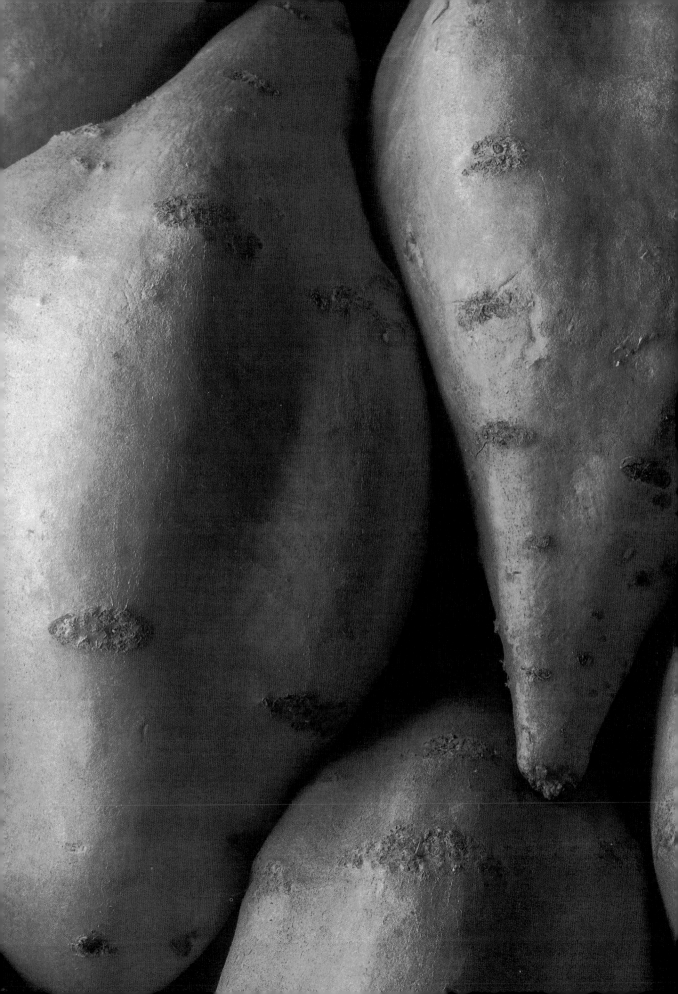

Good digestion

The process of digestion is an everyday miracle, as the foods we eat are efficiently used by our body to maintain health and provide energy. It is a process we often take for granted until something goes wrong, so it is worth understanding the basics. The digestive system is a collection of glands and muscles and, like any other part of the body, responds to your diet and lifestyle.

Digestion begins when you put food into your mouth. Saliva is the first of the digestive juices to prepare your food for processing by your body; chewing food thoroughly allows it to come into contact with as much saliva as possible and gets digestion off to a good start. Swallowing sends the food down the gullet, or oesophagus, the tube that leads to the stomach. The average adult stomach can hold about one and a half litres/two and a half pints, and can take from two to seven hours to process a meal. In the stomach, food is churned with different digestive juices to become a smooth, acidic paste. When the paste is at the correct consistency and acidity it passes, a little at a time, through the pyloric sphincter, a muscular ring at the base of the stomach, into the duodenum, the first part of the small intestine. Here, the pancreas adds its digestive enzymes and insulin, the gall bladder adds bile (for the digestion of fat), and the food is helped on its way by waves of involuntary muscular contractions known as peristalsis. Most of the digestion of food and absorption of nutrients takes place along the six metres/twenty feet of the small intestine, where further digestive enzymes are secreted. Digestion is completed in the large intestine (colon or bowel). But the bowel is not just the last stage in the process; it houses bacteria which synthesize energy, vitamins and minerals. More recently scientists have found that these bacteria, along with certain foods, help the body to produce substances that protect it against cancer and heart disease. Finally, any leftover matter is shifted to the rectum, ready for expulsion.

It takes between two and thirty-six hours for food to pass through your body, depending on the type of food and its fibre content, your water intake and whether you have also been drinking alcohol, coffee, tea or other caffeine-containing drinks. Your general body environment also affects the digestive process; this is partly genetic – some people's guts are just more sluggish than others – partly hormonal, and also related to your mood, exercise habits and whether you are taking any form of medication.

Vomiting

Sometimes, unfortunately, food does not stay in your gut very long. Vomiting is often caused by bacterial or viral infection; it is your body's way of rejecting the bugs before they gain a foothold. Overindulgence in rich or spicy foods or alcohol is another common cause of vomiting; again, your body is rejecting what it cannot handle. Nausea may also be caused by hormones, as pregnant women are well aware; and we have all heard tales of actors or musicians being physically sick before a performance because of stress hormones.

Unpleasant as it is, remember that most bouts of sickness are soon over. Don't force yourself to eat, but if you feel you need a little something to avoid feeling weak, try nibbling plain bread or an oatcake. Some people find that sucking a fruit sweet helps. Take frequent sips of water to rehydrate yourself. If you are losing a lot of fluid, try sipping a rehydration fluid, available from your pharmacist, or make some yourself (see margin, opposite).

If you feel 'sick with nerves', the homeopathic remedy aconite 6 is good for calming anxiety on occasions.

Some medication can also make you nauseous; consult your doctor to find out whether it would be possible to adjust your prescription, because if you are ill it is important that your intake of nutrients is maintained.

Because of their immature digestive system, unweaned babies seem to vomit small amounts of milk quite frequently – and happily. It is only when vomiting is profuse, usually accompanied by other symptoms such as fever or diarrhoea (see below) that you need to take further action.

Diarrhoea

Diarrhoea is often associated with vomiting, in that it can be a sign that your body needs to get rid of an unwanted substance quickly. Hormonal changes can also cause diarrhoea – many women experience it once a month as part of their natural menstrual cycle (see the chapter on Learning to live with periods). Sometimes your gut simply reacts badly to being overloaded, whether it be with fruit, dairy produce or sugary, fatty or spicy foods; a well balanced diet with a variety of different foods should help prevent this. There are a number of things you can do to help your body get over a bout of diarrhoea:

- Remember that, as with vomiting, diarrhoea causes your body to lose more water than usual, so if you're not careful you can become dehydrated. Try to drink at least two and a half to three litres/four to five pints of water a day.
- Avoid caffeine-containing drinks such as coffee, tea and cola. Caffeine can irritate the gut; it also inhibits the absorption of vitamins and minerals, which is the last thing you need when you are losing them rapidly through diarrhoea.
- Although you might think that high fibre foods would be the answer, the fibre acting as a 'sponge' within your bowel, in fact they can be difficult to digest, so the gut expels them. Natural binders include lower fibre white rice, pasta and potatoes, so base your meals around these foods.

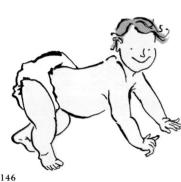

Feel good

Rehydration fluid
Cheaper and just as effective as commercially available drinks.
Take 4–8 g/½–1 teaspoon of glucose powder and a pinch of salt and dissolve them in 100 ml/3½ fl oz of hot water.

- Raw fruit and vegetables can be tough on a sensitive gut, but you may find you can tolerate baked or poached fruit, boiled, steamed or puréed vegetables. However, a banana is usually a good snack when you have diarrhoea.
- Fatty foods are particularly difficult to digest, and if fat builds up in the bowel it can cause or aggravate diarrhoea. Keep to naturally lower fat foods such as bread and other cereal products, potatoes, fish, shellfish and lean proteins.
- Spices can irritate the bowel; instead, use fresh herbs to flavour your foods.

TODDLERS' TUM

Diarrhoea is a common problem in babies and young children. It may simply mean that their gut is a little immature. Mothers of breastfed babies sometimes think that their child has chronic diarrhoea because the motions are so liquid and regular. I always advise them that as long as the stool hasn't changed and the baby is otherwise well, there is no need to worry. But if there are other signs of illness such as pain, excess wind or vomiting then you should consult your doctor; the diarrhoea may signal a minor problem such as an ear infection, but it could be the start of a stomach infection or a more serious illness.

There is no specific age at which a child's gut will mature; with some children it can occur when they are two, while others don't manage to produce a well-formed stool, or suffer from bouts of unexplained diarrhoea, until they are four. We call this 'toddlers' tum', and it can be down to the foods they eat. When a child is born the gut is very sensitive, and it takes longer to tolerate some foods than others. I most frequently see toddlers' tum in families who eat a healthy, high fibre diet with a lot of wholemeal bread, fruits and vegetables. This diet is fine for adults, but for a young child you need to make a few adjustments, as their body cannot cope with too much fibre. Give them white bread, rice and pasta as well as the wholegrain versions, with a few vegetables and fruits alongside sources of fats and proteins.

It is most important to consult your doctor if your baby has acute diarrhoea. With an infant under the age of four months I suggest you contact a doctor after twelve hours of vomiting or diarrhoea. With older children it is usually fine to wait for twenty four hours, but if you are worried, seek medical advice.

The most serious problem with diarrhoea is dehydration. Nutritionally the best way to deal with diarrhoea is to stop all milk and solid foods for twenty four hours. However, it is vital to make sure that the body is getting enough fluid. For babies and small children I always recommend a commercial rehydrating fluid such as Rehydrat or Dioralyte, as their bodies need very finely tuned quantities of sugars and salts. Aim to give a baby the same volume as the quantity of feed you normally give them, or more if they still appear to be thirsty. Reintroduce a baby to his or her usual feed, made up at half strength. If this is tolerated for a day you can go back to a full strength feed. Continue replacing lost fluid with extra water. It is possible to continue breastfeeding a baby with diarrhoea, but you must make sure they are given extra water. If the diarrhoea and/or vomiting reappears, return to clear fluids. If things don't settle down in another twenty four hours, seek the advice of your doctor.

For older children, you may need to encourage them to drink water, diluted fruit juices or fizzy drinks, taken in small mouthfuls. If the diarrhoea and vomiting stop, reintroduce solids gently: a piece of toast, a plain biscuit or a little mashed potato. If the symptoms recur go back to plain fluids.

INFECTION

Mild cases of stomach upset, or gastroenteritis, usually correct themselves within a few days. Children seem to suffer more frequently, partly because their immature gut finds it more difficult to cope with infection, and partly because they don't understand the importance of washing their hands. Bugs can spread like wildfire through playgroups because the most common mode of transfer is from an unwashed hand to food. Always wash your hands after you have used the lavatory or changed a nappy, and before you deal with food. If children are taught this by example from infancy, they will not have to be nagged later on.

Severe gut infections, known as dysentery, produce frightening symptoms such as raging diarrhoea, which can be caused by bacteria (or occasionally amoebae) invading the gut.

The drugs your GP prescribes will depend on whether the upset is caused by a bacterium or a virus. The majority of stomach upsets are caused by viruses, so antibiotics will not be any use. You should never give a child anti-diarrhoea drugs meant for adults, such as kaolin and morphine, Imodium or Diocalm.

If your child is aged one or older and is prescribed antibiotics it is a good idea, if they are able to tolerate dairy products, to give them some live yoghurt, containing bifidus and acidophilus, every day, as these will promote the growth of 'good' bacteria in their gut. Sometimes a bout of gastroenteritis can cause a child to become intolerant of certain foods. If you suspect this, I suggest you read the chapter on Managing allergies.

ALCOHOL

When diarrhoea is caused by bacterial or viral pathogens, the French believe that claret (red Bordeaux) or Beaujolais act as cures. They also believe that travellers' diarrhoea, where a traveller is caught out for not being immune to the local organisms, can be prevented by drinking these red wines. In 1995 an American report suggested that red wine, even when diluted, can help prevent food poisoning from organisms such as E. Coli and salmonella.

However, not all alcohol suits people with bowel problems. Irritable bowel syndrome (IBS), a multi-symptom disorder that causes diarrhoea in some people, constipation or even both in others, is often aggravated by alcohol. With IBS it seems to be the type of alcohol that determines the effect: darker drinks such as port, brandy, whisky, red wine and beer all seem to have more of a laxative effect than white wine, champagne or clear spirits.

Constipation

While vomiting and diarrhoea are, for most people, occasional occurrences, constipation seems to be a constant concern. Constipation, the condition of infrequent or difficult emptying of the bowels, with a hard stool which is painful or sometimes impossible to pass, has a number of causes, but in most cases responds extremely well to a few adjustments to your diet and lifestyle. Unfortunately, the dread of constipation makes some people spend a small fortune on laxatives, and parents worry that there is something seriously wrong if their child is not passing a stool every day. In our weight-obsessed society some people take laxatives regularly to help their bodies feel light and cleansed, or even undergo colonic irrigation.

In many cases, this worry is unnecessary. In order to work out whether you have a problem, the first thing to do is to keep a food and symptom diary (see page 85), plotting when you feel constipated or bloated and when you open your bowels. If after a couple of weeks you can see a regular pattern, you can be reassured that the problem is not as bad as you think. People consider themselves constipated when in fact their normal bowel habit is every three to four days. The timing between movements is not that crucial, as long as you feel well. If you are in pain or your bowel habits have changed, you should mention this to your doctor, so that he or she can investigate and ensure that nothing untoward is happening. At worst, constipation may be a symptom of an underlying disorder, such as an obstruction of the bowel by a tumour or structural deformity. However, it is more likely that the problem is simply that the bowel has become lazy, losing its normal, ripple-like, propulsive ability. It needs a nutritional overhaul to get it going.

You cannot really expect the bowel to behave and feel well if you don't look after it properly. Patients come to me with chronic, crippling constipation, but when we look at their eating habits we usually agree that it is hardly surprising. Going for long periods without eating and then having a huge meal in the evening, eating foods with very little nutritional value and full of non-nutritious additives, or bombarding your body with antibiotics every time you get a cold, are typical lifestyle habits that will hinder the bowel.

There are a number of common causes of constipation – and once you know the cause you are halfway to a cure. In many cases laxatives and other medication can be stopped or at least reduced once the bowel receives the nutrients it needs and is not filled with foods that compromise its performance.

LACK OF FIBRE

This is the most common cause of constipation in adults. Fibre in the presence of water forms a soft stool, which stimulates the bowel into action. A soft stool prevents strain when it comes to expelling the waste; straining can lead to piles and start off another cycle of problems and remedies.

If fibre is the answer to preventing or curing your constipation, it clearly must form part of your daily eating plan: try to have some fibre provider, five times a day. Fibre is part of the cellular structure of plants: grains (cereals), nuts, seeds, fruits, vegetables and pulses. In order to gain maximum benefit from the fibre, the plant cell wall needs to be intact: the highest fibre foods are those which have not been heavily processed. For example, wholemeal bread has more fibre than white bread, fruit has more fibre than fruit juice.

There are plenty of delicious ways to include fibre in your daily diet. The best way to begin is simply to eat more fresh fruits and vegetables, wholemeal bread and pulses (lentils, beans and peas), and fewer ready-made foods. The Taste Good section of this book is packed with recipes for high fibre meals, from breakfasts to main meals and desserts, and there are also some healthy snack ideas on page 66. Fruit is a perfect snack: fresh, poached, stewed, mixed into a fruit shake, or enjoyed with a small piece of cheese.

Look afresh at the vegetables in supermarkets and on market stalls. They are simple to cook, full of vitamins and minerals as well as fibre, and you can ring the changes by serving them with a variety of sauces and dressings (see page 312). Grilled, baked or barbecued, they are delicious with herbs and a good olive oil drizzled over the top. Pop vegetables into soups or bake them with a rich tomato sauce (page 313) to make a hot pot. Leftover hot pot can be liquidized and turned into a high fibre soup, adding some beans or pasta shapes to boost the fibre content further.

Don't be drawn to ready-made food – breakfast cereals are a good example – just because the manufacturers have decided to label it 'high fibre'. In many cases there is so much sugar and salt in high fibre cereals that they are not altogether healthy.

Consider having a family health day (page 81), as this can give a good start to your new lifestyle, in which you and your family learn to enjoy fresh foods, especially fruits and vegetables, as part of your daily eating habits.

If there is a drawback, it is that high fibre foods contain substances that tend to bind vitamins and minerals in the gut. However, as long as you have a good balance of different foods – they don't all have to be high fibre – your nutritional requirements should be met.

One final point to remember is that high fibre foods tend to be relatively low in calories. For most people this is a bonus, as they will feel healthier all round, but children and anyone who is underweight needs to balance their intake of fibre with energy-giving foods. Simple ways to increase the calorie level of your healthy meals include: sprinkling extra grated cheese on a vegetable or pasta dish; enriching a sauce with a few tablespoons of cream; serving fruit puddings with custard, thick yoghurt, cream or real dairy ice cream.

LACK OF WATER
The second most common cause of constipation is lack of water. Central heating and air conditioning can cause our bodies to lose water through evaporation

without our realizing it: you don't need to sweat profusely. Constipation is one of the first signs of an imbalance in the amount of water in the body.

Many people eat some fibre, but they don't drink enough water to enable the fibre to swell within the gut, form a soft stool and stimulate the bowel into moving. Fibre is useless unless the water is there to help it swell. If your fibre intake is high and yet you still feel constipated, check that your water intake is at least two and a half litres/four to five pints every day. Children should drink as much as they can in excess of the recommended half a litre/just under a pint for two-year-olds and three-quarters of a litre/one and a quarter pints for three-year-olds. If you boost your fibre intake you need to take in extra fluid.

Get into the habit of having water on your desk at work, carry a small plastic bottle around with you and always have a glass by the bed at night.

Increase your water intake gradually, so that your bladder does not complain, and you will be amazed at how great you feel.

EXCESS CAFFEINE
Although coffee can help correct constipation as a short-term measure (see page 152), the caffeine it contains is a diuretic. Diuretics make your body lose water and hence aggravate constipation, so try to stick to no more than two or three cups a day. It's not just coffee that contains caffeine: tea, cola drinks and hot chocolate all do too, so any of these drinks, taken in excess, can have a similar effect. Experiment with herbal teas and see page 343 for alternative hot drinks.

LACK OF EXERCISE
Exercise tones up your whole body, including your bowel muscles. Make some form of exercise part of your weekly routine. Thirty to forty minutes of aerobic exercise three days a week must be considered the minimum; four or even five days would be ideal.

EMOTIONAL AND PHYSICAL TENSION
Some adults suffer from stress-related constipation. Since the bowel is a muscle, it is very receptive to stress hormones such as adrenaline. Fluctuations in the levels of stress hormones can upset your normal bowel function. Some people find that when they are stressed or upset their bowel goes into 'shut down' and they become constipated. While the nutritional advice given above can help minimize the adverse effects, the underlying stress issue needs to be addressed if there is to be real improvement.

INAPPROPRIATE USE OF LAXATIVES
People who use laxatives on a regular, even daily, basis are making a big mistake; instead of helping their bowel muscle to work efficiently, they are encouraging it to be lazy, which can actually cause constipation. When laxatives – including the plant or fruit-based preparations sold in health food shops – are overused, the

- *Soak prunes in Armagnac
  and serve with shortbread
  biscuits and thick yoghurt*
- *Stew prunes with peaches
  and serve with vanilla
  custard*
- *Add prunes to a hearty
  meat stew, such as beef,
  game or oxtail*
- *Spread prune jam on slices
  of warm wholemeal toast*
- *Rub plump prunes with
  Kirsch and coat with good-
  quality dark chocolate sauce*

bowel can start to rely on the laxative to stimulate it into action. Overuse can also cause diarrhoea, which may ultimately result in malnutrition.

Only if all avenues of the diet have been explored should one turn to laxatives. They should never be given to children unless prescribed and supervised by a paediatrician. Even adults should seek medical approval, for reasons I shall now explain.

The choice of laxative is very important, as an inappropriate choice can potentially aggravate rather than help. It all depends on the cause of your constipation and your general diet. There are three types of laxatives:

- The gentlest are the bulking agents, which contain gels that swell within the bowel. Their action is very similar to the way in which fibre works. These can be useful for adults who are unable to eat a high fibre diet, for instance if they have a gut problem or certain food sensitivities.
- Irritant-based laxatives work by irritating the bowel and making it expel the food; examples are the laxatives made from the leaves or pods of the senna plant. Too many irritant laxatives can cause your bowel to become very sensitive, which can ultimately lead to haemorrhoids (piles) and bleeding.
- Propulsive laxatives affect the muscle function of the bowel; they cause the muscles to contract and relax, like normal peristalsis.

Irritant or propulsive based preparations are more appropriate if you know that you do not lack fibre, but your doctor will be able to assess your specific needs.

WEAK BOWEL MUSCLES

As with any other muscle in the body, it is important to 'train' the bowel. You can keep your bowel muscles strong by allowing them to empty when they give you the signal. Constipated people have often developed the habit of ignoring their urges. Don't 'hold on' too long, as this can cause increased pressure in the rectum, which can ultimately lead to problems such as incontinence and piles.

SHORT-TERM MEASURES

Many people ask me what they can do nutritionally to get over a bout of constipation. The best short-term cures are prunes and coffee.

You can nibble the delicious, moist, ready-to-eat prunes or chop them into yoghurt or have a glass of prune juice (for other ideas, see margin).

Prunes have no side effects, but you have to be a little careful with the coffee. A cup of strong black coffee causes the smooth muscles to relax and kicks the bowel into action, but if you come to rely on it it may have adverse side effects such as decreased absorption of iron and other nutrients, which may in turn cause anaemia and palpitations. Keep your intake of coffee to a minimum.

In cases of severe and chronic constipation I see no harm in occasional colonic irrigation, as long as it is done under strict medical guidance and no more than two or three times a year.

CHILDREN'S CONSTIPATION

Most children are constipated from time to time. It is especially common after a bout of illness, even a cold. It can be self-perpetuating; if a hard stool causes a child's anus to rip, going to the loo can be painful, and they put it off. Sometimes it is more of a psychological problem. Some children just don't feel relaxed about using the loo, especially if they feel it is something to be rushed before they go out. Let them take their own time, and try not to make them feel they are being watched and their bowel habits noted.

In the worst scenarios, untreated constipation can go on for weeks, and can cause serious problems. If a child becomes severely constipated, such a mass of matter builds up that their bowel muscles become distended and they fail to recognize the feeling that they need to go to the loo. If they then soil their pants they may be told off, as parents think they are being careless or naughty. Before scolding them, take the time to remember when they last opened their bowels. A food and symptom diary (see page 85) can be useful, as this will help you to stay objective. If you are worried, seek your doctor's advice; the child may need to be admitted to hospital so that their bowel can be emptied carefully and good toilet habits established.

TREATING CONSTIPATED CHILDREN

Nutritionally, as with adults, you need to encourage them to eat plenty of high fibre foods. Try to make these foods tempting to eat (there is a selection of high fibre puddings in the Taste Good section of this book); if meals become a chore or a battle the child will become more uptight, which won't help them relax and go to the loo. Don't forget that children also need plenty of energy-giving foods, so balance their intake of high fibre foods with white bread and pasta, eggs, milk, cheese and other dairy products, fish, poultry and meat.

Make sure that they drink plenty of fluids, as dehydration can cause constipation, especially during the summer months. Encourage them to drink fresh fruit juices, possibly diluted with sparkling water. Some canned drinks contain so much sugar that the sugar slows the gut down and aggravates constipation. Never give a child laxatives, except under the guidance of a doctor.

Wind

Wind can be excruciating. After an operation, the pain can be so severe that you need to take medication to help relieve the pain of trapped wind. When people suffer from wind they usually put it down to eating pulses or vegetables such as cauliflower and broccoli, but there are other reasons why it occurs, and therefore different nutritional measures to help relieve it.

HOW TO PREVENT WIND

- Keep a food and symptom diary (see page 85) for a couple of weeks. This can help you discover whether particular foods seem to trigger the wind.

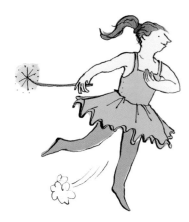

Eliminate the suspected foods for a few days and see if you notice any difference. If this simple step solves the problem, I suggest you keep the diary going for a further two weeks and then compare your overall intake with the information in the chapter on Understanding your nutritional needs, to make sure your body is receiving all the nutrients it needs. If you remove foods, you need to replace them with suitably nutritious alternatives. For instance, if you remove pulses you should eat plenty of other sources of protein (if you are vegetarian), fibre and B vitamins (see pages 27–39). Alternatively, you may like to experiment with different cooking methods, or different pulses, as some people find these just as effective in relieving flatulence.

- Your fat intake may be contributing to the problem: large loads of undigested fat cause wind in the gut. The enzymes that digest fat are produced by the liver and are normally stored in the gall bladder. In young children, these fat-digesting enzymes are slow to develop. Older people do not escape: anyone who has their gall bladder removed or is born without one (as I was) relies on their liver to secrete bile directly into the gut, which it does at a constant rate; they can only tolerate small amounts of fat. The best way to deal with this is to cut down your intake of fatty foods, and to accompany the small amounts you do eat with a fibre provider. For example, eat cheese with an apple or an oatcake, accompany fried foods with a slice of wholemeal bread. The fibre holds the food in the stomach for longer, allowing the bile to digest it gradually.

  Another scenario, which applies to everyone, is that the body regulates its production of fat-digesting enzymes according to the food you eat. Periods of abstinence from fatty food cause your liver to reduce the amount of bile it produces, and after a while the gall bladder will reduce the amount it stores. Fat leaving the stomach enters the small intestine, where it sends a message to the gall bladder to release bile. If the bile is not available, the undigested fat irritates the wall of the small intestine, causing food to pass quickly into the colon before it is fully digested, where it whisks up wind. This explains why many people feel 'windy' after an unusually rich, fatty meal, and also why some people suffer unduly when they temporarily lapse from a low fat diet. The problem is sometimes – in very rare cases – the result of an enzyme deficiency, for example if you suffer from cystic fibrosis.

  The majority of people can avoid wind by staggering their intake of fat in a well balanced diet, which naturally includes small amounts of fat (dairy products, eggs, oil for cooking, hidden fats in meat and oily fish).

- Consider whether your gut bacteria are healthy. The bowel is home to a colony of good bacteria that help your body in several ways, but if bad bacteria gain the upper hand they can produce wind and bloating. You could be encouraging the bad bacteria by eating foods high in additives, preservatives, sugars or fats, or by taking medication unnecessarily, rather than allowing your body to recover naturally from minor ailments. To help redress the bacterial balance, try taking a daily dose of acidophilus and bifidus, the bacteria found in live 'bio' yoghurt; a small pot a day would be ideal. If you cannot tolerate dairy products you can take these two flora as tablets, available from health food shops.

- Sparkling drinks can aggravate wind in some people. Try replacing them with fruit juices and still mineral waters.
- Wind can be due to a food intolerance, such as wheat or dairy products. If your food diary suggests this, I recommend that you read the chapter on Managing allergies, so that you can learn about eliminating certain foods.
- Eating too quickly is a common cause of wind; you end up swallowing a lot of air. Slow down and relax when eating. The earlier you instil this good eating habit in your children, the healthier they will stay.
- Allowing your body time to digest food and not rushing around after you have eaten can alleviate wind, because the gut is very sensitive to the 'fight or flight' stress hormones.

WHAT TO DO WHEN YOU HAVE WIND
- Taking a painkiller can sometimes help, but various herbs can calm the intestine and reduce the production of wind. Mint (see margin, next page) and camomile are two of the most successful herbs, and are easily made into soothing teas, using either the whole herb, or herbal tea bags.
- Some people find that a tot of a certain alcohol, such as brandy or Scotch, can help reduce wind.
- Don't drink coffee or tea, as the caffeine and tannins in these drinks irritate the gut, and can further aggravate wind.

Indigestion

Sales of indigestion remedies continue to rise, as we bombard our bodies with food and eating habits that hinder rather than help digestion. Adults carry mints or antacid remedies around with them, fall into bed at night feeling heavy in the stomach and awake far from rested, children complain of tummy ache. The symptoms of both chronic and acute indigestion can be frightening; people may feel as if they are having a heart attack, that they've dislocated a shoulder, or as if their gut is going to explode. Indigestion is a symptom of many stomach and intestinal problems, some more serious than others. If you or your child regularly suffer from indigestion or tummy ache or have any other symptoms, you should consult your GP, who will investigate the cause; there may be something that needs to be corrected surgically or treated with medication.

Once you have established that there is nothing more sinister than simple indigestion, you will be relieved to hear that a lot can be done, both nutritionally and in your general lifestyle, to reduce the symptoms. Medication has its place, for occasional relief, but if you rely on indigestion tablets and take them every day, they can interfere with the absorption of vitamins and minerals from the gut, as they neutralize the acid these nutrients need for their absorption. If, after

Mint

The mint family contains many herbs, peppermint and spearmint being the most well known. Mint has a relaxing, calming effect on the gut. The distilled essential oil is used in confectionery and various pharmaceutical products; you can buy mint oil capsules, which can aid digestion and prevent wind. To soothe a troubled gut, make mint tea: pour boiling water over the leaves and leave to infuse for a few minutes.

following the advice in this chapter, you still find yourself having to chew them regularly, see your doctor to ensure nothing more serious is happening. Don't encourage children to rely on indigestion remedies.

The term 'simple indigestion' usually means that you become uncomfortably aware of the acidity of your stomach; you may also tend to suffer from wind or belching. The acidity may either be felt in the stomach itself, in which case it is called gastritis, or further up the oesophagus, the feeding tube that leads to the stomach. The latter condition is called oesophagitis, but is more commonly known as heartburn. The reason for this name is that the pain is felt round about the area of your heart; if you experience this it is most important that you get the 'all-clear' from your doctor and not simply suffer in silence, assuming that it is indigestion. Heartburn occurs because the acid contents of your stomach leak up into the alkaline environment of the oesophagus. This may be the result of a hiatus hernia, in which part of the stomach protrudes through the diaphragm at the oesophageal opening. Heartburn can occur either before or after eating, as a reaction to something you have eaten or drunk, or as a result of not eating. Indigestion can also cause an acid taste in the mouth, which in extreme cases can cause you to be physically sick.

HOW TO AVOID INDIGESTION
- Make sure that your main meals are high in fibre. Fibre helps to keep the food within the stomach for the maximum amount of time, hence reduces the time the stomach is left empty and prone to acid attack. When planning your meals you should try to include some wholegrain bread, brown rice, wholewheat pasta or another high fibre cereal, along with fresh vegetables or fruits. However, some people find large amounts of vegetables or fruits hard to digest. If you find this, try eating regular smaller amounts.
- Avoid having fatty foods on an empty stomach. Fatty foods can cause the valve at the top of your stomach to become lazy, allowing stomach acids to leak upwards. This happens because the hormones released when you ingest fat make the muscles in this valve relax. Instead of crisps or chips, look to lower fat snacks such as wholegrain crackers. If you do want to eat something fatty such as cheese, make sure you eat it with a high fibre food, such as wholegrain bread, as this diminishes the adverse effects.
- Eat a little something every three to four hours. Eating something, even if it is a light snack such as a biscuit, a slice of bread or a scone, will help keep the acid produced by the stomach away from sensitive areas. For those of you who worry that you will put on weight if you start eating every few hours, remember that you need less at main meal times if you have regular snacks. Over a twenty four hour period your intake does not increase.
- Avoid foods that you find hard to digest. This may sound an obvious thing to say, but some people don't put much thought into what they are eating, especially if they are under stress. When pushed for time it's tempting to fill

up with a fatty takeaway meal at the end of the day, only to regret it during the night. Choose something light like a bowl of soup, or a plain, starchy food such as a potato, pasta or rice dish. Some people find bread or acidic foods such as citrus fruits upset them, others find that a huge salad of raw vegetables can be a little hard to digest. Either avoid these all the time, making sure your diet is still well balanced, or just when you are feeling under pressure.

- Try to eat slowly; do not gulp large amounts of food, water or air. Forcing food, air or fluid into your stomach will disturb the gentle digestive processes. People who dine out on business can be prone to rush through their food, as can children who want to dash off to play. Sitting still and eating slowly helps reduce indigestion. Remember that your digestive system needs oxygen to work efficiently. Rushing off after a meal leaves the stomach lacking in oxygen and prone to cramps and indigestion. All you need is a few minutes to relax.

- Avoid spicy foods. It will come as no surprise to many people that spices such as chillies and ground coriander can aggravate and inflame the stomach. However, there are many other flavours you can use to enhance the flavour of your food. Try fresh herbs such as dill or mint, or some roasted or baked garlic, which has a subtler effect than raw or fried.

- Avoid excessive coffee, tea and other caffeine and tannin-containing drinks, such as cola and hot chocolate. These irritate the stomach lining. One of my patients had been suffering tremendously with oesophagitis, but when he removed caffeine from his diet he said goodbye to the pain. Include plenty of other drinks such as herbal teas, especially camomile and mint (see margin opposite), or see pages 342–3 for other caffeine-free drinks, especially the ginger tea, which is a good after-meal digestive.

- Avoid drinking large amounts while you eat. Lots of liquid sloshing around the stomach makes it more likely that the acid contents will leak up into the oesophagus. Take small sips to help the food go down and to refresh your palate. Some people find that fizzy drinks upset them, so choose still rather than sparkling mineral water.

- Avoid excessive amounts of alcohol. Too much alcohol irritates the muscular valve that separates the stomach from the oesophagus, causing acid to leak up into the oesophagus. Alcohol can also irritate the stomach, especially if you are stressed, have an empty stomach, or have eaten something which could also aggravate the stomach. Heavy drinkers sometimes skip meals, which increases their risk of digestive problems, including indigestion. The effect of alcohol is very individual: some people cannot take stronger spirits such as whisky and brandy, whereas others find them helpful as an after-meal digestive; some people find lighter drinks such as champagne or white wine irritating. I suggest that you avoid drinking on an empty stomach and choose small amounts of your favourite drink with food.

- Give up smoking. Smoking severely aggravates the stomach and oesophagus, weakens the stomach valves and aggravates indigestion.

- Make sure that you are not carrying too much fat. Excess body fat around your middle can squeeze your stomach and cause acid to be nudged into your oesophagus. Frequently, if you lose this excess fat you will find that the indigestion disappears; see the chapter on Achieving your ideal weight. Don't crash diet or starve yourself for long periods of time; either way you will aggravate your indigestion.

WHAT TO DO WHEN YOU HAVE INDIGESTION
- Resist the temptation to drink milk. Milk can seem the natural, perfectly inoffensive, cooling drink, and many people with a tendency to indigestion believe they should spend their days eating milk puddings and having endless glasses of cold milk. This is outdated and potentially very damaging. Substances within the milk cause the stomach to produce more acid, which means that the initial cooling effect is quickly followed by extreme indigestion. Therefore, in the majority of cases, milk is best avoided. However, a small number of people have an ulcer in the jejunum, an early section (after the duodenum) of the small intestine. In these cases milk can help, but I suggest you avoid it unless you have been given this diagnosis. Instead, try to have small, regular, starchy snacks (see page 66 for some ideas), which don't have the same 'knock-back' acid effect.
- Peppermint and ginger are very soothing. Try drinking boiling water infused with mint leaves or a slice of fresh ginger, or you could use a mint or ginger tea bag. It is best served warm, rather than very hot or icy cold, as extreme temperatures can cause the stomach to go into spasm. Camomile is another calming tea, especially as a bedtime drink.
- Large amounts of fruits, vegetables, fatty or sugary foods are difficult for the body to deal with, so avoid these when you have indigestion. You would be better off with a starchy snack such as potato soup or a sandwich.
- Avoid highly spiced foods when you have indigestion. Spices irritate the stomach wall and valves leading into and out of the stomach, making it much easier for acid juices to leak where they are least wanted.
- Eat slowly and take small mouthfuls and sips of food and drink. Try not to gulp, as air inside a sore stomach can be very painful.
- Have a rest. Rushing will aggravate your acid stomach and encourage the contents to leak into your oesophagus. Resting in a comfortable chair should help to keep the acid down in the stomach. Reading or playing some calming music will help. Tell a story to a child, and discourage them from playing taxing games, where they run around or become competitive.
- Try applying a little warmth over your stomach. Warmth can help the stomach muscles to relax and become less painful. Use a hot water bottle, or have a warm bath. Aromatherapy oils such as lavender, rosewood, orange and ginger can relax the body and ease the pain. Add a few drops to the warm bathwater, or use an aromatherapy burner while you're soaking in the suds.

24 HOUR BOOKSHOP

www.waterstones.co.uk

24 HOUR BOOKSHOP

Ulcers

Stress undoubtedly increases the body's tendency towards indigestion and ulcers of the digestive system. Simply speaking, an ulcer is an open wound on the surface of the muscle lining. Through the lens of an endoscopic camera, it looks very similar to a mouth ulcer. Ulcers can be very painful and, if untreated, can burst and cause internal bleeding. However, there is much you can do to avoid getting ulcers, and with improved medical understanding and treatment the situation of a burst ulcer shouldn't arise.

When stress is constant, acid levels in the stomach tend to be rather high, which can make the stomach more sensitive than usual; poor eating habits, which you may have got away with for years, suddenly start to cause problems. In times of extreme stress the stomach becomes severely inflamed. The inflammation is made worse if the stomach is left empty for long periods, which can easily happen if you have other things such as work or family on your mind. If this situation develops one stage further, an ulcer can appear, as a result of the acid wearing away the protective lining of the organ, whether this is the stomach, oesophagus, duodenum or elsewhere in the intestine. Astonishingly, ulcers can occur in young children, especially if they are being bullied, or are really worried about school work.

Ulcers can also plague people taking strong anti-inflammatory medication for conditions such as rheumatoid arthritis. I advise that this medication should not be taken on an empty stomach, and you could ask your doctor whether it could be taken by suppository to avoid affecting the stomach.

Traditional remedies for ulcers relied on decreasing acid production or neutralizing the acid. Medical treatment of ulcers has improved dramatically since the discovery that the bacterium *Helicobacter pylori* is frequently found at the site of ulceration. This means that doctors can now prescribe antibiotics to kill the bacteria and enable the ulceration site to heal. Killing *Helicobacter pylori* also decreases the risk of stomach cancer.

The nutritional and lifestyle guidelines for indigestion and ulcers are very similar. You may feel that some of the suggestions in the preceding section do not apply to you, but consider them individually and you could save yourself a lot of pain. Above all, try to find ways to relieve your stress. Exercise is one of the best stress busters, either in the fresh air or in a gym or workout class.

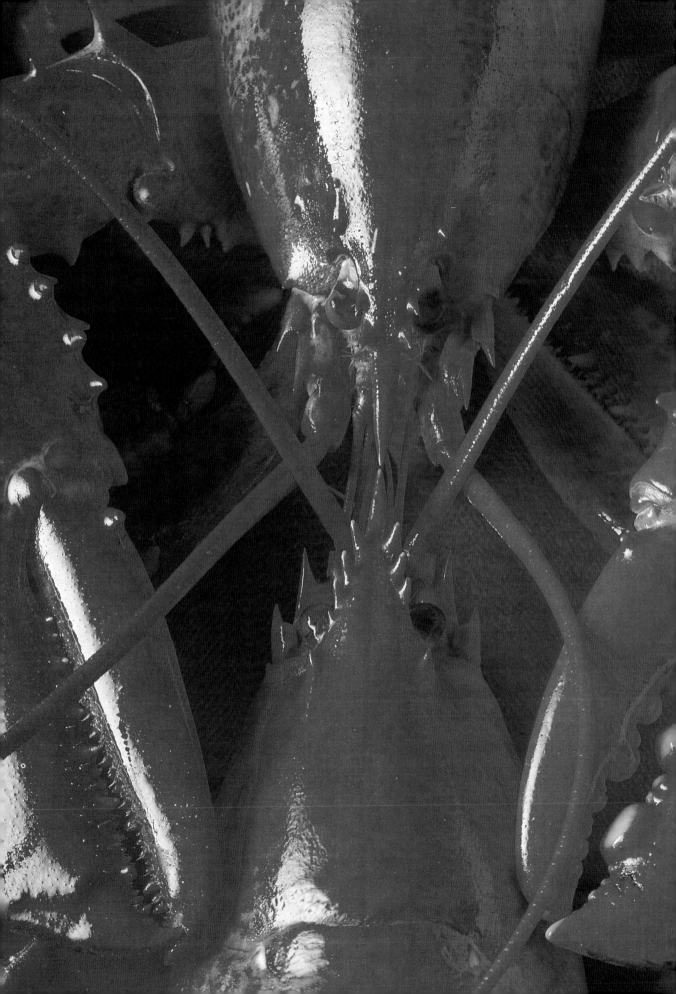

A happy, healthy sex life

There are a great number of nutritional factors that can affect your sex drive. Although low libido can be caused by many non-food factors, including stress, depression and ill health, all of which need addressing in their own right, if you are suffering from a low sex drive it is well worth exploring the nutritional cures. If nothing else it can be delicious fun!

Mention sex and food to most people and the word aphrodisiac will spring to mind. Nothing has been scientifically proven as to whether certain foods such as oysters, caviar and champagne can increase your libido. It is more often one's perception that makes a so-called aphrodisiac food a real 'turn on'. Swallowing an oyster, peeling prawns, or sucking asparagus spears can elicit many a sexy thought. The aphrodisiac qualities of the food have more to do with mouth feel than with any secret ingredient.

Tips to help your sex life
MAKE SURE YOUR DIET IS RICH IN ZINC

Low zinc levels have been linked with poor libido in women and low sperm counts as well as low sex drives in men. Foods rich in zinc include the classic aphrodisiac, seafood, but also less sexy items such as wholegrain bread and brown rice, green leafy vegetables, lean red meat, and crumbly cheeses such as Cheshire or Lancashire. If you suspect your zinc intake is low, boost your intake of these foods (see page 45 for more sources).

KEEP YOUR WEIGHT WITHIN THE IDEAL RANGE

Excess weight hinders more than your physical ability to perform. Men with beer bellies are more likely to be impotent, and women who are overweight are less likely to conceive. However, there is no benefit to be had from being at the other end of the weight spectrum. Underweight women with a Body Mass Index of less than 17 or 18 and low body fat percentages (see chart on page 109) can have a problem metabolizing the sex hormones oestrogen and progesterone, which can affect both their libido and their ability to conceive.

There is also a psychological relationship between the way you feel about your body and your ability to have fulfilling sexual relationships. People with low self-esteem may avoid sex or they may seek excessive sexual encounters because they need to be with someone and feel cared for. The ideal scenario is to accept your body the way it is, preferably keeping it within or close to the ideal weight range, as this will help your body manufacture and circulate the hormones it needs to feel sexy.

SLOW DOWN AND PAY ATTENTION TO YOUR BODY

Some people find that the act of paying attention to their life, eating habits and body's needs helps boost their self-confidence and that this frequently manifests itself in the bedroom (or wherever else takes your fancy!).

KEEP YOUR CHOLESTEROL LEVEL WITHIN THE IDEAL RANGE

There is a link between cholesterol levels and sex hormones. Cholesterol is the major carrier hormone of testosterone and oestrogen. Men who lower their cholesterol levels very quickly or take them below the recommended range can suffer from low levels of circulating testosterone and hence a low libido. This is a common occurrence in men who become obsessive about their eating and try to exclude fat from their diet, or among those who suffer from digestive complaints that cause fat malabsorption, such as cystic fibrosis, Crohn's disease, ulcerative colitis, or when part of the gut has been removed in surgery. Men who have medical reasons why they cannot absorb fat efficiently should seek the advice of a dietitian. For those men who have started rigorous non-fat diets – if you lighten up a little you should find that your libido will improve. A similar thing can happen with women – if the cholesterol level falls too low, oestrogen levels can drop and your libido can disappear. However it is not the case that the higher your cholesterol level, the higher the libido! It is a question of balancing cholesterol within a healthy eating plan. See the chapter on High blood cholesterol for more information.

DON'T OVERLOAD YOUR BODY

Learning to eat just enough and not too much is important. Sex on a full stomach is not much fun. After a heavy meal, the body produces sleep-inducing hormones that antagonize the sex hormones – making sex rather like swimming against the tide. You can also get indigestion if you have eaten too much.

WATCH YOUR ALCOHOL INTAKE

Temporary impotence after a night's heavy drinking can be the result of stupor, but it is more likely that the alcohol has had an anaesthetizing effect on the peripheral cutaneous nerves leading to the penis and the nerve supply to its blood vessels. The traditional view that excess alcohol only adversely affects men is untrue – a woman who has drunk to excess may reduce not only her ability to orgasm, but also to be enthusiastic and energetic in bed.

The long-term effects of drinking are even more significant. Long-term heavy drinking can cause testicular atrophy, shrinkage of the penis, loss of body hair and enlargement of the breasts in men. This is due to hormonal changes – the liver fails to metabolize the oestrogens that naturally flow throughout men as well as women, and testosterone is metabolized differently. Testosterone levels decrease and oestrogen levels increase. The body shape can change too: out pops the beer belly. Some studies have linked a pot belly and impotence.

Of course, there are also some positive aspects: drinking champagne in bed or a gorgeous wine with your meal can bring out the sexiness in both of you – it's just a question of not drinking too much. Drinking plenty of water as well as the alcohol can reduce the potential negative effects and help your body stay hydrated and sober.

Remember that drinking on an empty stomach can cause your appetite to increase, which may mean that you overindulge and then feel stuffed, not sexy. It can also send your energy levels crashing and can make you sleepy. The presence of food keeps the alcohol in the stomach and slows absorption. Enjoy wine with your meal or prepare some simple hors d'oeuvres to nibble with the aperitif. Why not have sticks of crisp raw vegetables and dips, sliced tomatoes with torn basil on thin slices of bread, or small pieces of charcuterie or smoked fish on wholewheat crackers?

TRY TO EAT A WELL BALANCED DIET

To achieve a healthy, sexy body, eat a varied, well balanced diet (see the chapter Understanding your nutritional needs). People normally run into problems when they are cutting corners with their diet, eating lots of fast food, sweet snacks or heavy restaurant meals, going for long periods of time without eating and then eating too much, or drinking excessive amounts of coffee or tea. This is when the body feels sluggish and far from sexy. A well-nourished body devoid of artificial stimulants can find great pleasure in physical stimulants.

DON'T GET STRESSED ABOUT FOOD

Whichever foods you decide to eat to help your sex drive, it is important not to become obsessed with ways of increasing your sexuality. Stress itself can reduce your enjoyment of sex. Sexual arousal can diminish if you are worried about work, money, relationships and equally the food you eat or don't eat. Relax and choose foods you will find easy to prepare and fun to eat. Simple pasta dishes, or a platter of fresh seafood with some fresh bread and salad don't take much preparation. For a special meal, think about foods that you can prepare before-hand, or that can be left to simmer. If you have a strong flavour such as garlic in the meal, make sure that both of you eat it, and remember that curries and spicy foods can irritate the gut, causing flatulence; not the sexiest thing! Think about the food's presentation and sex appeal, as well as your own. Choose foods that look appetizing, with a variety of colours, shapes, textures and temperatures, as this helps stimulate all the senses.

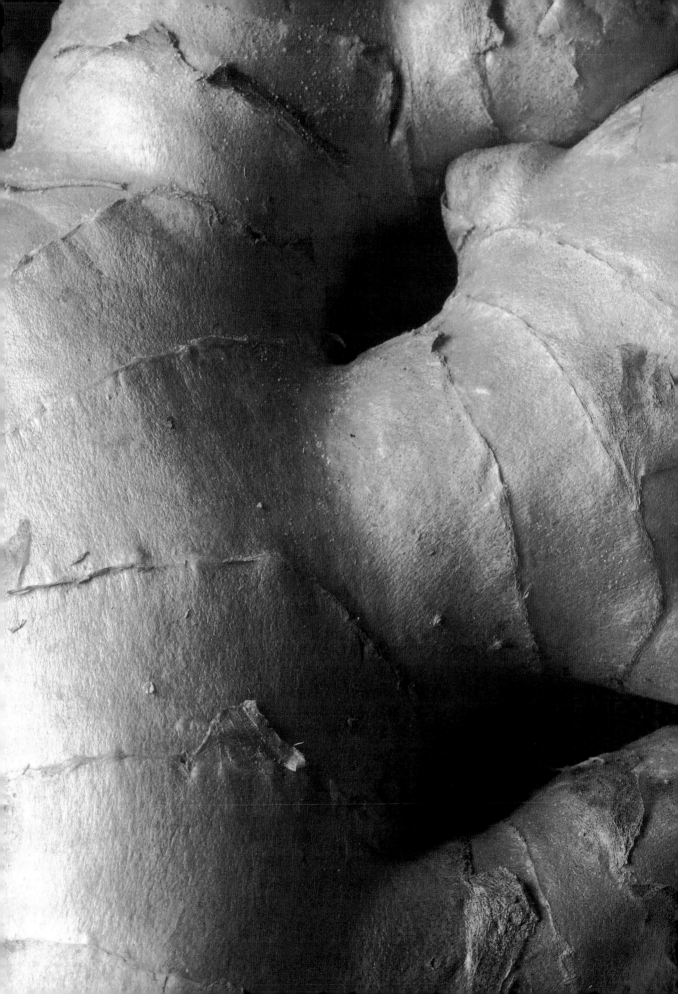

Tackling headaches and migraine

No one seems to escape the occasional headache. Thousands of children and teenagers suffer from headaches to the extent that their education is disrupted. Stress headaches are affecting increasing numbers of men and women. Migraine differs from other headaches in a number of ways, but there are several nutritional principles which can help both. By looking at the food you eat and the way you live your life, you can help your body eradicate headaches and migraines or at least become far less reliant on medication.

In order to understand how food can help, you first need to understand a little of the physiology. The brain itself doesn't have any pain receptors, but the blood vessels and membranes surrounding the brain do feel pain. Either of these can produce a headache. The majority of headaches result from changes in the blood vessels, which may be due to hormones or other chemical substances produced in the body or introduced in our food and drink. Tension, stress, anxiety, overwork, irregular eating habits, caffeine and alcohol can all contribute to a headache.

If you are experiencing regular headaches and feel generally unwell, don't just pop a painkiller, consult your doctor, as there are rare occasions when the headache signifies something more serious such as meningitis or a brain tumour. Children and babies with headaches, particularly if they are off their food or drowsy, or if they also have a stiff neck, should be investigated by their doctor straight away to ensure that they are not suffering from meningitis. Meningitis is an inflammation of the meninges, the membranes that cover the brain and spinal cord. Bacterial meningitis can be fatal, or can result in brain damage, blindness and deafness, but if diagnosed and treated early the outlook is good. Viral meningitis may follow a virus infection which has hit another area of the body, such as mumps. Luckily children usually recover completely. Don't panic if an older child or a friend has the symptoms of meningitis – stiff neck and a headache – especially if they are well in all other ways, as meningitis is, thankfully, quite rare.

Migraine

The point at which a headache becomes a migraine is a controversial point. Migraines can cause pain in the head and neck, nausea, vomiting, loss of balance and disturbed vision. The severity varies from a thumping headache to complete incapacity. Other migraine sufferers have disturbed vision – black spots, flashing lights or lines – without any particular pain. Young children can find it hard at school and changes in their behaviour and ability should be investigated by your doctor. Some people, particularly young migraine sufferers, vomit profusely without appearing to suffer pain in the head. It is usually as they get older that head pain becomes the prominent symptom. Migraines are more commonly suffered by women than men, but more than half of all female sufferers cease to be troubled by migraines after their menopause.

What causes a migraine headache?

A neurologist will tell you that the causes of a migraine are extremely complex. In simple terms, there are two phases. First, the blood vessels become constricted; secondly, they react to this narrowing by overly expanding (dilating). If the sensitive blood vessels in the head constrict for a period of fifteen minutes to an hour and then rapidly expand, it causes pain. The narrowing of blood vessels that starts off the cycle is triggered by the release of serotonin, a substance produced in the blood. Serotonin can be released by eating certain foods and drinks, by stress or even by oversleeping. As your kidneys process the serotonin and the level drops, the blood vessels dilate rapidly, pressing on surrounding nerves and causing inflammation and a pulsating pain, usually on one side of the head. The pain can last for days as the swelling takes time to go down, even when the blood vessels have returned to normal.

The foods that lead to the release of serotonin include sugary and carbohydrate-rich foods such as white bread (see page 140 for more details), and also foods that contain substances known as vasoactive amines, which I shall come to later. Such foods include chocolate, hard cheeses and red wine.

FLUCTUATING SUGAR LEVELS

Headaches and migraines can also occur when your blood sugar level swings from very low to very high and vice versa. Your body reacts badly to lower and higher levels than it is used to, or, more importantly, dramatic changes in level.

When trying to stabilize blood sugar levels, the worst thing you can do is to take a sweet food when you feel 'low'. This causes the blood sugar level to rise too quickly; the body reacts by producing more insulin, the hormone that breaks down sugar and thus causes the blood sugar level to fall too low.

The solution when you feel weak and low in sugar is to eat something that is both sweet and high in fibre, for example a banana or a wholegrain biscuit such as a piece of flapjack: the fibre slows the release of sugar into the blood. If your sugar level goes very high quickly, there isn't a specific food that can lower the level slowly; soon afterwards you should try to eat a high fibre meal or snack (vegetables, wholegrain cereal products such as oatcakes, brown rice or wholemeal bread), drink plenty of water and try to relax. This should help your blood sugar level to drop gradually.

General guidelines

Taking a good look at your food and lifestyle may shed light on a number of ways in which you can help your body avoid and deal with headaches and migraines.

KEEP A FOOD DIARY

The most important aspect of any form of self help is to keep detailed notes of what you're eating, drinking and doing, and the resulting effect on your body (see page 85). You may have come to some conclusions already, but when things are written down a pattern may fall into place that wasn't obvious before. The cause and effect don't necessarily occur within a short period of time. Triggers such as eating cheese can cause a migraine within twenty minutes, whereas other triggers such as extreme exercise or a stressful meeting may not cause a migraine for a few hours.

The question of food intolerance and migraine is slightly controversial. I find that following sensible principles of living and eating well cures the majority of patients. However, there are instances where elimination diets help to reduce migraines. In this case food diaries are of paramount importance, as it can be the smallest quantity of food, such as milk in a sauce, that triggers a migraine.

HAVE SMALL, WELL-BALANCED MEALS

'Little and often' is the best eating plan. This might mean changing your habits of a lifetime, but it could also mean freedom from headaches. Skipping breakfast as you dash out in the morning and then expecting your body to last until a late lunch, or going from lunchtime to eight or nine o'clock in the evening before you eat again, are recipes for disaster. Some people say they 'can't face food' early in the morning, but eating something small such as some fruit and yoghurt can be enough to stave off the headache or migraine. Eating regularly doesn't mean you have to overeat, but keeping your stomach happy with satisfying snacks can reduce the likelihood of headaches. See page 66 for some ideas.

KEEP YOUR FIBRE INTAKE HIGH

High fibre foods 'cushion' the effects of sugar in your food and help the body control blood sugar levels.

ACT QUICKLY

The key to getting rid of a migraine quickly is to stop the pain as soon as possible. Once the migraine headache takes a strong hold it usually becomes more difficult to treat. Don't just ignore it and hope it goes away.

I am not saying that you always need to take medication, although if you do, take it on time to lessen the pain. Sometimes, by eating a high fibre snack and resting, preferably in a room without artificial lights, or just taking a few minutes to breathe properly and concentrate on relaxing your muscles, the headache may disappear. Some people find that a warm hot water bottle around the neck can help reduce the constriction within the blood vessels. Others find an ice pack (or a bag of frozen peas) more effective.

BE PREPARED

It is a good idea to have some simple nutritious snack foods close at hand – carry them in your bag or briefcase and keep some at the office – for when you recognize the early signs of a headache or migraine. Good snack foods include fresh and dried fruits, wholemeal biscuits and wholemeal cakes. Encourage children who suffer from migraines to carry a little 'survival pack' around with them. Teach them that it is important to eat something healthy when they feel the first signs of a headache or migraine-related tummy ache coming on.

AVOID CARRYING TOO MUCH BODY WEIGHT

Try to keep your weight within the correct range for your height (see page 109). Carrying too much fat, especially around the middle, presses against the chief blood vessels leading to and from the heart, which causes blood pressure to rise and increases the risk of developing a migraine or headache. Don't crash diet as this can really cause your head to complain. The chapter on Achieving your ideal weight has advice on controlled weight loss.

TRY NOT TO GET TOO STRESSED

Stress aggravates and indeed causes both headaches and migraines. Some researchers believe this is due to the effects of stress hormones such as adrenaline in the blood. Try to build some stress-relieving techniques into your regular routine; this could mean listening to music or a soothing relaxation tape, reading a good book, having a massage or going for a brisk walk in the open air.

Dentists have found a fascinating link between stress and migraine headaches. Some people often grind their teeth as they sleep, as a result of stress or tension; in doing this they damage the surfaces of their teeth. The treatment is to wear a dental plate at night. The majority of patients reported that wearing the plate either eliminated migraines altogether or drastically lessened their frequency. If you know you grind your teeth at night this is an area worth investigating.

SLEEP

Disturbed sleep patterns, lack of sleep and, perhaps surprisingly, excess sleep can all cause headaches and migraines. Regular sound sleep is far more beneficial than disturbed or irregular rest. See the chapter on How to sleep soundly.

TRY NOT TO BECOME CONSTIPATED

Some people find that constipation over a number of days can cause toxins to build up in the body, which can cause headaches. If you have a tendency to be constipated, see the section within the chapter on Good digestion, page 149.

Food and migraine headaches

Having established the principle that little and often is the best way to eat, it is worth looking at the types of foods you eat.

Many people who suffer from severe headaches and migraine know that the classic trigger foods are caffeine (coffee, tea, hot chocolate, cola), red wine, cheese, chocolate and citrus fruits, particularly oranges. Avoiding these foods completely isn't easy and for some people is unnecessary, as everyone reacts differently to different foods.

I have been able to help many patients to manage some of these foods, either by experimenting with different types of red wine or cheese, or by being careful with the timing, quantity and the combinations of foods. Fibre and water will usually cushion the effect of the trigger food. For instance, eating cheese with wholemeal bread and fruit usually causes fewer problems than eating a plate of cheese on an empty stomach and with little else apart from a glass of red wine. Some people can take a couple of glasses of red wines which are low in flavonoids (see below, under Alcohol), but not a rich claret. Children and chocaholics can enjoy a small amount of good quality chocolate after a meal that contains a lot of fibre, but not a chocolate bar as a mid-afternoon snack.

Certain other foods have proved to trigger headaches or migraine in some people, so it is sensible to watch out for them, and make a special note if you are keeping a food diary. They include processed meats such as cured hams, sausages and hot dogs, lentils, chicken livers, citrus fruits, mangetout (it is the pods that can cause problems, so regular peas should be fine), and the flavour enhancer monosodium glutamate (MSG, food additive number 621). MSG is often found in bottled sauces, ready-made meals, crisps and in Chinese restaurant food. Sticking to fresh and unprocessed foods will mean that you avoid MSG. The best Chinese chefs do not use MSG, but to be on the safe side, get into the habit of asking restaurants to leave MSG out of your food when you order it.

VASOACTIVE AMINES

These substances are found in chocolate and mature red wine, hard cheeses and sour cream, and in a range of other foods: hams such as Parma ham, dry cured sausages such as salami and chorizo, preserved fish such as rollmop herrings and smoked salmon.

Rather than feeling deprived, I suggest looking for alternatives to smoked and preserved foods: fresh cream rather than sour; soft goats' cheese or ripe Brie instead of mature Cheddar; cold cuts of meat such as boiled or baked ham or turkey, fresh poached salmon rather than smoked.

COPPER

Research shows that the metabolism of people who suffer from migraines is slightly different from those who don't suffer, and it seems that foods that are high in copper can cause problems. These include shellfish, fish paste and taramasalata, liver, nuts, chocolate, wheatgerm (found in wholemeal bread and some breakfast cereals) and dried fruits. My advice is to limit your consumption of these foods rather than avoiding them altogether.

Some foods, particularly citrus fruits such as oranges, grapefruit, lemons and limes, cause the body to absorb more copper. They can therefore aggravate your tendency to have a migraine. Try to avoid having a lot of them, especially on an empty stomach; a glass of fresh orange juice in the morning is a habit best avoided. Choose other fruits such as papaya, mango, banana, kiwi fruit.

TYRAMINE

Tyramine is a substance that releases a hormone called noradrenaline, which causes a rise in blood pressure and can lead to headaches. Tyramine is found in cheese, game, meat extracts, and in wine and low alcohol beers and lagers, which is why some people find a glass of red wine with a chunk of cheese causes the most horrendous headache.

ADDITIVES

Besides monosodium glutamate, mentioned above, other additives can trigger headaches. The worst culprits seem to be nitrites, traditional preservatives in meat products. Nitrites are found in most fresh and preserved meat products, including sausages, salami, chorizo, hot dogs, pastrami, mortadella and corned beef. Most of these are also very high in fat, so they should not be a regular feature of any healthy eating plan. In terms of avoiding headaches, stick to unadulterated meats. Include as many organic foods as possible in your diet, as the fewer additives, preservatives and pesticides your body has to deal with, the less likely you are to suffer either headaches or migraines.

Aspartame, an artificial sweetener, can trigger headaches and migraines in some people. It is usually found in diet drinks and sweets as it provides a sweet taste with very few calories. Avoiding these items can only be good for your body, as they are frequently high in additives and preservatives.

CAFFEINE

Caffeine is one of the commonest trigger substances for people with sensitive heads. Coffee is the obvious culprit here, though caffeine is also present in tea. Caffeine intake in general should be no more than three cups a day and this should be significantly reduced if coffee affects you adversely. Interestingly, there is less caffeine in espresso (and hence real cappuccino) than in filter coffee, as the water is forced more quickly though the grains. If you find that coffee does seem to trigger your migraines, save your coffee drinking for special times and make a treat of it.

Note that if you decide to cut caffeine out of your diet entirely, you may initially suffer from a withdrawal headache. This may develop after about eighteen hours without your usual caffeine fix. Stick with the abstention (drinking plenty of plain water will help) and the headaches should disappear after twenty six to thirty six hours. You might prefer to lower your caffeine dependence, cup by cup, over a few days. I promise you your body will thank you for it, and think of all the other delicious drinks you can enjoy: herbal teas such as jasmine and peppermint; ginger and orange blossom teas; fresh fruit punches and shakes (see page 342).

ALCOHOL

Ask the majority of headache and migraine sufferers which drinks they can and cannot tolerate and the majority will either say red wine or acidic white wines, including champagne. Sadly some cannot tolerate any alcohol as they find that its dehydrating action is what causes the headache.

There is a huge range of individual components (and additives) in beers and wines; some people's bodies react violently to one or more of these. Tyramine (see previous page) is one such substance. Recent research suggests that some flavonoids can also cause migraine and headaches. Red wine has more flavonoids than white and it is worth experimenting with white wines if you find red wine a problem. Many white wines, such as 'big' Chardonnays and New World mature Semillons, can hold their own when paired with traditional 'red wine' foods.

Some red wines these days are made using a substance called PVPP. This reduces the tannin levels to produce a drinkable wine at a greatly accelerated rate. It also reduces the quantity of flavonoids, which means that headache sufferers may be less affected by wines made using this process.

Some scientists have put forward the theory that certain wines containing large amounts of free histamines can cause an allergic reaction which culminates in a headache or migraine. Italian wines have been highlighted as being rich in free histamines, although the Italian wine industry denies this.

As you will now appreciate, it is not just the red or white issue that affects your body. If you really want to enjoy wine or other alcoholic drinks I suggest that you explore a range of grape varieties and countries of origin and keep a food, drink and symptom diary (see page 85), recording as much detail about the wine as possible. Drink plenty of water to reduce the dehydrating effects of the alcohol. Avoid drinking on an empty stomach, as this can cause a drop in blood sugar and hence a headache.

LACTOSE

Lactose (the type of sugar found in milk) is one of the less common trigger ingredients, but it can cause severe headaches in some people. In many cases, all that needs to be done is to avoid having too many foods that are particularly high in lactose: milk, cream, butter, yoghurt, cheese, ice cream. If you suspect that these foods make your headaches worse I suggest that you read the chapter on Managing allergies, to find out how you can reduce your lactose intake without compromising your calcium status.

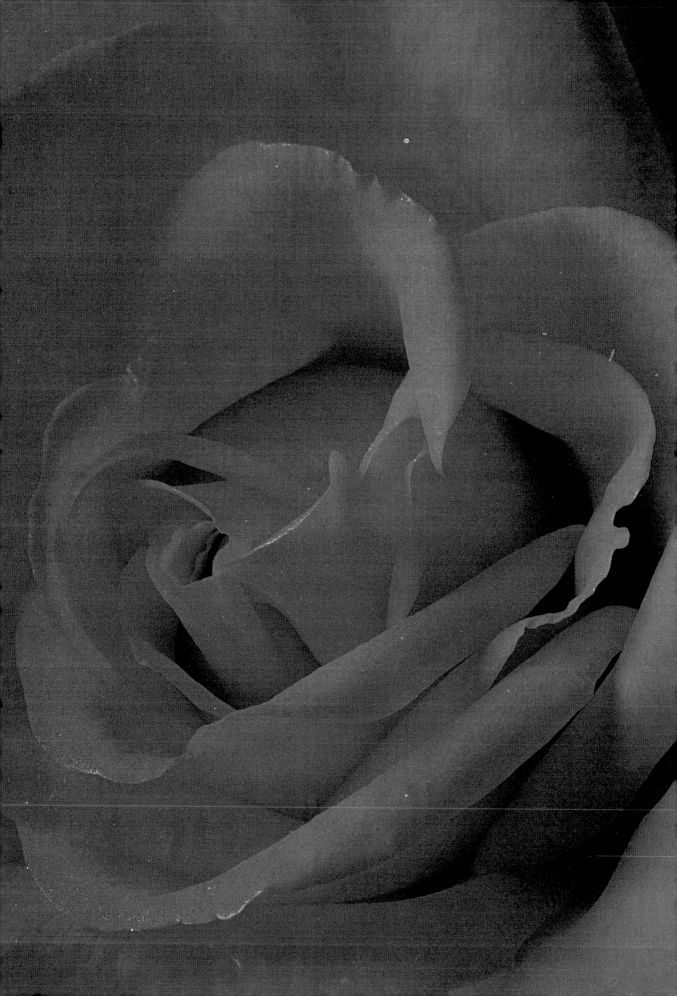

Managing allergies

Allergy in one form or another affects at least forty per cent of the population at some point in their lives, and more and more potential allergens are emerging every day. Allergies take numerous guises. They may affect the respiratory system and cause asthma, which is reported to affect three million people in the UK – one in seven children carries an inhaler. Our guts can react silently or violently to allergens in our food, causing bloating, vomiting, diarrhoea, or anaphylactic shock, which can be fatal. The number of cases of people suffering severe reactions (for example from nut allergy) is small compared to the number of people whose bodies do not tolerate wheat, dairy products, eggs and other foods. Most people experience discomfort and other symptoms, which, while inconvenient, are not life-threatening. Simply by avoiding the offending foodstuffs they are able to feel perfectly well. This chapter will take you through the jungle of how to reduce the risk of developing a food allergy, how to identify an allergy or intolerance and how to adjust your diet accordingly.

What are allergies and intolerances?
Although there is a physiological difference in the body's response to allergies and intolerances, the symptoms are similar. The immune system is designed to rid the body of bacteria, viruses, microscopic parasites, cancer cells – anything that has no business being inside us. Allergies and intolerances are what happens when the system becomes oversensitive to certain foreign substances. Usually allergies are more severe than intolerances, but both can be measured by looking at symptoms and reactions within the blood. In this chapter I shall group them in terms of their treatment, referring to them both as food sensitivities.

If you suffer from symptoms such as diarrhoea, constipation, bloating of the stomach, eczema or other skin conditions and rashes, migraine, irritability or extreme tiredness, you may well have a food sensitivity. Other less common symptoms include asthma, recurrent ear infections, and swelling of the lips, mouth and tongue. Seek immediate attention in cases of swelling of the throat, as this can cause breathing difficulties. If you have any of the above symptoms it is worth exploring your food intake, to see if any relief can be gained. With all these symptoms, I suggest that you also consult your doctor to rule out any non-food cause.

Sometimes aversions or cravings are signs of food sensitivity. For instance some people who don't like milky products are diagnosed as being sensitive to lactose (found in milky foods). Others find the opposite: they crave the thing to which they are sensitive. I therefore look for any out-of-the-ordinary food likes or dislikes. Your body's reaction to an unwanted food has three likely causes:

- The release of histamine. This substance is overproduced by the body when it is faced with a food which is rich in an unwanted substance. A severe histamine reaction normally occurs with food allergies, rather than intolerances. Shellfish is a well known example; some people cannot eat certain types of shellfish without being violently sick.
- An enzyme defect. This is when the body does not produce sufficient enzymes, substances that break down various foodstuffs, such as lactose, the sugar found in dairy products. The symptoms are sickness, diarrhoea and gut pain. Some people completely lack a particular enzyme, whereas others just seem to have a small amount of the enzyme. This can account for why some are able to eat a small amount of the offending food on occasions.
- Irritant effect. The gut can become irritated by certain foods, such as spices or monosodium glutamate (MSG).

Our digestive system undergoes natural changes throughout our lives. When we are born it is immature and, at first, cannot handle solid food. Elderly people may find that their body becomes poorer at dealing with certain foods. In addition, a food sensitivity can occur at any age as the result of an accumulation of foods or toxins, which the body rejects once a specific threshold is reached. For other people, hormonal changes can drastically affect the bowel. These may be natural hormonal changes that are most pronounced during puberty and later middle age, or artificially introduced, for example in women taking a contraceptive pill or hormone replacement therapy. In the latter cases it is worth asking your doctor to change your prescription; a simple adjustment of the hormones sometimes does the trick.

Some people have a mild food sensitivity and can eat a small amount of the offending item without experiencing any symptoms, whereas others with an extreme sensitivity need to remove the offending item completely from their diet in order to avoid serious symptoms. While a sensitivity should be treated seriously, becoming obsessive and neurotic about what you eat will not help you.

Genuine food allergies and intolerances can make life difficult. You need to see a reputable health professional who can make an accurate diagnosis and offer constructive advice as to how to eat healthily and how to avoid the potential allergens. I see far too many people who have either received an incorrect diagnosis, or have diagnosed themselves and are eating very unbalanced diets. I also see children whose parents are so worried that they might have or develop a food allergy that they restrict their child's diet to such an extent that the child becomes malnourished and unhealthy.

Why are more people suffering from allergies and intolerances?
Our grandparents didn't seem to have them, so what has changed? It may be that we are increasingly aware of food allergies and their symptoms, so that more people are receiving a correct diagnosis for symptoms that in the past would have been missed or not taken seriously. Alarmingly, more people are diagnosing themselves as having an allergy when they don't – they are either suffering from another medical condition that should be treated differently or they have a psychological problem that manifests itself as symptoms that seem to respond to changes in the diet.

However, it is undoubtedly true that food allergies and intolerances are increasing, for a number of reasons:

- We are eating fewer fresh foods and more foods that have been highly processed and contain additives, preservatives and pesticide and other chemical residues from the production process. Our bodies aren't equipped to deal with these high levels of foreign substances.
- We push our bodies to work and play hard, stress is rife and the gut takes the brunt of the strain.
- We are not giving our bodies enough time to recover from illnesses. In the past we would have taken to our bed and allowed our body to recover in its own time. Now we expect our body to get better immediately and bombard it with drugs.
- Antibiotics interfere with the natural balance of flora in the gut. Some people believe that the use of antibiotics in the production of meat and other livestock and vegetables can also cause the gut to become 'florally unbalanced'.
- We are not feeding our bodies the correct nutrients. People have lost confidence in their ability to choose wholesome unprocessed food, and are skipping meals.

Food allergies and intolerances are one of the most common ways the body exhibits a very simple message: that it cannot cope with the stress and strain of modern living. However, dietary changes can make a great deal of difference.

How to avoid developing a food allergy or intolerance
One of the major worries parents have with their children is how to reduce the likelihood of their developing a food allergy. Allergies and intolerances are bad enough for adults, who can understand why they are avoiding something and how to avoid it, let alone for children, who want to eat what everyone else eats. Luckily there are positive steps you can take.

The most sensitive time for the digestive system is the first eighteen months of life, as this is when the gut is not particularly well developed and the immune system can have problems dealing with allergens. Babies who develop allergies early in life often grow out of them once their bodies become mature enough to cope, which is usually around two years of age.

There is a great deal of research to show that breastfeeding helps to reduce the risk of developing a food allergy, as the baby's immature immune system is much more likely to react favourably to breast milk than cows' milk protein. This is particularly true in families with a strong history of food allergies, rhinitis, asthma or eczema. When your baby is relying on breast milk, you shouldn't restrict your own diet unless your baby has symptoms such as profuse diarrhoea, vomiting, rashes or swelling of the eyes or lips or you have a family history of allergies to food. If you notice any symptoms, the way to react is to remove the most common food allergens one by one from your diet for a week or two, to see if things improve.

Because the gut is so sensitive, it is best not to rush the weaning process. Start your child on solid food between the ages of four and six months, introducing common allergens one at a time, in small amounts. The most common food triggers are cows' milk and dairy products, eggs, fish (especially shellfish), nuts, foods containing gluten, and some fruits.

- It is best to continue to breastfeed or use a modified infant formula until your child is one year old, or at least until the baby is taking drinks from a cup. Whole fat pasteurized cows' milk, provided it is fresh and has been kept in a refrigerator, can be given occasionally, for instance used in mashed potatoes, after your child is six months old. Yoghurts and cheese can also be introduced after the age of six months, but try them a little at a time to see whether the child reacts adversely.

  However, if you or your partner has a history of asthma, eczema or hay fever it is best to discuss the introduction of cows' milk with your doctor or a dietitian specializing in this field; they may advise you to use an alternative such as goats' milk or soya milk. Some children are sensitive to these milks also; seek the advice of a professional.

  Some questions have been raised over the level of pasteurization that milk receives. If you want to be extra careful, I suggest that you boil the milk and let it cool before giving it to your child.

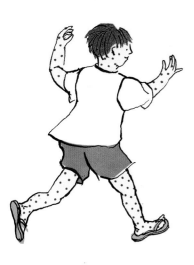

- Avoid giving egg whites before the age of one year. Cooked egg yolks may be given once your baby is stabilized on a mixed diet at the age of eight or nine months.

- Fish are best introduced after the age of eight months, a little bit at a time. It is best to avoid shellfish for the first couple of years.

- Nuts in any form, whether ground or as peanut butter, should be avoided for the first eight months. Remember that older children can easily choke on whole nuts.

  Although some manufacturers are beginning to label foods containing nuts, many products are not labelled. Mothers can be alarmed to find that the most obscure things can contain the potential allergen. For example, the cream they rub on their nipples when they are sore from breastfeeding can contain peanut oil, as do several brands of formula milk.

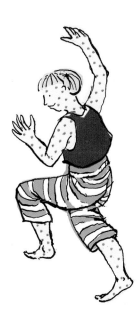

New research seems to show a correlation between pregnancy and nut allergies: peanut oil based creams and nuts consumed during pregnancy are thought to increase the risk of nut allergies in children. It is thought that this applies particularly in families where allergies are rife. I don't want you to think 'Oh no, not another thing I can't eat', but if allergies concern you, see your doctor.

- If you have a family history of gluten sensitivity, it is best to avoid all forms of gluten until your baby is at least six months old. As a safeguard I normally suggest that ALL babies avoid gluten for the first six months.

  Gluten is found in products containing wheat, rye, barley and oats. Alternatives include: rice, millet and potato flours, which are useful in thickening sauces and making bread and cakes; corn; buckwheat and rice noodles. Read the labels on ready-made baby foods as many contain gluten.

- Some babies have an adverse reaction to berry and citrus fruits such as strawberries, raspberries, oranges and tangerines. Since these fruits are rich in vitamin C, an essential growth and development vitamin, it is important to find another source in fruits such as blackcurrants, kiwis and rosehips (in the form of rosehip juice). Pears, apples, peaches, apricots, especially stewed or poached, puréed and mixed with yoghurt, are easy fruits to feed your child. Look at your consumption of the suspect fruits, as it may be that you are passing on antigens that upset your baby.

Identifying food sensitivities

I cannot stress enough the importance of keeping a detailed food diary (see page 85). Noting everything that you or your child eats, including details of ingredients of ready-made foods, will enable you to start deciphering the most likely causes of your symptoms. Write down all symptoms such as bloating, skin condition, mood swings, energy levels. I tell my patients to imagine I am a parrot on their shoulder taking notes of everything that is happening in their body and mind.

Some people find that their bodies react differently at different times of the month. Women can experience bloating and skin rashes during their premenstrual week and have absolutely no problems during the rest of the month. Extreme work pressures can bring out symptoms which stay away when people are relaxed at home. If your symptoms seem to come and go, keep the diary going for a few weeks, so that you can pick up patterns over a wide spectrum of situations.

If you are keeping a diary for a child, try to get hold of information about what they eat outside the home as well as what you are feeding them. You should also try to keep secret the fact that you are recording their behaviour symptoms.

A useful first step would be to analyze your diet to make sure it is well balanced and contains all the nutrients your body needs (see the section beginning on page 25). A number of symptoms occur for no other reason than that there is something not quite right about your eating habits or general life-style: are you drinking plenty of water and eating at least five portions of fresh fruits and vegetables a day, or do you regularly skip meals, drink too much tea or coffee, or rely on sweet snacks? A healthy lifestyle is a lot easier to manage than an exclusion diet of any sort.

If you are reasonably happy with your diet and suspect that a particular item may be causing problems, try removing the item from your diet for one or two weeks. You will need to check labels carefully if you suspect you are allergic to an additive. If your symptoms disappear, you can probably assume that you have a sensitivity related to this item. If they persist, seek professional advice before proceeding any further, as once you start removing more than one food, things can become complicated.

Give your body a chance to improve; a week or two is usually the sort of period you should allow. A day or two won't normally give you a realistic result, although some people notice dramatic results in a few hours.

Treating food sensitivities
Once you have found that you are sensitive to a particular food, you need to make sure that your body is not going to become malnourished by removing it. Psychologically you also need to ensure that you are not going to feel deprived. Find other foods that provide the same or similar beneficial nutrients without the offending ingredients. Also, seek the advice of a dietitian who will check whether you require any vitamin or mineral supplements. This is especially important with growing children.

By far the most common food sensitivities I see are: cows' milk protein and lactose; egg; wheat and gluten; additives. Do not experiment with food allergens if your symptoms are very severe, and if your child has an allergy, don't tackle it alone. Always seek professional advice.

EATING OUT
Eating out can be difficult for people with food sensitivities, as it is hard to know what has gone into the food. Remember that simple food such as fish, good quality meat, pasta, rice and unadulterated food is less likely to contain hidden ingredients. Try to choose restaurants where the food is prepared fresh, and not somewhere where you can have your meal in two minutes: the likelihood is that the food in fast-food restaurants has a lot of additives and preservatives. In restaurants never be afraid to ask how things are cooked and tell them that you are allergic to something. You could even ask the chef to make a sauce without cream, for instance, if you are milk sensitive. Most good restaurants will take your requests seriously.

Milk sensitivity

There are two main types of milk sensitivity: cows' milk protein and lactose sensitivity. Both cause symptoms such as bloating, diarrhoea, sickness, stomach and abdominal cramps, headaches, and can aggravate skin complaints such as eczema. Some scientists believe that half of the world's population is unable to tolerate cows' milk. Children are commonly lactose sensitive until their gut becomes more mature, usually around two years of age.

Lactose sensitivity is mainly due to a deficiency in the body's production of lactase, the enzyme that digests lactose, the sugar found in all milk products, particularly cows', sheep's and goats' milk. Without sufficient lactase, lactose cannot be broken down and absorbed by the body, and therefore there is a build-up of undigested lactose in the gut.

If you are lactose sensitive, you need to avoid all forms of milk, other than soya milk. This includes cream, butter, yoghurt, cheese, skimmed milk powder and products containing any of the above as well as lactose, casein and whey, which might be present in baked and processed products such as biscuits and cakes. You need to look out for foods containing monosodium glutamate (sometimes labelled as MSG or 621), as these frequently contain lactose.

Cows' milk protein sensitivity is slightly less common than lactose sensitivity, but it can occur at any age. In this case the sensitivity is not due to an enzyme deficiency, but the body is unable to tolerate any form of cows' milk. However, it may be able to tolerate sheep's or goats' milk and products made from them, such as yoghurt and of course the many delicious sheep's and goats' milk cheeses.

Many food manufacturers refer to cows' milk protein and lactose-free products as 'milk-free'. All products marked 'milk-free' should be suitable for both lactose and cows' milk protein sensitive people.

Always consult a doctor or dietitian if you suspect that your child is lactose sensitive, as it is vital that you do not deprive their body of essential nutrients such as calcium and protein once you remove milk and milk products from the diet. The adult body also needs calcium throughout life, and there are a number of ways to obtain it in a varied and balanced diet.

Soya milk and soya products such as margarine, cheese and yoghurt are often calcium-enriched. Other calcium-containing foods include oily fish such as sardines, anchovies, mackerel, pilchards; green leafy vegetables such as spinach and broccoli; sesame seeds and tahini (sesame seed paste, used to make hummus), almonds and dried apricots. See page 42 for more information on calcium sources. However, these foods, especially the green leafy vegetables, contain 'salts' that stop the body from absorbing the calcium efficiently. This means that you need to eat a lot of them to meet your daily requirement for calcium. See them as an added extra, not an equivalent – you will probably need to take a calcium supplement. It is vital that you don't choose calcium lactate as this is obtained from lactose. There are plenty of other types, such as calcium oxalate, so ask your dietitian or pharmacist.

Many cheeses contain only a trace of lactose, which makes them manageable for adults with mild lactose intolerance. You may like to include some of these in your diet to see whether your body reacts adversely. Lower lactose cheeses include Brie, Camembert, Edam, Gouda, soya cheese and vegetarian Cheddar.

Egg sensitivity

Egg sensitivity is slightly less common than milk sensitivities, but it is more often associated with severe symptoms. Some people suffer from unpleasant bouts of diarrhoea, others from acute and chronic episodes of constipation and stomach cramps. Egg sensitivity can also aggravate eczema, cause mood swings, and disturb sleep.

If you suspect that you have an egg sensitivity, you need to avoid eggs, foods containing whole egg, egg yolk, albumin, egg lecithin and dried egg. Some people may be sensitive to either egg yolk or egg white, but not both. People with mild sensitivity may find they can tolerate small amounts of egg, or can tolerate cooked eggs. I suggest that you avoid all eggs for your trial period, and then if you conclude that there is an intolerance, re-introduce yolks or whites only and see what happens.

Avoiding egg and its derivatives is relatively straightforward as long as you steer clear of store-bought biscuits, cakes, meringues, mayonnaise, egg pasta and other manufactured foods unless they are free of the offending ingredients. If in doubt, check the label. This doesn't mean that cakes and biscuits are completely out of bounds: but you will have to look quite hard for suppliers and recipes. Apple flapjacks (page 331) are one idea for an easy egg-free biscuit; instead of apple purée you could use chopped dried apricots, figs or raisins. You can also enjoy shortbread and other biscuits, fruit desserts, pies and tarts, as long as the pastry is not made with egg. I wouldn't recommend the egg replacers on the market, as the result is less than ideal.

Wheat and gluten sensitivity

These sensitivities are very common, and the severity and symptoms vary greatly. Some people simply feel that by avoiding the ingredient as much as possible they feel more energized, less bloated, or have less pain with rheumatoid arthritis. Others need to avoid offending foods completely or risk severe pain, diarrhoea, or internal bleeding, symptoms often associated with coeliac disease (see page 182). The first step in managing a wheat or gluten intolerance is to establish whether your sensitivity is to wheat or gluten. Wheat is a grain, whereas gluten is the protein found in wheat and other grains: oats, rye and barley. If you are sensitive to wheat, you may be able to eat oats, rye and barley. If gluten is the offender, you must avoid all sources of gluten.

If you are sensitive to gluten, you need to avoid wheat, barley, oats and rye grains and products containing them. You additionally have to avoid products containing flour, starch, food starch, edible starch or modified starch, unless the

**Five ideas for
gluten-free breakfasts**

- *Rice pudding, warm, with
honey and sliced banana or
dried fruits*
- *Rice pudding, cold, with
hot stewed plums*
- *Cornflakes with yoghurt
and sliced peaches*
- *Rice cakes with sliced
tomatoes and Parma ham*
- *Gluten-free bread (see
recipes, page 329), toasted,
with avocado, lemon juice
and cracked black pepper*

label clearly states that it is gluten-free. In practice this means avoiding bread, crackers, cakes, biscuits, pasta, sauces containing flour and stuffings made with bread. You need to look at labels to see whether bread is used as a 'filler': sausages, salamis, pâtés and other meat products commonly fall into this group. Mustard powder, white pepper, gravy thickening, stock cubes and pickles sometimes contain gluten. Soy sauce usually contains wheat, but tamari, the Japanese naturally brewed soy sauce, does not. Many baby foods and infant formulas contain gluten. The Coeliac Society (address on page 352) produces a list of products that are free from gluten.

The above sounds a long and forbidding list, but think positive. Rice and potatoes are gluten-free, and rice and potato flours can be used in cooking; you can also use soya flour, buckwheat flour and cornflour. Rice cakes can be an alternative snack to bread and crackers. Instead of pasta, base meals on rice and potatoes; think of risotto, paella, Chinese and Thai rice and rice noodle dishes, stuffed jacket potatoes, fishcakes, potato gratins, hot pots and potato bakes (see recipes, page 327). You might like to look at some Italian cookbooks, as there are a number of traditional Italian cakes made with rice, cornmeal (polenta) or chestnut flour, available from Italian delicatessens. If you are allergic to wheat but not gluten you will be able to use oats and rye: make oaty crumble toppings, oat muffins (page 328), oatcake or rye bread (pumpernickel) snacks.

Try not to see wheat or gluten allergy as a handicap. Look for ways round it and think of all the things you can eat that will not make you ill. This is especially important for children; instead of making them feel isolated and different from their friends, look for treats that they can all eat.

GLUTEN-FREE SAUCES

You can use potato flour as a direct replacement for the wheat flour in a white or béchamel sauce. Potato flour is a little more inclined to thicken in lumps if you stop stirring or have the heat too high. I use an electric hand blender in the saucepan as I heat the sauce gently.

Sauces can also be thickened at the last minute by whisking in a little arrowroot dissolved in about 2 tablespoons of water.

Don't forget the reduction method for making sauces. Good quality stock, or stock and wine, or a sweet juice such as orange, apple or strawberry, can be left to simmer gently in an uncovered saucepan until it reduces down to a thick syrupy consistency. The flavours are then concentrated in the syrup. If you like you can whisk in a little more wine, some fresh cream or yoghurt, just before serving. Fish stock reduces beautifully, and is delicious if you add cream and some chopped fresh herbs such as dill, parsley or coriander.

GLUTEN-FREE BREAD

Be aware of the difference between breads labelled 'yeast-free' and 'gluten-free'. Yeast-free breads may contain wheat or gluten. Gluten-free bread doesn't contain the supportive characteristics of gluten, which means that it tends to be heavy and dense. I think that the shop-bought versions are nowhere near as nice as homemade. Try making your own (see pages 328–9); the recipes are not difficult, especially if you have a food processor or blender. It's best eaten fresh and still warm from the oven, but is also delicious toasted, and it freezes well.

The secret to making delicious gluten-free bread is to use a wide variety of sources of starch. Millet, sorghum and buckwheat flours are good for baking, especially when combined with rice or grain flour. Sweet chestnut flour is one of my favourites for making a light, soft, sweet bread. Apple, banana or tofu, beaten to a purée, help to make the bread lovely and smooth-textured. The lack of gluten prevents the carbon dioxide produced by the yeast in normal bread from being retained in the usual way; instead the use of bicarbonate of soda and tartaric acid helps the loaf rise. Sprinkling seeds such as pumpkin, sesame and poppy seeds on top of the breads gives a crunchy variation in texture.

DRINKS

Beers are gluten free as long as they are not home-brewed or cloudy beers. Wines and spirits do not contain any gluten.

Malted milk drinks, milk shakes and milk drinks from vending machines usually contain gluten. If it is modified starch (used to thicken milk drinks), some people can tolerate this small amount – it depends on the severity of the allergy.

COELIAC DISEASE

A severe intolerance to gluten is known as coeliac disease. This condition can be diagnosed only by a surgeon taking a small 'nip' of the lining of the intestine and studying it under a microscope. If coeliacs eat gluten, their gut becomes inflamed, which results in severe pain, diarrhoea and in some cases severe malabsorption problems. Babies double up with pain and in extreme cases the malabsorption causes growth retardation.

The good news is that once you remove gluten from the diet, the gut frequently returns to normal. It is generally necessary to avoid all forms of gluten for life, but some people may be able to tolerate some oat or rye-based products. The gluten content of these is lower than wheat, but you should ask for professional guidance before you experiment. In some cases the reaction can be so severe that the body goes into shock. It is especially important to remember this when dealing with young children with coeliac disease. The nutritional management of coeliac disease is the same as for gluten intolerance, you just have to be that bit more careful to avoid gluten.

Additive sensitivity

There are thousands of different additives in foods. As a fast-track society which imports food from all over the world we couldn't survive without some of them. However, in today's overprocessed food world, when packets and tins take up far more supermarket space than fresh foods, our exposure to additives is much greater than the body can reasonably be expected to tolerate. Nobody benefits from eating additive-filled foods, but some people experience severe reactions to food additives. Symptoms include headaches, rashes and other skin complaints, mood swings and depression.

The most common culprits are the antimicrobial preservatives sulphur dioxide and its related salts, or sulphites (E220–E227), yellow azo dyes (tartrazine/E102, Yellow 2G/E107, Sunset yellow/E110) and the flavour enhancer monosodium glutamate (621). All these additives have to be declared on food labels either in their true name or as an E number.

In the US sulphites have been banned for use on fruits and vegetables, but that is not yet the case in Europe. If you suspect that you have a sulphite sensitivity, look at the following list of foods, as they frequently contain sulphites:
• Wines, cider and beer
• Canned and bottled soft drinks
• Dried potatoes, including packet mashed potato, crisps and savoury snacks. French fries used in the catering trade have usually been dipped in metabisulphite solution.
• Dried fruits and vegetables. Most dried fruits are treated with sulphur dioxide; this does not have to be declared on the label. However, dried fruit that has not been treated will usually be labelled unsulphured, so hunt these out.
• Fruit salad, fruit juices, glacé cherries
• Canned soups and sauces, ready made meals, sausages
• Frozen prawns
• Cod may be treated with sulphites to bleach and preserve it.

Remember, the simpler and fresher you keep your diet and the less you rely on processed foods, the fewer additives you will consume. Whenever you remove items from your diet you need to make sure you are still eating healthily and getting all the nutrients you need, but where it is an additive you are investigating, this is relatively easy; you just need to focus on fresh, unprocessed foods. For example, instead of a ready-made chicken dish in a sauce full of additives and preservatives, look at the simple recipes on page 325; or just grill chicken and serve it with one of the sauces or dressings on pages 312–313.

Antibiotics
Both long and short courses of antibiotics can render the gut temporarily or permanently intolerant to a particular food. Many people cannot tolerate milk, lactose, wheat or gluten during or immediately after taking a course of antibiotics. This sometimes results in a permanent food sensitivity, but more commonly, if you allow your body a couple of weeks to recover from the infection and the antibiotics, you should find you can start to reintroduce these foods in small amounts and your gut will tolerate them.

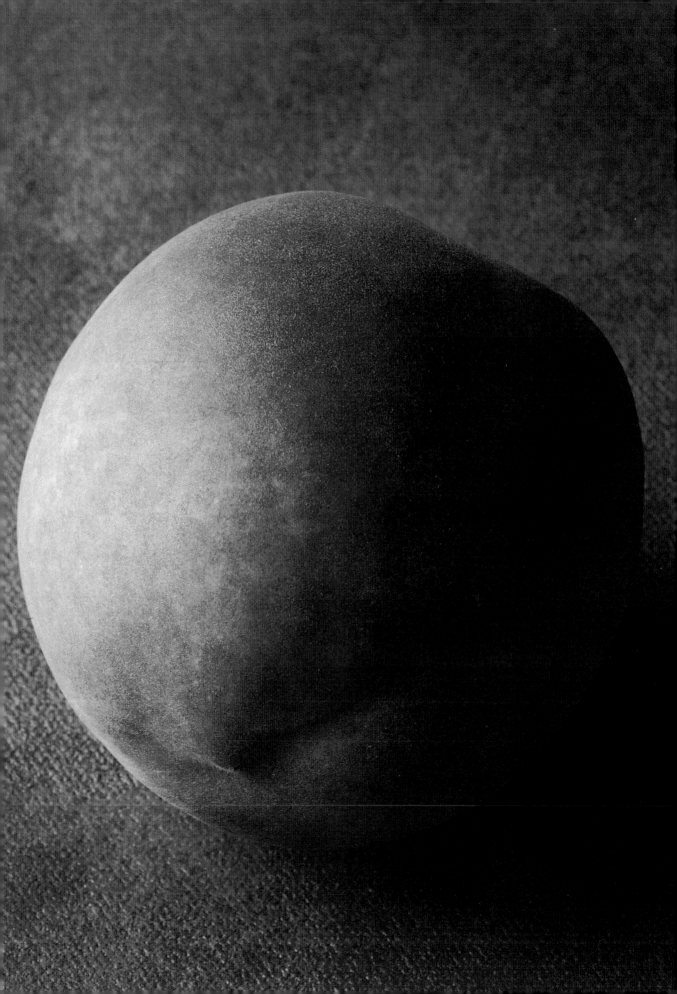

Helping hyperactive children

Several terms are used when discussing children who literally 'can't sit still': hyperactivity, hyperkinesis, hyperkinetic disorder, overactivity, and Attention Deficit Disorder. The official name for the problem, hyperactive child syndrome, was described by *The British Medical Journal* in 1975 as: 'a chronic level of motor activity relative to the age of the child, occurring mainly in boys between one and sixteen years, but characteristically around six years, accompanied by short attention span, impulsive behaviour or explosive outbursts causing substantial complaints at home or in school.' Although hyperactivity is challenging to parents, phenomenal improvements in behaviour can be achieved by changing a child's diet.

Symptoms and causes

Boys are more frequently diagnosed as being hyperactive than girls, but this may be due to the fact that girls usually don't exhibit such extreme symptoms. Boys are louder, whereas girls more commonly suffer from mood changes, lack of attention and in some cases speech disorders. Most children aren't diagnosed until they are a few years old, but it is worth bearing in mind that hyperactive babies often suffer from colic and need very little sleep. They may also be very restless, fidgety and perpetually rock in their cot. Children can have poor control and coordination and are generally clumsy, and they leave a trail of destruction behind them. Other common symptoms include learning, social and behavioural problems, aggression, poor eating and sleeping habits and temper tantrums. Some hyperactive children also suffer from headaches, asthma or hay fever.

One of the problems with the diagnosis of hyperactivity is that children have such different personalities, and adults' perception of their behaviour differs. A boisterous child may appear lovable and full of beans to one adult, while to another, the same child seems like a hyperactive pain in the backside. It may also be the case that a child 'acts up' for more attention in certain circumstances, for example when a younger sibling is in the room. Try keeping a record of your child's behaviour, noting the other people present and whether the child has a spurt of energy about half an hour after a sweet drink or snack (which is perfectly normal). Some people grow into adults before they are diagnosed, so mood swings and behaviour problems can be due to hyperactivity even in your later years.

The cause of hyperactivity is still unknown. It was once thought to be caused by brain damage, but research does not support this theory. What we do know is that it is genetically determined, in other words it is passed down from parent to child. It is also known that certain foods can influence hyperactivity, either by causing an allergic reaction or because an enzyme deficiency in the child's digestive system means that certain compounds found in foods/food additives cannot be broken down by the body; instead they become toxic and cause behaviour problems.

Before you start treating your child you should seek professional advice to ascertain whether he or she is hyperactive or is suffering from another type of psychological or sociological problem.

Food and hyperactivity
Once your child has been diagnosed as hyperactive, the treatment frequently involves a modified diet, possibly in conjunction with drug and/or behavioural therapy. It is better to help your child by changing their eating habits than to put them on medication or simply to ignore the potential healing effect of food.

When treating hyperactivity with dietary changes, there is a fine balance between controlling your child's diet while at the same time making the dietary changes appear normal. If you overplay the message that their food is being controlled, children may start to use the situation to their advantage.

Managing your child's diet
The first stage in managing hyperactivity is to keep a diary of everything your child eats and drinks, how they are behaving, and whether they suffer from any physical symptoms such as diarrhoea, upset stomach, a blotchy red rash, or colour draining from their face. It is important to make notes and not to rely on your memory. Time-consuming as it is, you need to keep details of food packaging and to question the school about what they eat and drink there. In the long run, it will help everyone if you can be specific about the foods they can eat and the foods they should avoid. See page 85 for notes on keeping a food diary.

The only way to investigate the relationship between certain foods and behaviour is to follow a type of exclusion diet, but this has to be managed in a way that does not isolate your child. It is important to replace excluded foods with something equally delicious and nutritious.

You may find your child is hyperactive even when they are still being bottle or breast fed. Your doctor or dietitian can help you to find more suitable milks and infant formulae. If you are still breastfeeding, you could apply the advice in this chapter to your own food.

The main types of foods linked to hyperactivity in children are food additives and colourings, sugary foods such as sweets and chocolate and, occasionally, particular ingredients such as wheat or dairy products (this is more common in families where there is a history of asthma, eczema or migraine).

ADDITIVES

Additives are chemicals – natural or artificial – added to manufactured foods to make them last longer or taste and look as the food producer thinks people will find most appealing. Not all additives are potentially harmful chemicals; some are vitamins and preservatives that are essential to prevent food poisoning. However, the following additives have been most strongly linked to hyperactivity in children:

- Colourings: E102 Tartrazine; E110 Sunset yellow; E124 Ponceau 4R; E127 Erythrosine
- Preservatives: E210; E219 Benzoic acid and the salts of benzoic acid; E320, E321 Antioxidants BHA and BHT

In most European countries, the majority of additives and preservatives are shown on the label with an E number: this is a code number recognized within the European Union. In the wake of bad publicity about E numbers, food manufacturers sometimes list technical names rather than E numbers. Remember that just because there is not an E number on the label, doesn't mean an additive isn't there. Flavouring additives do not have to be specifically listed on the label. Additives also include processing aids, chemicals used in food manufacture for technical reasons. For example, they are used to stop ingredients sticking to machinery or to help foods chill or freeze quicker. These additives do not have to be listed on the label.

The best way to ensure your child has an additive-free diet is to feed them food that has not been processed by a food manufacturer. Use as much organic produce as possible, to keep chemicals out of your food. Stick to plain fish rather than fish fingers or fish coated in breadcrumbs or batter, lean meat rather than ready-made sausages or burgers. Give your child fresh vegetables and fruits rather than tinned or frozen, unless they are of a reputable make and state on the label that they are free of questionable additives. Buy natural, unflavoured yoghurt and add your own fresh fruit, either cut into tiny pieces or puréed. Instead of ready-made sauces, pickles and salad creams, stick to homemade mayonnaise, dressings and sauces (see recipes on page 312). Keep a stock of homemade sauces in the refrigerator and freezer for occasions when time is short.

SUGAR

Keeping to pure, unprocessed foods is the best way to manage a child's diet, because even foods that can claim to be additive free may be high in sugar, which can also aggravate bad behaviour. Sweet foods, such as chocolate, cakes, biscuits and drinks, send blood sugar levels shooting up, resulting in a rush of energy. If the energy rush can be slowed down, behavioural problems will be less severe.

Some high fibre foods contain a fair amount of sugar, but the fibre inhibits the absorption of sugar into the body. Conversely, foods with smaller amounts of sugar but no fibre will be rapidly absorbed; potentially, these foods are worse

Organization is the trick in managing a child's diet without resorting to 'convenience' foods, full of additives and preservatives. Why not coordinate your child's diet with a healthier lifestyle for the whole family, by arranging a family health day (see page 81)?

for your hyperactive child. Look to the fibre content as well as the sugar content of the food.

With sugar, as with additives, labelling can get a little tricky. Under current legislation it is difficult to check the amount of sugar added to a drink or food because quantities are seldom given. The list of ingredients gives you no idea as to whether the food contains a small amount of sugar, which won't aggravate behaviour much, or – as is the case with a can of cola – as much as seven teaspoons of sugar, which will cause havoc!

You may think that it is easier to stick to products labelled sugar-free, no added sugar or low-sugar, but there is usually a catch. Sugar-free products may contain artificial sweeteners (and quite likely a host of other additives). No added sugar probably means the product is naturally sweet. Low-sugar may simply mean that the food has less sugar than the standard version of the product. There are also many different forms of sugar. Words to look for on a label include sucrose, glucose, dextrose, fructose, glucose syrup, corn syrup and invert sugar. Many parents think that if something contains fructose (fruit sugar), it means it is healthy. Fructose, like any other form of sugar, can aggravate hyperactive behaviour. Unrefined brown sugar and honey can have just as destructive effects on behaviour as refined white sugar.

Fresh or dried fruits, as long as they are free of preservatives and additives, will not have the same effect. This is because the fibre within the cell walls of the fruit slows the absorption of fruit sugar into the body and therefore your child doesn't experience sugar swings, closely linked to behaviour swings.

One of the major problems for parents of hyperactive children is finding suitable puddings. It is all very well to say that fresh fruit is the ideal dessert, but you need to find ways to make it special. In the Taste Good section of this book I have created some versatile, fruit-based desserts that can be enjoyed by the whole family. Even chocolate can be enjoyed, if it is the right sort of chocolate and is eaten as an occasional treat. By the 'right sort' I mean one that is high in cocoa beans and therefore has less sugar. Specialist chocolate companies make chocolate with at least 60% – better still, 85% – cocoa solids.

I do not recommend substituting artificial sweeteners for sugar for a number of reasons. I have seen some hyperactive children behave badly after they have eaten artificially sweetened foods, as it is the sweet taste that sets off the behaviour, through a learned association, rather than a rise in blood sugar level. Children don't need sweet-tasting foods. They should be able to get all the energy and nutrients they need from fruit and from foods that are not naturally sweet (see page 66 for some healthy snack ideas). Some artificial sweeteners can irritate your child's gut and cause diarrhoea.

CAFFEINE AND COLA DRINKS

Another association between food and behaviour lies with caffeine. This chemical is found not only in coffee, but also in tea, cola drinks and chocolate; it affects the pancreas and the body's ability to control sugar levels. Some children go wild when they are given cola drinks, or tea or coffee. Instead, I suggest healthy, fruit-based drinks (see page 342) and plenty of water to maintain steady blood sugar levels.

EATING HABITS

As well as eating the right foods it is important to look at the frequency of eating. Regular small meals help to keep blood sugar levels steady and the digestive system primed to deal with foods efficiently. Encouraging your child to eat breakfast, even if it is as simple as some fruit and yoghurt, is a good start to the day. Fruits and healthy (not-too-sweet, fibre-rich) biscuits, packed in a little box for school break times, reduce the likelihood of them eating something inappropriate when their friends are tucking into snacks.

Taking time to sit at the table and relax at meal times is also very important. Hyperactive children are more sensitive to situations such as the television being on when you are trying to get them to eat their meals.

VITAMIN SUPPLEMENTS

Many vitamin and mineral supplements contain not only a lot of sugar, but also colourings and other additives. My philosophy is that children shouldn't need supplements if they are eating a well balanced diet, which you can achieve with the help of this book. If in doubt, ask your doctor or dietitian for advice.

Further investigations

Sticking to a well balanced, low sugar, low additive diet with lots of fresh fruit and vegetables, fish, meat, eggs and beans, and some bread, pasta and rice for about a month should give you time to note improvements. You will probably be so relieved you will find it easy to continue with the healthy eating regime.

If your child's behaviour is still a problem, it may be related to a specific food such as milk, eggs, wheat or tomatoes, to name but a few likely culprits. At this point I suggest you read the chapter on Managing allergies and experiment with cutting these foods out of the diet completely for no longer than two weeks. If you notice an improvement you should consult your dietitian or doctor to check that your child is receiving adequate nutrients.

Of course, you may find that your child's behaviour is not linked to diet. There are plenty of professionals who can help you cope, so don't struggle alone.

Growing out of it

The good news with hyperactivity is that your child may grow out of it. I usually suggest that you retest the foods after about a year to eighteen months and then at yearly intervals after that. Do this gradually, introducing small quantities, so that if there is a reaction it shouldn't be too severe. Don't tell the child when you are retesting, as some children play up to the situation.

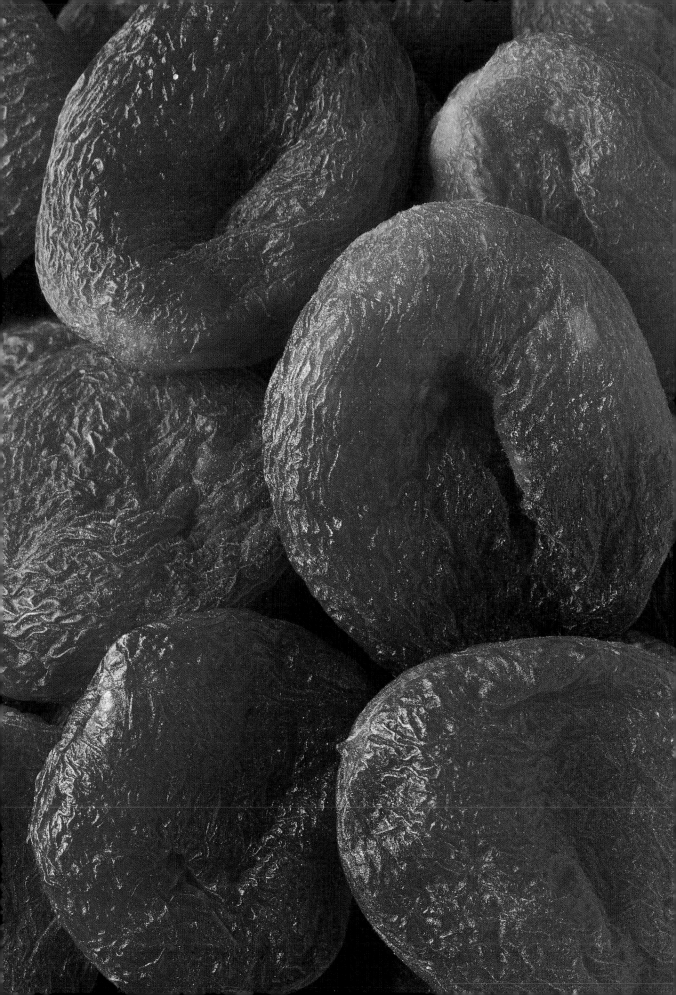

Managing hypoglycaemia

Hypoglycaemia means a low blood sugar level. When your blood sugar drops to a level you are not comfortable with, you can become weak, pale, shaky, moody, nauseous, acutely tired, have problems sleeping, headaches, and your body can break out in a cold sweat. In children hypoglycaemia can occur from birth, especially in small-for-date babies. They can appear pale, lethargic and can be difficult to settle. From toddlerhood onwards low blood sugar can cause hyperactivity and extreme moods, making children very hard to appease. Older hyperactive children may become violent and adults have been known to cause grievous bodily harm while suffering from a hypoglycaemic attack. Hypoglycaemia should be taken seriously, especially as there is so much that can be done to prevent and treat it.

One of the problems in diagnosing hypoglycaemia is that everyone is different. In some people symptoms appear even when their blood sugar level is above the point at which it is technically considered to be low. Your doctor may be unsympathetic, as medically there is apparently nothing wrong, but you still feel terrible and need to know what can be done.

There are two main types of hypoglycaemia: fasting hypoglycaemia, which occurs when you haven't eaten for six or more hours, and reactive hypoglycaemia, which occurs any time from thirty minutes to four hours after a meal. Either type suggests that your blood sugar regulatory system is not functioning effectively. A third scenario, periodic hypoglycaemia, is usually caused by hormonal changes in your body.

What causes hypoglycaemia?
Usually, when you eat a carbohydrate (sugar-containing) food, either in a simple form such as chocolate or ice cream or in a more complex form such as a piece of bread or potato (see page 25 for more information on carbohydrates), the body secretes a hormone called insulin. The insulin enables your body to use the sugar as fuel or store it as fat for later use. If your body secretes too little insulin the blood sugar level remains too high and you become diabetic. Hypoglycaemia is the opposite condition and is thought in many cases to be due to too much insulin being produced, which leads to the blood sugar level dropping too low.

Fasting hypoglycaemia is less common and more serious than reactive hypoglycaemia, as it can be a symptom of uncontrolled diabetes, a tumour of the pancreas (the organ that secretes insulin), liver damage, or starvation such as occurs with anorexia nervosa or cancer. See the chapter on Diabetes for more information.

Hypoglycaemia can also be a symptom of either an underactive or overactive thyroid gland. If you suffer from symptoms such as weakness or dizziness, seek the advice of your doctor. You should also be aware that some medication can precipitate hypoglycaemic symptoms, but when you stop taking the medication the condition usually disappears.

The majority of people who feel that they suffer from hypoglycaemia simply have a problem with the regulation of their blood sugar levels, which can be easily rectified by adopting good eating habits. The results can be astounding. A patient of mine suffered from extreme hypoglycaemic attacks, especially during the morning when he was stressed at work. These attacks caused him to lose his temper to such an extent that colleagues were complaining, and he felt so out of control that he thought he was heading for a nervous breakdown. On changing his diet, the symptoms completely disappeared.

Testing for hypoglycaemia

Many people feel as if they suffer from the symptoms of hypoglycaemia I have described. Although it is relatively easy to test for fasting hypoglycaemia, it is a little more tricky to test for reactive hypoglycaemia. The most common test used is the Glucose Tolerance Test (GTT). This entails taking a very sugary drink and testing the blood sugar levels at regular intervals, to find out whether your body reacts appropriately to the rise in sugar. If your sugar level behaves abnormally, your doctor may diagnose fasting hypoglycaemia, in which case other tests will probably be arranged to determine the cause. Alternatively, your doctor may tell you that although you don't suffer from fasting hypoglycaemia, your blood sugar level pattern indicates that you have a sensitivity to sugar, which causes your body to overreact to sugary foods. If there is no evidence of an abnormality, your problem could be periodic, or occasional, hypoglycaemia (page 195). Whichever situation you are in, you can do a great deal to eliminate the symptoms.

Eating to avoid and treat hypoglycaemia

The nutritional principles for managing hypoglycaemia are focused on keeping your sugar level as constant as possible. In people who don't have an abnormal GTT it is often the dramatic fluctuations – the rapid rises and falls in sugar level – that cause them to feel unwell, rather than the absolute sugar level.

EAT A WELL BALANCED DIET
The first and foremost guideline is to base your eating plan on fresh vegetables, fruits, wholegrain cereals, lean proteins, dairy foods, small amounts of fat and plenty of water. See the section on Understanding your nutritional needs. The best way to check whether your diet is well balanced is to keep a food diary (see

page 85); people are often astounded by the difference between what they think they eat and the facts that face them when they see it written down. Keep a note of your symptoms, so that any patterns and trigger foods can be identified.

EAT SMALL MEALS, OFTEN

Eating regularly helps stabilize your blood sugar levels. Try not to leave more than three or four hours between meals or snacks. This eating pattern serves two purposes: it prevents your blood sugar from dropping too low, and it helps you refrain from overeating at meal times, which could cause your body to become overloaded with various sugar-containing foods.

The majority of people I see find that they feel a lot better if they have five or six snacks, rather than two or three large meals a day. Some patients then worry about their weight increasing. You shouldn't put on weight if the total amount of food you consume throughout the day is not greater than you would consume in three normal meals. For instance, save your dessert until two or three hours later.

Of course, it is also important that the snacks you choose are neither high in fat nor in sugar. I have suggested some healthy snacks on page 66.

KEEP HEALTHY SNACKS CLOSE AT HAND

You can run into problems if you end up having to dash or stagger around looking for good snacks or leave yourself hungry for too long. Fresh and dried fruits and wholegrain biscuits can easily be kept in your bag or at work.

AVOID HAVING SUGARY FOODS ON AN EMPTY STOMACH

If you eat a sugary food on an empty stomach, the effects can be felt in minutes. The rapid rise in blood sugar level stimulates your body to secrete a large amount of insulin, which then causes your sugar level to fall very quickly. This is when you experience the horrible dizziness or other symptoms.

Note that there are various types of sugar in food, such as sucrose, glucose, fructose, brown sugar, molasses, honey, and they all have similar effects on blood sugar levels. The reason that I recommend fruit as a healthy snack is related to the beneficial fibre content; it still contains sugar, in the form of fructose, but the fibre cushions the rise in sugar level. Products labelled 'no added sugar' are by no means sugar-free; usually they are high in natural sugar of one kind or another.

If you feel that you can't live without sugary fats, or you really enjoy them as a occasional treat, have them after you have eaten a meal containing a lot of fibre: vegetables, wholegrains (such as brown rice, wholewheat pasta) or pulses. If you fancy something sweet, choose a dessert that contains some fibre; there are plenty of ideas in the Taste Good section of this book.

DON'T SUBSTITUTE ARTIFICIAL SWEETENERS

Although artificial sweeteners do not directly aggravate sugar levels in the body, I do not recommend them for several reasons. First, they don't taste very good, so you can feel dissatisfied after a meal or snack and therefore become tempted to eat something else. Secondly, substituting one sweet taste for another does not help our bodies, as we are still subject to the negative cycle of cravings; it's far better to try to wean ourselves off the desire for excessively sweet things. Finally, some people suffer from digestive complaints such as bloating, diarrhoea, wind or pain when they eat foods containing artificial sweeteners.

AVOID CAFFEINE-CONTAINING DRINKS

Avoiding caffeine (which is present in coffee, tea, cola drinks and hot chocolate) can have a positive effect on your hypoglycaemic body. Caffeine causes your pancreas to secrete more insulin, thereby aggravating symptoms.

Some people can tolerate small amounts of caffeine as long as it is not drunk on an empty stomach, but as an initial step I recommend you cut out all caffeine. Be prepared to suffer from caffeine withdrawal symptoms such as headaches and irritability for a day or two, but if you can ride through it, taking a headache-relieving pill if necessary, the results will be well worth it. Drink plenty of water, herb teas, fruit juices and see pages 342–3 for other caffeine-free drinks.

AVOID DRINKING ALCOHOL ON AN EMPTY STOMACH

Alcohol on an empty stomach causes your blood sugar level to drop rapidly after initially being absorbed very quickly. If you wish to drink alcohol, make sure you have it with a meal that contains some fibre, or prepare yourself with a high fibre snack (see page 66) before you go out; the fibre will help to cushion the adverse effects by slowing down the absorption of sugar into the blood.

TRY TO GIVE UP SMOKING

Nicotine, present in cigarette smoke, disturbs the production of both insulin and another hormone called glucagon. Glucagon is secreted by the liver in response to low blood sugar levels; it enables the liver to release glucose. If you smoke your body can find it very difficult to regulate its sugar levels, as it is forever reacting to a dose of nicotine. You will notice a vast improvement in your hypoglycaemia if you give up.

TRY TO MAKE YOUR LIFE HEALTHY IN BODY AND MIND

Hypoglycaemia can be aggravated by excess body weight, low weight and fluctuating weight; crash dieters often suffer from severe hypoglycaemic symptoms. Try to keep your body weight stable and within the ideal range; if you need to lose weight, see the chapter on Achieving your ideal weight.

Stress can also aggravate hypoglycaemia. Remember that hypoglycaemic symptoms decrease your ability to concentrate and perform, so taking the time to eat properly is time well spent. Skipping meals is counterproductive. This is an important point for parents to emphasize when children are revising for exams.

Periodic hypoglycaemia

Some women find that at certain times of the month their bodies become severely hypoglycaemic. This can cause mood swings, lethargy and loss of concentration. Men sometimes find that periods of stress can hit them hard; they become short-tempered and unpleasant to be with. Children sometimes become dizzy if they play a sports game on an empty stomach. These scenarios are often caused by fluctuating levels of hormones, such as oestrogen, adrenaline and cortisol. I have devoted a separate chapter to periods, but anyone who suffers from symptoms of hypoglycaemia should make an effort to implement the above guidelines, as they can make a significant difference.

If exercise is your problem area, for instance, during the after-work squash game or a morning gym workout, eat a high fibre, sugar-containing snack such as a banana or a few dried fruits about half an hour before you exercise.

Tackling a hypo attack

All of this advice should help to prevent further attacks, but just in case, here's the survival plan:

- Have a sweet, high-fibre snack to help bring your sugar level up to normal. Sweets and chocolates are the worst foods for you to take, as a rapid rise in sugar level will cause your body to produce a lot of insulin, which will then cause your sugar level to drop even further. Fruit combines sugar and fibre, so a fruit-based snack is ideal.
- Eat a well balanced meal as soon as possible.
- Rest. Vigorous exercise will make symptoms worse. Relax, keep warm and have a hot drink such as a mug of hot milk or camomile tea.
- Avoid caffeine. This will make things worse.

Diabetics should read the chapter on Diabetes, as the treatment of a diabetic hypoglycaemic attack is a little more complicated than this. People who have medical conditions such as a gut malabsorption problem like Crohn's disease should seek the advice of a professional dietitian.

Chromium

People who suffer from bouts of hypoglycaemia sometimes ask me whether they should be taking a chromium supplement. Chromium is a mineral which is needed in minute quantities in our body. It is essential for the production of insulin, the hormone that controls blood sugar levels. The body also excretes more chromium when you consume a lot of very sugary foods. Therefore if you avoid sugary foods your chromium level should remain at a satisfactory level.

Boosting your intake of chromium-rich foods such as cheese, shellfish (molluscs such as scallops, clams, oysters), baked beans and wholemeal products has in some cases improved hypoglycaemic symptoms. I wouldn't recommend a supplement, as the quantities needed are so small.

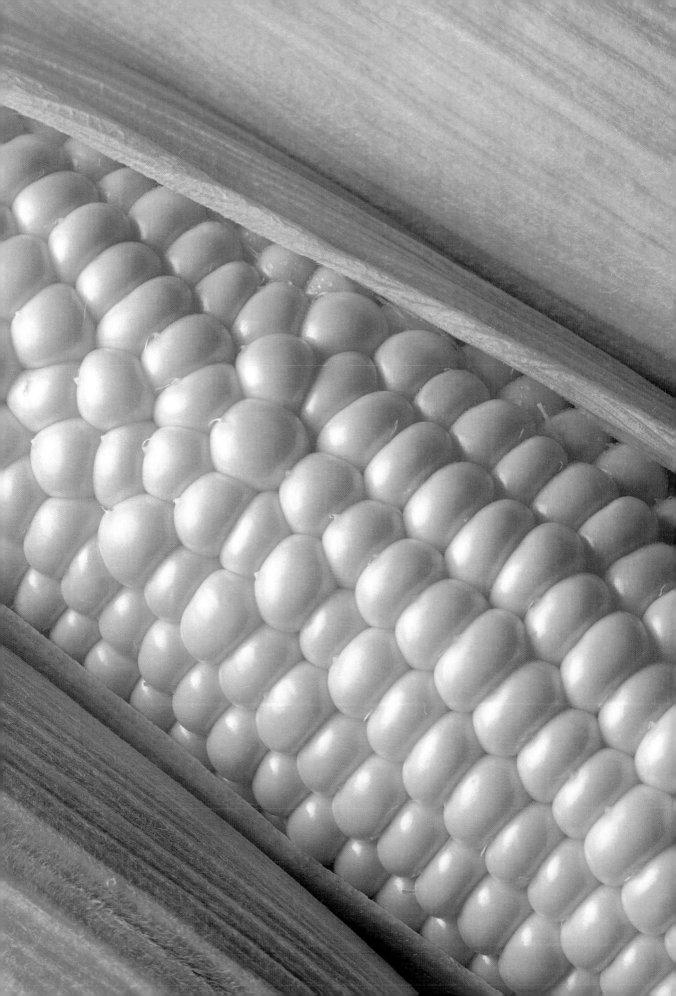

Learning to live with periods

The regular cycle of hormonal changes affects not only our reproductive capabilities, but also helps the body maintain strong bones, supple skin and muscles; one of the hormones, oestrogen, helps protect the body against heart disease. However, many women suffer some unpleasant symptoms during their menstrual cycle, including mood swings, breast tenderness, cramps and pains, fluid retention, bloating, food cravings, constipation, diarrhoea and in some cases depression: these symptoms are often classed together as pre-menstrual tension (PMT). While no particular food can cure period problems, what and how you eat can have a profound effect on the severity of the symptoms.

Food has a fundamental role in the progress of menstruation. Diet helps determine the time of the onset of menstruation in girls. It is usually the case that the healthier and better nourished you are, the earlier you start your periods, the more regular they will be and the longer you will have them. Scientists believe that a woman's body has to reach a level of 17 per cent body fat before the oestrogen and progesterone cycle kicks into action. Girls who keep their weight below the ideal Body Mass Index (see page 109), usually in the 16–17 range, either because they are very athletic, because they are on restrictive diets, or are suffering from anorexia, may find that the start of their periods is delayed.

If you lose too much weight at any time in your life, especially if you lose it rapidly through crash dieting, your periods can cease. Stress and shock can also cause your periods to disappear. If your cycle does not return after a few months, seek medical advice.

PMT

Pre-menstrual tension affects a huge proportion of women. If the pain, mood swings or symptoms are causing you distress I recommend that you see your doctor to find out whether there is any medically treatable cause. For example, heavy bleeding can be caused by fibroids or a hormonal imbalance. You should also seek advice if you experience a significant change in your period. Some women in their thirties start to suffer from bloating and severe constipation around the time of their period, which could be caused by irritable bowel syndrome.

Generally, women who eat a well balanced diet, rich in fresh fruits and vegetables, pulses, wholegrains, fish (but less meat) and plenty of water, seem to suffer less with PMT than those who eat lots of sugary and convenience foods and drink a lot of tea or coffee. Women with the healthier eating habits seem to produce more of the sex hormones oestrogen and progesterone. Since women with lower levels of these hormones generally suffer from PMT more than other women, it is worth boosting your intake of pulses, vegetables and fruits to see if you feel better.

It is easy to assume that you have a well balanced diet, but I recommend that you read the chapter on Understanding your nutritional needs and perhaps keep a food diary (page 85) for a couple of weeks.

Some studies have shown that PMT can be alleviated by taking vitamin B6. However, the studies are inconclusive and can at worst encourage women to take unnecessary vitamins and potentially cause toxicity (with symptoms of extreme lethargy and lack of appetite, numbness in the fingers and toes, and serious liver problems). Instead of taking vitamin supplements, I recommend that you eat foods rich in all the B vitamins. These include dairy produce, eggs, wholegrain foods and green leafy vegetables such as watercress and spinach.

Staying positive about your body and the way it changes is a crucial aspect of managing PMT. If your body insists on gaining a few pounds prior to a period and then loses it afterwards, accept it. Our bodies change throughout our lives. If you fight these changes, stress hormone levels will escalate and PMT will too.

Energy levels

Many women find that during the week leading up to their periods they are sluggish, want to sleep and find it very hard dragging their bodies through the simplest of tasks. Getting stressed out about it, kicking your body to get going by having a 'quick fix' sweet food is the worst thing to do as the sugar boost will be followed by an energy crash, making you feel even worse. Accept that this is going to be a slower week than your other three, adapt your life around it, and eat foods that give you a slow but sustainable energy intake.

Weight gain and bloating

Many women suffer from the feeling that their stomach has swollen and their clothes are uncomfortably tight. This affects a woman's moods, making her feel unattractive, and it can worsen other symptoms of PMT. Before changing your diet, you need to find out whether the swelling is fluid, fat or gas; some women unfortunately suffer from all three.

FLUID RETENTION

The most common cause for the weight gain is a temporary increase in fluid retention – which disappears when the period starts. Fluid retention can make your whole body feel puffy, although the worst affected areas are usually the face, waist, feet and hands. In rare cases fluid retention can be caused by a lack of protein or a deficiency of a particular vitamin or mineral, but this is rarely seen in healthy women who eat a reasonably well balanced diet. If you are

Small pots of herbs can be grown very easily. Be careful not to overwater them or strip them of all their leaves at once (buy two plants and take a few leaves rather than stripping one plant bare). Freshly chopped herbs can be frozen in small portions, such as in an ice cube tray, so you can easily pop them into sauces and soups.

Arabic mint tea is delicious. Use whole peppermint leaves (about ten leaves to a large cup or small pot) and infuse in boiling water for 5-7 minutes.

worried by your fluid retention and suffer from any other symptoms, such as pain in the chest and kidney area, seek the advice of your doctor.

- Keep your salt intake low. PMT fluid retention occurs because there is a temporary rise in the body's sodium level, which causes the body to retain excess fluid to dilute the sodium concentration in the tissues. Reducing your intake of salt helps your body redress the balance. Avoid blatantly salty foods and watch the amount of salt you use on food and in cooking; herbs and spices can enhance flavours just as well. If you reduce the amount of salt in your diet during the week or ten days leading up to your period, your fluid retention should decrease.

- Drink plenty of water. Don't think that the less water you drink, the less your will retain: the opposite is true. Providing your body with extra water helps to dilute the salt level in your tissues and enables the body to excrete more salt and fluid, thus reducing fluid retention. You should aim to increase your water intake to three litres/five pints a day during the week leading up to your period. Don't make the mistake of thinking that alcohol or caffeine-containing drinks such as coffee and cola serve the same purpose; they can dehydrate your body further.

- If you reside in or are going away to a hot climate, it is important not to restrict your salt intake excessively. A body that sweats a lot loses a lot of salt, so you need to replace some in your food. Just keep to a sensible intake and make sure you drink plenty of pure water.

- Think potassium. Potassium and sodium exist in tandem throughout the body. The levels of the two fluctuate constantly, but if you boost your intake of potassium-rich foods, your sodium and hence retained fluid level comes down. Foods rich in potassium include bananas, tomatoes, and in fact most fruits and vegetables, including dried fruits and fresh fruit juices. You should not take a potassium supplement for fluid retention unless your doctor has prescribed it.

- Keep your caffeine intake low. Although caffeine is a diuretic, it acts by stimulating the kidneys to produce more diuretic hormone and makes you lose water too quickly; it impedes the excretion of excess salt and fluid from your tissues. It also upsets the natural hormone changes, so mood swings and breast tenderness increase. Removing caffeine can have a tremendously positive effect on PMT. Just be aware that you might experience caffeine withdrawal symptoms such as headache and lack of energy for a few days.

- Avoid diuretics as far as possible. They can be useful on occasion, for example to help you feel comfortable in a party dress, but they should not be used long term. The body can become accustomed to them, and you will swell up badly when you stop taking them. They can also cause a drop in blood pressure.

- Exercise can help reduce fluid retention by maximizing your circulatory and tissue drainage mechanisms. Keeping active helps keep the fluids moving in the right direction and helps reduce puffiness. Exercise also produces endorphins, the body chemicals that make you feel happy and exhilarated.

COMBATING CRAVINGS

If you notice an increase in appetite leading up to your period, your additional weight is likely to be fat. See the chapter on Achieving your ideal weight for healthy ways to control the tendency to put on weight.

Mention food to many women during their PMT week and the majority will say the word chocolate! Many women crave sweet foods, others crave salty foods or indeed any food just prior to their period. This is caused by fluctuating levels of hormones and other body chemicals. Some people believe that women who crave chocolate are trying to get a fix of phenylethylamine, a substance that makes you feel comforted and happy. However, the phenylethylamine cycle is both an addictive and negative cycle; the more you have, the more you need to satisfy yourself, and it can worsen mood and energy swings.

• Try not to have the first mouthful. Once you eat the first little bit of chocolate, the body will be set off on its cycle. The ideal way to boost your energy is to choose a sweet food that has some fibre in it. Fibre helps your body glean the sugar from the food slowly, evening out energy levels.

• I have given many recipes for high-fibre fruity desserts which should satisfy any cravings for sweet foods. You could bake a fruit and malt loaf or a batch of oat muffins, raspberry bars or flapjacks to keep you going for a few days, or you could make a big bowl of fruit compote using fresh or dried fruits. See also page 66 for healthy snack ideas.

• If your craving is for salty foods, remember that although salt doesn't upset blood sugar levels, it can still set up its own cycle of 'the more you have the more you want', and can aggravate fluid retention (see previous page).

• Boost your intake of chromium and magnesium rich foods during your pre-menstrual period. These can help some women stave off sugar cravings. Foods rich in chromium and magnesium include wholewheat bread, oats, brewer's yeast (which can be sprinkled on breakfast cereal), green leafy vegetables, winkles, shrimps, prawns, cheese, calf's liver, soya beans and black pepper.

BLOATING

A common symptom of PMT is bloating. Your tummy fills with gas, which makes you feel uncomfortable and windy, and can cause pain, because any distension in the bowel presses on your already tender womb.

There are two main reasons why many women develop more gas at this time of the month. First, the intestine reacts to fluctuations in hormone levels. If you keep a detailed food diary, you will be able to see whether certain foods upset you more than others; many women report that bread or dairy produce are the prime suspects. If so, remove them for a few days before your period, making sure they are replaced by equally nutritious alternatives. Secondly, you may eat different foods during your PMT time, sugary or salty foods in particular, which change the bacterial balance in the gut; the good bacteria are driven out and the bad bacteria take charge and produce wind.

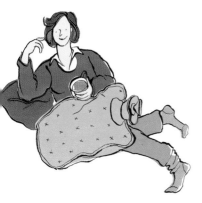

- Try redressing the bacterial balance in your gut by putting some good bacteria back. If you eat a small pot of live yoghurt every day for the week leading up to your period, this might solve the problem.
- Some women find broccoli, cabbage, cauliflower and pulses particularly hard to digest during the PMT days. Choose alternative vegetables such as French beans, mangetout, asparagus, parsnips, carrots, broad beans.
- Rushing your food, and eating at irregular times can increase bloating. A gut left for a long time with nothing in it slows down its production of digestive juices. When you come to eat, the enzymes are not around in sufficient quantities, so the food lies heavily in the gut and frequently causes bloating. Slow down your eating, relax and eat small meals often.

Diarrhoea

Hormonal changes can sometimes affect the tone of the intestine so that it cannot hold on to food for long. Period pain can also cause your body to produce substances that relax the smooth muscles in the intestine. When you have diarrhoea you need to treat your gut gently to help it deal with the foods you put into it. Most importantly you need to replace lost fluid by drinking plenty of water. See page 146 for further advice.

Constipation

Women may find that in the week before their period constipation becomes a problem. It can be prevented by eating plenty of fibre-rich foods (see page 28) and drinking lots of water. If it's too late for prevention, turn to page 149 for some suggested cures.

Breast and period pain

Tender breasts can be caused either by excessive fluid in the tissues, or because the breast tissue itself becomes inflamed. Fluid retention is discussed on pages 198–9, but if you have followed this advice for a month or two and still find that your breasts are tender there are some additional things you can try. A sore womb can also be helped by following this advice.

- Reduce or cut out caffeine-containing drinks. This simple step can bring dramatic improvements for many women, particularly with breast tenderness.
- Increase your intake of oily fish. Oily fish such as salmon, herrings, tuna and sardines contain omega 3 and 6 fatty acids, which can help the body produce natural painkilling substances and reduce inflammation. Keep your saturated fat intake low as saturated fats (see page 32) interfere with the metabolism of these beneficial oils.
- Consider taking evening primrose oil. This contains gamma linolenic acid (GLA), which enhances the production of prostaglandin, an anti-inflammatory substance produced by the body. As with fish oils, GLA can only help reduce breast and womb pain if your diet is low in saturated fats.

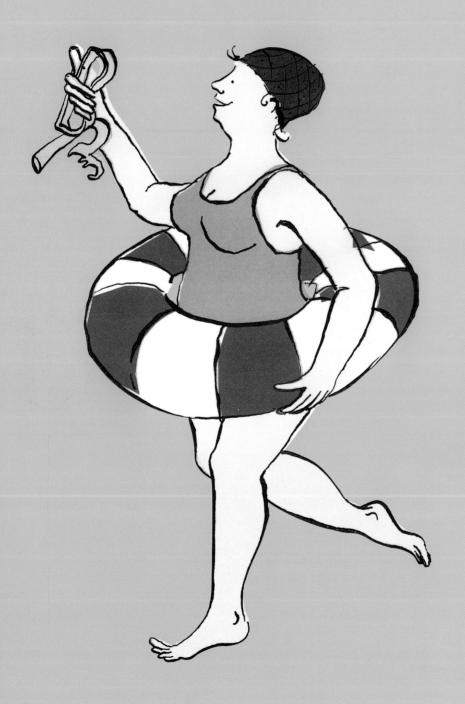

4

stay good

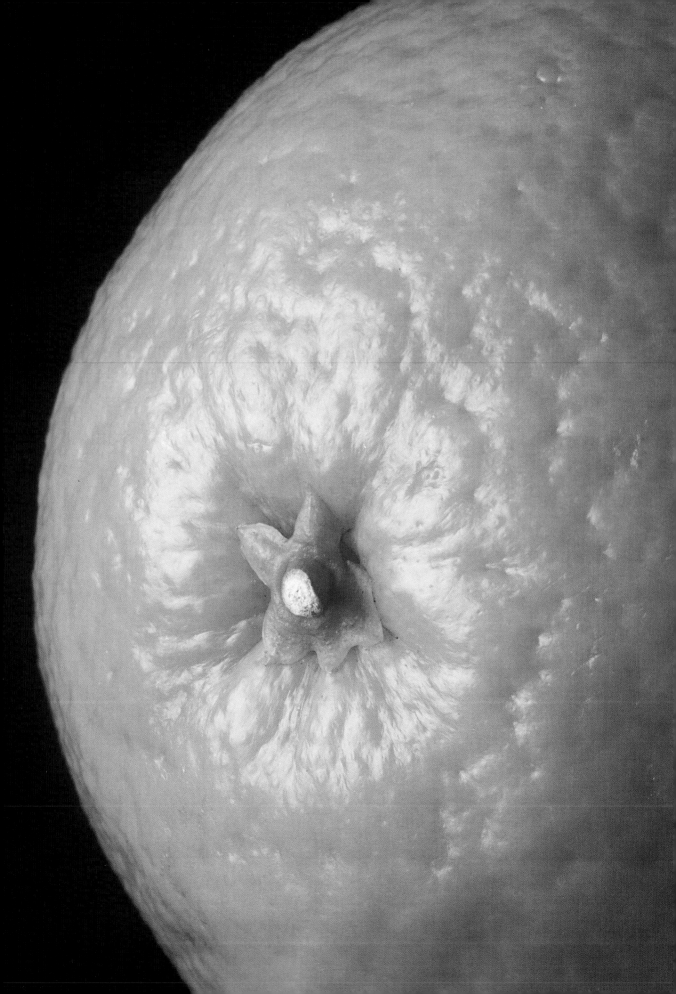

Pregnancy; issues of infertility

Pregnancy is not just about your baby – it can also be a turning point in your own life. Parents-to-be start to realize they can no longer get away with skipping meals, pushing the body until it collapses in exhaustion, not really thinking about the food they eat. By ensuring that both parents are fit and healthy before and during pregnancy, you will not only be giving your baby the best possible start in life, but also be giving yourselves an early helping hand in dealing with a newborn baby. The aim of this chapter is to help you to prepare for a healthy pregnancy, to enjoy the experience of carrying a baby, and to lay the groundwork to feel well after the birth.

One important point I would like to make is that food is best assimilated in a relaxed body. Becoming obsessive about every morsel of food you put into your mouth will not help you or your baby. While food safety guidelines are designed to reassure expectant parents that they are doing the right thing, food should always be seen as something enjoyable.

Pre-conceptual care

If you are hoping to have a baby, you should begin preparing for the pregnancy at least three months before you start trying to conceive. This allows your body to stock up on vital vitamins and minerals, such as folic acid, and also to cleanse itself of less desirable substances, such as prescription drugs or nicotine from cigarette smoking. For more information on diet and its relation to fertility, see page 214.

If your pregnancy wasn't planned and there has been no time for pre-conceptual care, don't worry. If you begin taking extra care of your health as soon as you know you are pregnant, your baby will still get the best start in life.

- If you are taking hormonal contraceptives, such as the pill, you should change to a barrier method, such as the condom, for at least three months. This allows your body time to re-establish its own cycle and hormonal balance.
- An unborn baby exposed to rubella (German measles) during the early months of develop-ment can be born severely handicapped. If you are not sure whether you are immunized against rubella, consult your doctor, who may recommend that you are immunized and then wait a month before you try to get pregnant.

*Life's aspirations come
in the guise of children.*
Rabindranath Tagore
(1861–1941) Fireflies

- Give up smoking. Smoking creates a greater risk of miscarrying and developing problems during the pregnancy. There is also a risk of sudden infant death syndrome (SIDS) among babies whose parents or carers are smokers.
- If possible avoid taking medication before conception and during pregnancy. Check with your doctor about the safety of any prescription medications.

For both men and women, the key nutritional issues that directly affect your ability to conceive and enjoy a healthy pregnancy are body weight, vitamin and mineral intakes and alcohol.

BODY WEIGHT

Before trying to conceive, it is helpful to bring your weight into the ideal range (see page 109). If you are overweight, a healthy weight loss plan will enable you to lose weight without sacrificing crucial vitamins, minerals and other nutrients. Avoid crash diets, which can upset your hormonal balance and inhibit conception.

Certain complications, such as high blood pressure and pregnancy onset diabetes, are more common if you are overweight before you get pregnant. However, if you are overweight, don't panic. Just be aware that you need to be careful not to put on excess weight during pregnancy (see page 211).

Being underweight can also affect fertility and the progress of the pregnancy. If you are naturally slight but are healthy and eat well, you have no need to worry. However, if you have been dieting and have a body mass index below 20 (see page 109), think about nourishing yourself a little more and putting on a few pounds. This will not only help you become pregnant, but will also allow you to have a more positive pregnancy experience and leave you stronger after giving birth. Remember that excess weight can come off after the birth – it is more important that your body receives the nutrients you and the baby need.

VITAMINS AND MINERALS

A varied, balanced diet (see the chapter on Understanding your nutritional needs), including fresh, unprocessed foods, preferably organic, should contain adequate vitamins and minerals. Certain of these nutrients are particularly relevant.

FOLIC ACID

A diet rich in folic acid has been shown to decrease the chances of giving birth to a baby with neural tube defects, such as spina bifida. It is therefore advisable to boost your intake of folic acid at least three months prior to conception and continue to do so for at least the first three months of pregnancy.

Foods rich in folic acid include: green leafy vegetables such as spinach, broccoli, Savoy cabbage, curly kale, Brussels sprouts and asparagus; citrus fruits such as oranges and grapefruits; pulses such as black-eyed beans and chickpeas; dairy products; yeast extract (spread it on bread or dissolve it in hot water and use in cooking); cereals and breads fortified with folic acid.

The folic acid content of foods decreases with time, so the amount in freshly picked asparagus is far higher than in asparagus that has been in transit for several days. Folic acid is also lost through heating, so a spinach salad or broccoli stir-fry is better for you than the boiled vegetable.

In addition to eating folic acid-rich foods, the Department of Health in the UK recommends that women planning a pregnancy also take a supplement of 400 micrograms of folic acid for three months before conception and throughout the first three months of pregnancy. This adds an extra safety net.

Certain drugs may decrease the amount of folic acid you store within your body. These include some indigestion remedies (antacids) and antihistamines. Alcohol also interferes with the storage of folic acid.

Since folic acid is absorbed in the small intestine, any disease that affects the lining of the small intestine, such as Crohn's disease, coeliac disease or ulcerative colitis, can cause a folic acid deficiency. If you suffer from any of these conditions, discuss the issue of folic acid with your doctor or dietitian, since any change in diet may trigger some symptoms.

IRON

For both men and women, iron-deficiency anaemia can adversely affect fertility. In women it is often related to a diet lacking in red meat. In men it is most likely to arise either due to a digestive complaint such as Crohn's disease or ulcerative colitis, or if you are taking strong medication such as anti-inflammatory drugs. See the chapter on Anaemia for advice on how to improve your iron intake.

ZINC AND MANGANESE

Deficiencies in these two minerals can lead to sexual problems for both men and women. Low zinc and manganese levels are related to decreased libido, sterility and birth defects. Zinc deficiency is particularly common in women who have been taking the contraceptive pill, so if you have just come off the pill I suggest you try to include plenty of zinc in your daily healthy eating plan. Foods rich in zinc are discussed on page 45. Try not to rely on a supplement as excess zinc can expose you to an increased risk of bacterial infections. Manganese will be found in adequate quantities in a balanced and healthy eating plan.

ALCOHOL

Excess alcohol intake in both men and women adversely affects the ability to conceive. A small amount of alcohol may be relaxing, but in excess it can lead to decreased sensitivity in both men and women, reduced fertility in women and in men penile shrinkage and testicular atrophy that can lead to impotence. In addition, excessive drinking can lower the levels of folic acid in the blood.

Try to keep your alcohol intake down to no more than one unit a day. Men should stick to a maximum of 28 units a week. A unit means a glass of wine, half a pint of beer or a single measure of spirits.

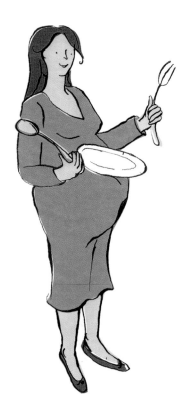

What to do when you are pregnant

The first thing to do is to evaluate your diet and see whether improvements are needed. Keeping a food diary (see page 85) is a good start.

Many women make the mistake of over-nourishing. You may think that because you are supporting two people your requirements double, but a baby is very small! Your body does have an increased demand for vitamins and minerals, both to maintain your health and to build a strong, healthy baby but during pregnancy your body becomes more efficient, absorbing more of the nutrients and using more of the calories you take in. You may initially think that you need to take a vitamin and mineral supplement, but other than folic acid there is no need, and indeed some supplements could be harmful to your baby. The developing baby's nutritional needs can easily be met as long as the mother follows a healthy, well balanced diet. It needs to be:

- rich in high fibre carbohydrates, because these foods contain energy, vitamins, minerals and fibre.
- low in fats and refined sugars. Try to avoid eating sugary, buttery or chocolaty snacks and fizzy drinks, and keep junk foods down to a minimum.
- moderate in lean proteins. Meat, fish, eggs, nuts, beans and lentils supply protein as well as vitamins and minerals. Milk and dairy products such as yoghurt and cheese also provide calcium. Note that in families with a high incidence of allergies, including eczema and hay fever, there is a risk of passing a nut allergy to your unborn child if you eat nuts during pregnancy. Pregnant women are advised not to use peanut oil-based creams for the same reason. If you are concerned about allergies, discuss the issue with your doctor.
- rich in fresh fruits and vegetables (at least five servings a day), because these contain vitamins, minerals and fibre.

Remember that everything the mother eats is passed, to a greater or lesser extent, to the baby. By keeping your diet as varied as possible, you will not only be benefiting your health, but also influencing your baby's taste preferences; if the mother's diet exposes the baby to many different flavours, he or she is more likely to be an adventurous eater. Try to stick to as many unprocessed, natural foods as possible, as the fewer additives you take in, the healthier you and your baby will be. If you have been used to existing on ready-made meals, try to make a fresh start now. The effects that many chemicals in common use in the food industry may have on your developing baby are as yet unknown. Organic products are best, because they have not been chemically treated.

Alcohol can be dangerous to the developing foetus. As soon as you know you are pregnant try to either cut out alcohol altogether, or to limit your intake very strictly to a unit a day. Foetal alcohol syndrome can be caused by drinking more than 10 to 12 units a week. Alcohol also lessens the amount of folic acid in your body.

ENERGY AND CALORIES

Although you don't need to 'eat for two', you do need to eat enough not only to ensure that your baby grows, but also to make sure that you remain strong during the pregnancy and after the birth. It is estimated that the total energy required during the nine months of pregnancy is in the region of 80,000 calories (kcals,) compared with the usual figure of around 55–60,000 calories needed by a non-pregnant woman over the same period. If you met this need by simply increasing your intake, you would need to take in an extra 150 calories a day in the first trimester and 350 calories during the second and third trimesters. However, since many women expend less energy when they're pregnant, especially in the late stages, this is not really necessary. I generally say that you should follow your appetite, and eat what you fancy.

Many women worry that they won't be able to lose the weight they put on while pregnant, even after birth. I can assure you that this is not the case: you will be able to get rid of the unwanted weight after you have stopped breast-feeding if you follow a healthy weight-reducing diet, as recommended in the chapter on Achieving your ideal weight. If you stick to a healthy eating pattern of three small meals a day, with fruit snacks in between to maintain your blood sugar and energy levels, you should not put on too much weight while you are pregnant.

IRON

You need to make sure that you take in enough iron, in order to help create new tissues and prevent iron deficiency anaemia. Every woman should maintain a good iron intake by eating a portion of a rich, well-absorbed source of iron once a day. Lean red meat is the best source of iron, but there are alternatives. These include eggs (as long as they are well cooked), baked beans, green leafy vegetables such as spinach, broccoli and sorrel. Although liver is very high in iron, it is not recommended during pregnancy because it is high in vitamin A, which is toxic in excess amounts and can harm your baby. Pâté and other liver products are best avoided while you are pregnant. You should also not take any vitamin or mineral supplements which contain the retinol form of vitamin A.

The iron in non-meat foods is not as easily absorbed by the body, so you need to eat more of them to gain the equivalent amount of iron. See page 44 for more details. In addition, caffeinated drinks, such as tea, coffee, hot chocolate and cola inhibit the absorption of iron, so cut your intake down to no more than two of these drinks a day. Better still, cut them out of your diet completely to give your baby a good start in life.

Even if you eat a diet rich in iron, you may develop iron deficiency anaemia in the last few weeks of pregnancy. Let your doctor or midwife know if you are feeling acutely tired or a bit depressed. They can carry out a blood test and if necessary arrange for you to take an appropriate supplement.

VITAMIN C

This vitamin is needed for the growth of healthy body tissues and also to help your body absorb iron and other important nutrients. See page 40 for more information. Good food sources include fresh citrus fruits such as oranges, lemons, grapefruits, tangerines; kiwi fruits; rosehips; tomatoes; green leafy vegetables.

CALCIUM

This is needed for the development of healthy bones, and is very important for pregnant women. You should ideally have 600 ml/1 pint of milk or its equivalent of cheese or yoghurt every day (see page 42). Don't forget that you can mix your calcium sources and use them in cooking. Women who are intolerant of dairy products should boost non-dairy sources of calcium, such as green leafy vegetables, and discuss calcium supplements with their doctor or dietitian.

Food poisoning

When you are pregnant, food poisoning can be serious. It is important to follow basic food hygiene rules (see page 77). Wash your hands carefully after you have touched any animal. Wash all vegetables and fruits thoroughly before you eat them. Keep cooked and raw foods separately in the refrigerator. Use separate chopping boards for cooked and raw meat, fish and vegetables/fruits.

Certain foods should be avoided during pregnancy:

- Soft cheeses, such as cream cheese and Brie, and blue cheeses such as Stilton, carry the risk of listeriosis, a food poisoning illness caused by a bacterium called *Listeria monocytogenes*. It produces flu-like symptoms and in pregnant women may cause miscarriage. There are so many wonderful hard cheeses, both pasteurized and unpasteurized, that you should certainly not feel deprived of cheese for these nine months.
- Soft whip ice cream carries the risk of listeria infection. Fruit sorbets are a safer option.
- Prepared salads such as shop-bought potato salad and coleslaw are other sources of listeria bacteria. Make your own salads, washing all vegetables well.
- Pâtés and ready-made chilled meals may carry listeria bacteria. You may have to forgo pâté, because it is also advisable to avoid liver when you are pregnant.
- Undercooked eggs can be a source of salmonella, a particularly virulent strain of food poisoning bacteria. It causes diarrhoea and vomiting, as well as head-ache and fever, between 24 and 48 hours after eating infected food. Any egg dishes should be thoroughly cooked. Avoid homemade mayonnaise, which is prepared from raw eggs (commercially bottled mayonnaise is safer).
- Undercooked meats and poultry, and unpasteurized milk, are other sources of salmonella.
- Raw meats or fish: it is best to steer clear of any uncooked meat, such as steak tartare and some salami, fish (such as sushi), or seafood (such as raw oysters). All meats, fish and poultry should be thoroughly cooked.

For acid stomach, try a quarter of a teaspoon of bicarbonate of soda dissolved in water, at least an hour before or after eating.

Dealing with common pregnancy problems

NAUSEA AND MORNING SICKNESS

Morning sickness is a feeling of nausea and, in some cases, vomiting, which often occurs in the morning, but can happen at any time of the day. It is caused by hormonal and metabolic changes and usually lasts no longer than the thirteenth or fourteenth week. However, some women can spend a whole nine months feeling and being sick. If you go for more than a day without being able to keep anything down, consult your doctor or dietitian.

To lessen the feelings of morning sickness, try the following:

- Check your iron supplement. Sometimes stopping these also stops the nausea. Ask your doctor or midwife first. Obviously if you do this you should make doubly sure that you are eating plenty of iron rich foods (see page 44).
- Don't go for long periods without eating, even if it's just a biscuit, oatcake or crispbread. An empty stomach can make nausea worse, so even if it's just a little something, it can help.
- Make sure that you are not drinking too much tea or coffee. Caffeine and tannins (found in tea) aggravate nausea and vomiting.
- Try soothing drinks. One of the best cures for nausea is rice water. Just take small sips of the warm water in which you have boiled rice. Peppermint, ginger and camomile herb teas are also very soothing. Some fizzy drinks, such as ginger ale, are also good at relieving nausea – but do sip them slowly.
- Avoid fatty foods. These are particularly difficult to digest and can irritate the muscle that normally keeps food in the stomach. Starchy foods such as bread, pasta, rice and potatoes are far gentler on the system.
- Delegate the cooking if possible. If food odours get to you, and you have someone to cook for you, let them do the cooking and stay away from the kitchen.
- Try to get a little fresh air before eating. If you can fit in the time, or juggle your schedule, it is often beneficial to go for a stroll to get a breath of fresh air.
- Experiment with the temperature of your foods. Sometimes cold foods are more appealing when you're feeling sick. Try a little of your favourite hard cheese, or ham and melon. Or slice a tomato on warmed ciabatta bread and garnish with fresh basil.
- Have a stock of biscuits by your bed, so you can nibble something before you get up in the morning. Ginger biscuits would be a good idea as some people find that ginger helps reduce nausea. Resist chocolate, buttery or creamy biscuits as these often aggravate nausea.

WEIGHT GAIN

Excess weight during pregnancy can increase your risk of developing high blood pressure, leading to pre eclampsia, and pregnancy onset diabetes. It is not just the total amount of weight you put on during the pregnancy that concerns midwives and obstetricians but also the pattern of weight gain. It is best to gain weight steadily throughout the whole pregnancy, rather than putting it on in spurts, but every woman is different, and some do have fits and starts of weight gain. The best way to ensure your weight-gain pattern is a healthy one is to keep in touch with your midwife or obstetrician.

If you are gaining weight too fast, take steps to cut out 'empty' calories and concentrate on getting the nutrients you really need from a healthy diet:

- Try to drink water rather than sugary drinks
- Make sure that you're drinking at least two litres/four pints of water a day
- Try not to use additional sugar in drinks and cooking
- Stick to lean proteins rather than fatty savoury dishes
- Keep the amount of fat you use in cooking down to a minimum
- Aim to have at least five portions of fresh fruits or vegetables every day
- If you have a sugar craving, choose fresh, poached or dried fruits, on their own or with a spoonful of natural yoghurt or fromage frais
- Choose high-fibre (wholegrain, wholemeal) breads, rather than the white varieties, and include some starch such as pasta, rice or potatoes with each of your main meals
- Remember to eat slowly, concentrate on what you're eating and juggle tastes, textures and temperatures within your meals
- Ask yourself the questions 'Do you like it and do you need it?' If you do, then go ahead and savour every mouthful. If you don't, don't eat it.

INSUFFICIENT WEIGHT GAIN

Because of nausea or indigestion, some pregnant women find it hard to eat enough to put on sufficient weight. If you are concerned, here are some ideas to boost your food intake:

- Try to make sure that your meals are as full of energy as possible. Don't worry about the size of the portions, and concentrate on making sure that you are eating a variety of protein, carbohydrates and fat-containing foods rather than filling up with vegetables.
- Keep concentrated sources of nutrients in your diet, such as cheese, meat, milk, full-fat yoghurt, fish, butter and cream.
- Dried fruits such as apricots, figs and prunes are good sources of nutrients, and are also high in fructose, so keep a bowl around to nibble at.
- Don't serve one main large meal – have little meals often. Serve beautifully presented little dishes that stimulate your eyes, nose and taste buds.
- Buy a selection of bread rolls, perhaps flavoured with fresh herbs, olives, oils and spices, and store them in the freezer. They are quick to warm through, so you will have a good source of food 'on tap', ready to accompany meals or as a snack.

If you find you still can't gain weight after a few weeks of trying these tips, seek the advice of your doctor or dietitian.

INDIGESTION

This frequently occurs once the baby grows to the size at which its body starts pressing on your stomach. The hormone changes during pregnancy can also cause the muscles at the top of your stomach to over-relax, which makes it more likely that the acidic contents of your stomach will leak into your oesophagus (the feeding tube leading up to your throat). The presence of acidic juices in your oesophagus causes 'heart burn' and an acidic, unpleasant sensation. It is often worse at night when you are lying down. See page 155 for more on these conditions. Here are a few simple tips:

- Try not to eat too late at night
- Try propping your head up a little while you sleep
- Sip settling drinks such as iced water, ginger or peppermint tea
- Don't drink milk. Although this gives you an initial cooling sensation, it causes your stomach to produce more acid shortly afterwards
- Avoid antacid preparations, unless recommended by your doctor, midwife or chemist. Some contain high levels of aluminium or sodium, which are dangerous for pregnant women.

CRAVINGS AND AVERSIONS

Some women experience cravings for the strangest foods. Usually they pose no threat to either you or the baby as long as you still manage to consume a well balanced diet. Obviously you should try to make sure that they are not high in refined sugars and fats and don't pose any food poisoning risk.

Sometimes particularly strange cravings – for coal for example – are a sign of nutritional deficiency and should be mentioned to your doctor or midwife.

Many women also find that they develop a strong aversion to a few flavours during pregnancy. This is again due to hormonal fluctuations. The most common taste dislikes are coffee, English-style tea and fatty foods. If a food aversion helps you to give up caffeinated drinks, be grateful. For hot drink substitutes, see page 343.

CONSTIPATION AND PILES

Constipation can occur when extra hormones produced in pregnancy cause the intestine to relax and become less efficient. Over time, it can lead to the development of haemorrhoids (piles), an extremely uncomfortable condition that can cause intense itching and can even bleed. Eating plenty of fruit, vegetables, wholegrain cereals and drinking plenty of water will all help. Light exercise can also help to get the muscles moving. See page 149 for more advice.

INSOMNIA

It is often difficult to sleep during the last weeks of pregnancy, when it is difficult to get comfortable and you have a frequent need to urinate, as the baby sits heavily on your bladder. See the chapter How to sleep soundly.

Issues of infertility

Infertility is defined as twelve months of unprotected intercourse without conception, or the inability to carry pregnancies to live birth. Men are deemed infertile when their sperm are unable to fertilize the egg, women when they fail to become pregnant. Around one in seven couples has trouble conceiving.

Infertility has many causes, some of which are affected by the food you eat. Although some couples will never be able to conceive, despite eating well and adjusting their lifestyle to reduce obstacles, many couples feel that analysing their diets is a positive step. In addition, changing your diet for the better is an important part of pre-conceptual care (see page 205). Some simple fertility issues can be ironed out by boosting your nutritional status. For instance, women who have been taking the pill for years may have a poor zinc status, so boosting your intake of zinc-rich foods over a period of a few weeks can improve fertility. Men make new sperm every few days, so dietary changes have a virtually immediate impact on the 'quality' of sperm.

WEIGHT

The first thing to address is your weight. Excess body weight in either partner can decrease the ability to conceive. It lowers libido and can lead to a decline in sperm production in men and an interruption in ovulation in women. Being underweight can also affect fertility. In women who have a body weight below the ideal range, the amount of stored energy (fat) in your body becomes so low that periods can be irregular or disappear. Men who keep their body fat levels low can experience a drop in testosterone levels, causing infertility or impotence. Swings in weight, either up or down, can interfere with hormone levels and thus your ability to conceive. Try to reach your ideal weight range (see page 109) and maintain it for six to twelve months. This will allow your body to achieve a balance of hormones that will maximize your chances of conceiving.

Unfortunately many of the drugs used to boost fertility or as part of assisted pregnancy procedures such as IVF can cause your weight to increase. This is mainly due to hormonal changes, which can lead to cravings for sweet food, fluid retention and a general increase in appetite. Although some weight gain is inevitable with many hormone treatments, this should not reduce your fertility.

Concern about infertility can also lead you to comfort eating. Keeping tabs on what you are eating by keeping a food diary (see page 85) is a good way to ensure that your body is getting plenty of healthy foods.

ALCOHOL

Excessive drinking adversely affects male and female fertility. In men alcohol is a reproductive tract toxin; the more alcohol ingested and the longer the period of alcohol abuse, the greater the impairment in fertility. The same can be true in women. In addition too much alcohol can reduce fertility by increasing the level of the hormone prolactin; a prolactin imbalance can cause menstrual dysfunction and infertility. Both men and women should reduce their alcohol intake to a maximum of 21 units a week for women and 28 units for men. It may be a good idea to go without alcohol for a few weeks, to give your body a healthy boost.

CAFFEINE

There has been some interesting research regarding the amount of caffeine a woman drinks and her ability to conceive. Caffeine, found in tea, coffee and cola-based drinks reduces the blood prolactin level; any imbalance in the level of the hormone prolactin is associated with infertility.

B VITAMINS

Vitamin B12 deficiency, although rare, can lead to pernicious anaemia, which is associated with infertility. The only way to treat pernicious anaemia is to have a course of vitamin B12 injections. Once the vitamin B12 levels return, fertility is restored. Vitamin B6 has been shown in some women to increase levels of progesterone, a female hormone that is needed to maintain a healthy womb lining that can support the growth of a fertilized egg. Good sources of vitamin B6 include dairy products, dark green leafy vegetables such as broccoli, nuts and yeast extract. I would not recommend a supplement as an excess of vitamin B6 can cause extreme lethargy and serious liver problems. Lack of folic acid has also been linked to infertility; for more information on this vitamin, see page 206.

VITAMIN C

There is some evidence to support the theory that if a man increases his intake of vitamin C it helps to improve his fertility. When sperm enter a woman's body, antibodies directed against them cause the sperm to clump together (agglutinate), which renders them less likely to fertilize the egg. The presence of vitamin C helps reduce the agglutination process. Both men and women should ensure they have good levels of vitamin C in their diet. Fresh vegetables and fruit are the best sources of vitamin C, which is one reason why everyone is recommended to eat at least five helpings of fruit or vegetables every day.

ZINC

One of the key minerals involved in sperm production and male hormone levels is zinc. It has been shown that if a man is low in zinc, both the level of male hormone and the sperm count decrease. Zinc-rich foods include oysters and other seafood, meat and crumbly cheeses such as Lancashire (see page 45).

DON'T FORGET PROTEIN AND FAT

Low intakes of either protein or fat can impair fertility. For instance, inadequate intakes of the essential fatty acid linoleic acid can lead to infertility. Linoleic acid is found in vegetable oils, nuts and lean meat.

Approaching middle age

For many people middle age is a transitional period, a time of change. Women go through a distinct hormonal change, the menopause; men may not lose the ability to father children, but they are more likely to lose their hair, and are just as likely to experience weight gain, depression and lack of sex drive. As people are living longer, now is the time to make an added investment in your health, taking the time to boost your nutritional status and ensure that you are doing everything possible to ensure you stay fit. Don't leave it until a problem arises in your late sixties or seventies. The earlier you start looking after your body the better.

There are also more immediate issues to deal with. Physically, the body is going through changes in metabolism that may cause a change in the pattern of weight gain, digestive problems and sleeping difficulties. The ageing process most noticeably affects the appearance of the hair and skin. For many people these physical signs of ageing can be stressful.

The menopause

The menopause is a period in life when a woman's reproductive capacity ends, oestrogen and progesterone levels drop and the body enters a new phase. The onset is gradual in most women, but can in some cases be hastened or brought on suddenly by an emotional trauma or surgery. The process will usually begin between the early forties and mid fifties. Diet plays a role in the time of onset: the better nourished you are, the later the menopause will start.

It is good to be aware of the physiological changes that may occur so that you know what to expect, and hot flushes don't send you off to the doctor fearing you have an infection. Symptoms include hot flushes, dry skin, hair loss, mood swings, depression, tiredness, poor concentration, headaches, vaginal dryness and loss of sexual desire.

Pollution in the air, soil and water have been found to aggravate symptoms, while women who have always maintained a healthy diet, high in fresh and preferably organically grown vegetables and not so high in fats, high-fat dairy products and meat, seem to pass through the menopause more easily. A well balanced diet (described in the chapter on Understanding your nutritional needs), keeping the water intake high, alcohol intake moderate and caffeine intakes low, is the goal we should all aim for. There are also specific foods that can help with some of the problems frequently experienced during the menopause.

HORMONE REPLACEMENT THERAPY

To counteract the symptoms of the menopause, many women turn to a drug therapy known as hormone replacement therapy (HRT). During a woman's reproductive years, the hormone oestrogen provides protection against heart disease and osteoporosis, a condition in which the bones become brittle. As women enter the menopause and oestrogen levels drop, the protective effect is lost and therefore the risk of developing these conditions increases. So not only do you suffer distressing symptoms, you also expose your body to potential problems in the future. HRT replaces the hormones that the body has ceased to produce.

Like any other medication, HRT has its pros and cons. The hormones can be taken as a tablet or a cream, or worn as a skin patch or an implant just under the surface of the skin. HRT is associated with an increased risk of endometrial cancer and endometriosis, fibroids of the uterus. It is also associated with an increased risk of breast cancer, secondary malignancies and thrombosis. On the plus side, not only can HRT make you feel younger, it protects your bones against osteoporosis and reverses the increased risk of heart disease.

NATURAL HORMONE REPLACEMENT

Research carried out in the US by Dr John Lees of Portland, Oregon, suggests that it is the non-production of progesterone that causes oestrogen dominance and thus many of the painful symptoms associated with an imbalance of hormones. It is possible to boost the progesterone level in the blood through nutrition. The Mexican yam, or sweet potato, is said to be high in progesterone. Root vegetables such as carrots, parsnips, potatoes, beetroot, and pulses such as chickpeas and kidney beans, help the body produce progesterone.

Herbs can also be useful. Some herbalists suggest sarsaparilla, grown in the southern US. Chinese medicine has long recommended dong quai, schizandra and white peony as hormone balancers at this time of life.

Some women find that vitamin E, found in foods such as avocados, black-berries, mangoes, seeds and nuts (such as sunflower and peanut and their oils), and also evening primrose oil and star flower oil, can help reduce hot flushes. An advantage of boosting your intake of fruits is that they are rich in vitamin C, which has been found to help relieve menopausal symptoms.

Be aware that after a while the body gets used to the dietary hormonal boost and you can start getting symptoms again. If you find this I suggest you take a break of a few weeks, so that when you return to your dietary remedy you should receive the same beneficial effects. Taking breaks prevents your body from becoming dependent on its boosters.

FOOD CRAVINGS

Some menopausal women experience food cravings, similar to those during pregnancy. Women taking HRT often crave sweet foods. This may lead to

**Five things to do
with yoghurt**

- *Mix it with chopped or
  dried fruit and a little
  honey*
- *Layer it in a wineglass
  with fruit purée or
  compote; sprinkle the
  top with chopped nuts
  or toasted coconut*
- *Mix with fresh herbs
  to pop in a jacket potato*
- *Use it in salad dressings
  (see page 312 for ideas)*
- *Mix with orange juice
  and orange syrup (made by
  reducing freshly squeezed
  orange juice to a thick
  syrup) and serve with
  stewed blackberries or
  strawberry shortcakes*

weight gain, but also to problems controlling your energy levels and moods. Moods are affected because there is a link between the hormones oestrogen and serotonin. Serotonin is a hormone that creates positive moods, so if the level in your body drops you can feel very low and depressed. The body responds to this drop in serotonin by craving the foods it knows will provide it; sweets, chocolates, ice cream. Although sweet foods cause a massive initial rise in serotonin, which makes you feel good, a survival mechanism to prevent the sugar level from going too high soon kicks in. The result is that serotonin levels crash and you feel lousy. The way to get a boost in your serotonin levels which won't make you feel bad is to choose a slow-release sugar such as a piece of fruit. See the chapters on Feeling full of energy and Dealing with depression for more information.

Osteoporosis, or brittle bones

From around the age of twenty, our bones start a gradual process of deterioration. In women, this process accelerates with the menopause, making them more vulnerable to a condition known as osteoporosis, or brittle bone disease. Some men can also be affected by osteoporosis. When bone mass drops, the bones become fragile and at risk of fracturing easily. Whatever your age, it can be a severely debilitating condition.

The best defence against osteoporosis is to build up good bone mass during childhood and the teen years. Later in life, it is essential to do as much as possible to prevent bone loss. See the chapter on Building strong bones.

There is a clear correlation between nutrition and osteoporosis, which means there is lot you can do to help your body through the foods you eat. Throughout adult life, both men and women should ensure that their diet is rich in calcium, around 800 mg a day. Other important nutrients are vitamin D, vitamin K, magnesium, zinc, copper and boron. Regular load-bearing exercise helps to reduce the rate of bone loss. Everyone should exercise for at least twenty minutes on at least three occasions every week. Examples of load-bearing exercise are running, hockey, tennis and brisk walking.

Disease prevention

Everyone should examine their body at least every month to check that there are no changes, especially small lumps, which could be a sign of a medical problem. If you find anything unusual, don't worry unduly, but get it checked by your doctor as soon as possible. This advice applies to men as much as to women; unfortunately men are far less likely to examine themselves, and if they do find a lump, for example in their testicles, they may be too embarrassed to consult their doctor. Remember that if problems are discovered and treated early the prognosis is usually good. In any case, you should keep in regular contact with your doctor so that he or she can ensure that all of your health is being looked after.

Unless women take HRT, as they enter the menopause they lose oestrogen's protective effect against breast cancer. If you have a family history of this disease or are worried about it, I suggest you read the chapter on Cancer to help ensure that your risks are minimized.

As women enter the menopause their risk of heart disease becomes equal to that of men. It is therefore important for both women and men to address the nutritional and lifestyle issues surrounding heart disease: what you eat and drink, your body weight, blood fat level, exercise and smoking. The chapters on High blood cholesterol and High blood pressure look at these issues in detail. Women on HRT have a slightly reduced risk of heart disease, but this should not allow them to become complacent; the risks are there if you don't look after your body.

SMOKING

Research has proven that there is an increased risk of osteoporosis, 'brittle bone disease' in people who smoke. Of course, smoking also greatly increases your risk of heart disease and many forms of cancer; for example, lung cancer killed 37,714 people in the UK in 1993. Do try to give up; it's never too late to do so.

Digestive changes

Many people find that the gut changes quite significantly as they enter middle age. They begin to suffer from bloating, constipation, indigestion and diarrhoea, conditions that had never troubled them before. This occurs because the digestive system consists of a collection of muscles and glands, all of which are very sensitive to blood hormone levels. At certain times of life your gut varies in its ability to absorb and metabolize the nutrients in the foods you eat. To help you address these problems I suggest you read the chapter on Good digestion.

In more extreme cases some women, and less frequently men, may develop food allergies and intolerances. These generally appear either because the hormonal changes trigger the gut to respond differently to foods, or your body has had enough of one particular food; its tolerance level has been met. If you suspect you have a food sensitivity, see the chapter on Managing allergies.

Weight changes

Most people seem to accept that they will change shape as they get older; it is considered remarkable if someone can say that he or she has 'the body of a twenty-year-old'. There are a number of reasons for these changes, which are usually in the form of weight gain, or 'middle age spread'. The first is simply a natural change in metabolism, discussed above.

Some of my patients get very upset as they seem to be unable to eat the same foods as they did when they were younger without putting on weight. Although there is a change in metabolism, an increase in body weight, especially fat, can only come from an excess of 'unused' calories. Ask yourself – are you really exercising as much as you used to and not eating any more?

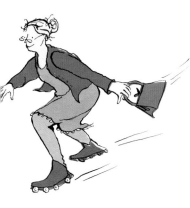

Many women find that when they start taking HRT, the weight piles on. There are two different issues here: oestrogen can change both your body fat levels and your appetite. Your appetite may change in degree and/or food preferences, and it may be that you are responding to food cravings, especially for sweet foods. See the note on Food cravings, page 200.

Men tend to put weight on around the middle, which is potentially more of a problem than women's tendency to put weight on around the hips. Excess weight around the middle can increase the pressure exerted on the major blood vessels around the heart, which can lead to hypertension (high blood pressure) and increase the risk of heart disease. If the excess weight is related to excess drinking, the characteristic beer belly can pop up. This occurs when the liver is suffering from a decreased ability to metabolize male hormones. This leads to a change in the ratio between the male hormone testosterone and the female hormone oestrogen. A rise in the female hormone causes the weight to accumulate around the middle and to disappear from the arms and legs. A side effect of the drink-related beer belly is that impotency increases and libido can plummet. Controlling your alcohol intake and losing excess weight can reverse this situation.

By adopting a healthy eating plan your weight problem should be minimized. I suggest that you read the chapters on Understanding your nutritional needs and Achieving your ideal weight to make sure that you are doing everything possible. I would encourage people who have a body mass index of more than 25 (see table, page 109) to do as much as they can to bring it down, as the more weight you carry into later years the greater your risk of heart disease, certain cancers and joint problems such as arthritis.

A word of warning about losing too much weight. It is not advisable for women to go below a body mass index of 19 or 20; below this the risk of osteoporosis increases. For both men and women, rapid weight loss can predispose you to an increased risk of stroke, heart problems and depression. It is above all essential not to allow your body to become malnourished by going on crash diets.

Fluid retention

Some women suffer from quite severe fluid retention, especially if they are taking HRT. Men who suffer from fluid retention usually do so as a result of circulatory problems. If you are worried about this I suggest you see your GP to check that there is no underlying medical problem.

Nutritionally you can tackle fluid retention in a number of ways:
• Firstly, and most importantly, you must not restrict your fluid intake. Instead make sure you drink at least two and a half litres/four to five pints of water a day.
• Try cutting out caffeine-containing drinks (tea, coffee, cola-based and chocolate drinks). Instead, drink herbal teas and fruit juices (and see pages 342–3 for alternative caffeine-free drinks).

- Make sure that you eat plenty of fresh fruits and vegetables. The potassium and other vitamins and minerals within these foods will help your body to deal with the unwanted fluid.
- Keep your salt intake down. Resist salty-tasting foods and use fresh herbs and spices to enhance flavours in your meals.

In addition, you should exercise regularly to maintain healthy fluid circulation and balance.

Don't take any diuretics unless they have been prescribed by your doctor, as these can seriously disturb your fluid, vitamin and mineral balances. This is dangerous nutritionally because if your body loses a lot of potassium, magnesium or zinc you could develop a deficiency, which would make you feel tired and run down and subject to muscle cramps. Even if diuretics are prescribed, you should make sure that your diet is well balanced, with lots of fresh fruits, vegetables and wholegrain products.

Sleeping problems

People are often puzzled by changes in their sleep patterns; these are usually caused by changes in hormone levels. The most common sleep problems are not being able to get to sleep and waking several times through the night. Other people seem to sleep throughout the night, but they don't feel refreshed in the morning. In this case it may be that your sleep hasn't been good quality sleep. In all these instances there are several things you can do:

- Stop drinking any beverage with caffeine in it after three o'clock in the afternoon. This includes tea, coffee, cola-based drinks and chocolate; the caffeine can stay in your system for far longer than you think. Experiment with herbal and fruit teas and look for caffeine-free soft drinks.
- Try having a glass of cold milk or a mug of warm milk before you go to bed. This can be both comforting and soporific. If you don't like milk, try a herbal tea such as camomile.
- Try to avoid having foods that cause swings in blood sugar level, especially in the evening. Rapid changes in blood sugar can cause disturbed sleep. Instead, choose higher fibre carbohydrate foods such as wholemeal bread and pasta, as these will give you a slow, steady release of restful hormones.
- Make sure that you're neither too full nor too hungry before you settle down. A full stomach can cause indigestion, while hunger can lead to stomach rumblings, neither of which help sleep.
- Avoid taking vitamin and mineral supplements late at night as they can affect sleep patterns.

Some people find that cheese gives them vivid dreams and disrupts their sleep. It is thought that substances within the cheese (vasoactive amines) trigger various neurotransmitters in the brain to go into overdrive and cause dreams. If this is a problem for you, try to eat cheese in the morning rather than the evening. For further suggestions on improving the quality of your sleep I refer you to the chapter on How to sleep soundly.

Loss of sex drive

Many men and women experience a lack of libido as they get older. The causes are quite complex: it is partly hormonal, but it can also be ascribed to society's expectations of the way older people 'should' behave. Some people worry (often needlessly) about being physically unattractive, while others may be suffering from the effects of long-term regular drinking. However, there is no reason why any healthy person should not enjoy sex into old age; for more information see the chapter on A healthy, happy sex life.

Hair loss and skin ageing

Finally, there are the outward signs of ageing such as hair loss (which can affect women as well as men) and the dreaded wrinkles. Although inevitable, we can minimize problems by eating well (see the section on Looking good). As your body enters a new phase of life, take these signs as a reminder to look after yourself, keep active both physically and mentally, and remain positive and full of vitality.

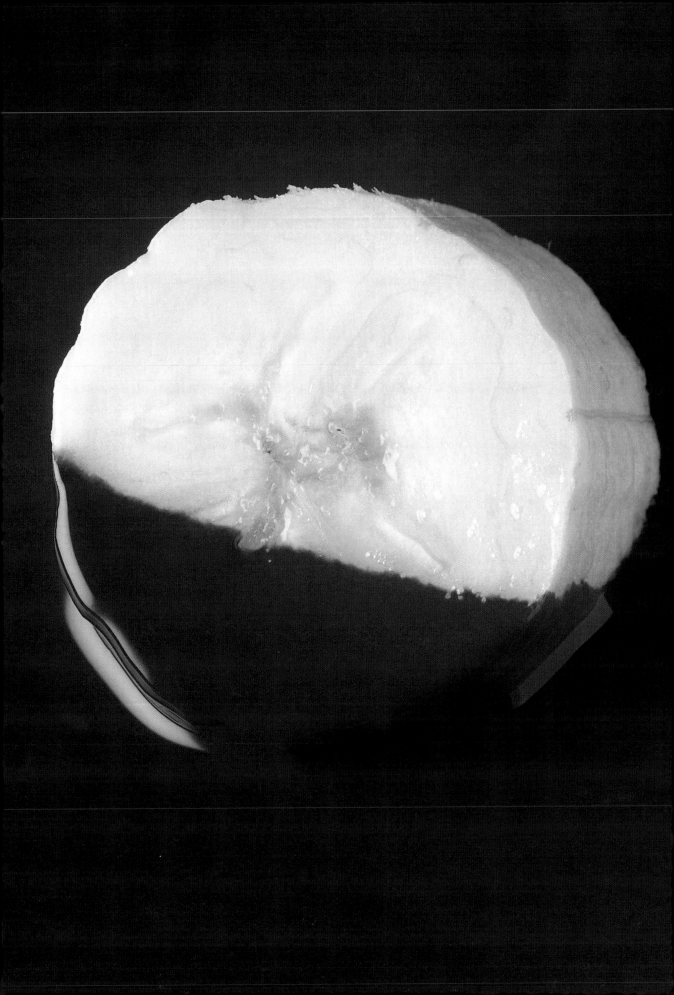

Problems of ageing

Advances in medicine and improvements in living standards mean that more and more people in Western society are living well into their sixties and seventies, an age previously considered old, but now just an extension of middle age. As discussed in the previous chapter, good nutrition helps the body deal smoothly with the ageing process.

One of the major problems I find among older people is keeping up their interest in eating. Sometimes this is because they have lost a partner, and the enthusiasm and routine of eating with someone else no longer exists. It is also easy to fall into the trap of thinking that you don't need as much food when you get older, and you don't need to pay as much attention to your diet. While there is some truth in the notion that you don't need to take in as many calories as if you were doing active work, your body still needs a regular and plentiful supply of nutrients. Without the right food, the body can become malnourished, weak and generally depressed. Minor cuts and sores are slow to heal, constipation becomes a long-term problem, and mustering the energy to take a walk can seem an impossible task.

In general terms an elderly person needs just as much protein, carbohydrate, vegetables, fruits, dairy products and water as a person in middle age. They may be less active, but the fact that the body is working less efficiently means that it needs more of a nutritional helping hand. Keeping a food diary (see page 85) for a couple of weeks is a good way of checking your nutrient balance. If you find you are 'living on tea and toast', make an effort to get more variety into your meals. Begin the day with porridge, have salad at lunchtime, and a piece of fish or chicken breast with a good helping of vegetables for your evening meal. If you stew some apples or pears with dried fruits like apricots or figs, you can have them warm on their own or with a simple crumble topping, or keep them in the fridge to eat cold, stirred into thick yoghurt. Never think it's not worth cooking just for yourself.

The best way to judge whether your body is getting the right amount of food is by your weight. If you are maintaining a steady weight then you have the balance right. If you are gaining weight it may be because of some medication you are taking (see page 227) or it may be that you are relying too heavily on high-fat foods. Ready-made, convenience and fast foods are often high in fat. Even if you do a lot of your own cooking, fat is very 'tasty' and it is easy to be tempted to fry things rather than using other cooking methods such as boiling and baking. If you are losing weight, you are clearly not eating enough for your needs. Lack of appetite is a common problem in older people, and it may be compounded by medication. For more advice, see below.

As well as keeping up your nutrient intake through a well balanced healthy eating pattern, there are a few specific nutrients and common health problems to which you should pay particular attention.

VITAMIN D

Vitamin D is primarily produced by the action of sunlight on our skin, but as we get older the amount of time we spend outdoors generally decreases. This can cause our bodies to become deficient in vitamin D, which is needed (along with calcium) to maintain strong bones. Since bone mass begins to deteriorate gradually from the age of twenty, you can see that by the time you are sixty your bones are at far greater risk of fracturing unless you get enough vitamin D and calcium from the foods you eat. Try to go for a stroll or sit outside every day so that your skin can synthesize some vitamin D. Alternatively, or ideally as well as this, you should boost your intake of vitamin D rich foods: herring, kippers and mackerel, canned salmon, sardines and tuna; cod liver oil; liver; margarine; eggs; full-fat dairy produce – milk, cream, butter, cheese.

DEHYDRATION

Dehydration is common in elderly people. Sometimes you just 'forget' to drink, especially the healthiest drink, water. When you remember, you tend to drink tea or coffee, both of which dehydrate the body. The fear of incontinence can also stop you from drinking. As distressing as incontinence can be, dehydration can cause serious health problems, such as kidney failure. Drinking water and other caffeine-free drinks (see pages 342–3 for some ideas) in small volumes throughout the day can help reduce incontinence. It is generally large volumes of liquid at a time that cause incontinence. I suggest you stop drinking a couple of hours before you go to bed, which helps prevent night-time incontinence. Take a glass of water to have at your bedside, just in case you wake up thirsty.

CONSTIPATION

Constipation is often a worry for older people. It is partly caused by the gradual slowing down of the metabolism, but is undoubtedly exacerbated by dehydration (see above) and the failure to drink enough water. Taking laxatives may seem the obvious solution, but it would be far better to correct constipation by increasing your fibre and water intakes. See page 149.

LACK OF APPETITE

Many elderly people seem to suffer from a lack of appetite. This is sometimes a side effect of medication (see next page) or can be due to a zinc deficiency. Depression can also cause you to go off your food. If you are feeling low I suggest you read the chapter on Dealing with depression – but remember, don't suffer in silence; ask your doctor if there is anything he or she can do to help you.

Don't think that you have to make a great effort to prepare and eat a large meal. It's far better for you to have lots of different snacks throughout the day (see page 66 for some healthy snack ideas). I have looked at ways to stimulate the appetite in more detail later in this chapter (under the general heading of dementia, but please don't let that put you off). First, here are a few hints:

- Boost your zinc intake. Try to include zinc rich foods in your daily and weekly eating plan: tinned sardines on toast; cheese, especially crumbly white cheeses such as Cheshire; a casserole of lean red meat (see page 45 for other food sources of zinc). If you cannot eat these foods, consult your doctor or dietitian, who may suggest a zinc supplement.
- Seize the hungry moments. Keep a small stock of biscuits in an airtight tin by your bed in case you wake up feeling shaky. Keep small pots of biscuits, nuts and dried fruits around the home to remind you to eat when you feel hungry.
- Have a little tipple. Alcohol can stimulate the appetite, so enjoy your favourite aperitif of sherry, gin and tonic, or a glass of wine or champagne – all best served chilled. You will probably find that it's quite easy to nibble at crisps, nuts or cheese while you sip your drink. Wine with the meal can also increase your appetite and nutrient intake.

Check with your doctor to ensure that alcohol is not contraindicated for any reason, and remember that excessive amounts of alcohol can put you off your food; moderation is the key. Sometimes alcohol can dry your mouth slightly, so intermingle sips of alcohol with sips of water.

Side effects of medication

The amount of medication we take in our twilight years can be astounding, ranging from indigestion remedies and laxatives to blood pressure pills and anti-inflammatories. These drugs can affect your appetite, eating habits and nutritional needs. What you eat can help or hinder the action of the drugs.

All too often people don't realize that the reason they crave foods or cannot manage to eat much is nothing more complicated than a side effect of medication. Some elderly people undergo needless medical investigations for symptoms directly attributable to a drug they are taking. This is not a direct criticism of the doctor; unless the person or an informed relative or friend tells the doctor or specialist about the medications they are taking, incorrect drug decisions can be made. In addition, elderly people often continue to take medication prescribed for a specific complaint way beyond the required time.

Sometimes people may have been on a certain drug for years, then quite suddenly they start feeling less well. As we get older our bodies change in composition and metabolism – we may develop more fat or become thinner, we store less water, and the functioning of our heart, liver and digestive system change – all of which can cause our body to react very differently to drugs.

People involved in preparing meals for elderly people need to be aware of the drugs they are taking and how their body can be affected. An example of this is tolbutamide, a drug used to manage diabetes by lowering blood glucose levels. In older people it can have an excessively strong hypoglycaemic action, causing the blood sugar levels to drop too low. This can make them feel shaky, tearful, depressed, weak and always wanting sweet foods. The reason why it affects older people differently is twofold: as we get older the composition of our blood changes, and our livers become less efficient at metabolizing foods and drugs. The result is that more tolbutamide will be left to work in the blood. Simply changing the medication can eradicate these symptoms. If there is no alternative to taking tolbutamide, you should make sure that you take it with or immediately after food, to lessen the risk of hypoglycaemia.

If you know how a drug is likely to affect you it can help you to juggle your food and drugs. Keeping a food and symptom diary (see page 85), noting the times when you take your tablets, should give you plenty of information upon which to act. For instance, splitting breakfast can help you feel better or increase your food intake if necessary. Having a simple biscuit and drink with the medication first thing and then leaving a couple of hours before having some breakfast cereal, eggs and toast can suit some people better than eating it all at once.

Many drugs make the appetite disappear. This situation can lull people into thinking that their body would tell them if they needed to eat; unfortunately this is not always the case. Drugs which decrease appetite include anti-cancer drugs, morphine, non-steroidal anti-inflammatories, theophyllines, biguanides, glucagon and the digitalis group.

On the other hand, some drugs can dramatically increase appetite, leading to excessive weight gain, which can aggravate, among other things, heart conditions and diabetes. Drugs which increase appetite include insulin, thyroid hormone, steroids, some antihistamines, sulphonylureas and psychotropic drugs.

Elderly and frail people are particularly vulnerable because certain nutrient needs take on a greater importance: they need to maintain their calcium intake to protect their bones, and their iron intake to prevent anaemia. The interactions and side effects of medication can make this a little tricky. Many drugs directly alter mineral and vitamin absorption and metabolism, which if unnoticed can lead to deficiencies. For example anti-cancer drugs can impair the absorption of food and affect thiamin (vitamin B1) status and biguanides (used to treat certain forms of diabetes) can reduce vitamin B2 and folate (folic acid) status. Prolonged aspirin treatment, commonly used for people with a history of thrombosis or heart problems, reduces the amount of vitamin C in the body. Ask your doctor to explain the nutritional implications of any drugs you are taking, and if necessary boost your intake of the relevant nutrients. See the chapter on Understanding your nutritional needs for lists of foods rich in specific vitamins and minerals.

Dementia

Dementia is defined as a state of serious emotional and mental deterioration. We all expect some mental deterioration, such as slight forgetfulness, as we grow older, but if this deterioration occurs before the age of sixty it is called pre-senile dementia. Relatives notice that the person starts to forget things, especially things that have happened recently. They can remember things from the distant past, but forget whether they have been shopping or received a phone call. Later there may be a widespread loss of intellectual functions. One of the symptoms which can cloud the diagnosis of dementia is the fact that the sufferer may become depressed, which in itself can cause a change in personality. It is likely that the individual is not acutely aware of the change in their mental and physical well-being, but to see someone you love slowly lose their mental capacity, which in turn affects them physically, can cause a great deal of strain in relationships. Many of my patients find one of the most stressful aspects of being in their forties and fifties is caring for a parent suffering from dementia.

There are many types of dementia, but one of the most common is Alzheimer's disease. Alzheimer's was named after the German scientist who first described the syndrome. With this condition, there are various biochemical disturbances which cause changes not only in the behaviour of the person, but also in their nutrient requirements. If you understand some of the ways in which the body changes, you can begin to understand why someone behaves as they do. From a nutritional perspective, some of the most important changes are:

- Changes in the levels of neurotransmitters, chemicals within the brain which recognize hunger and fullness.
- Reduced activity of the cholinergic systems, which leads to intellectual deterioration and poor memory function. This means they can forget when and what they have eaten.
- Deterioration in the ability to identify smells. This can have a profound effect on the types of food they want to eat. Patients can develop bizarre eating habits such as eating whole jars of marmalade.
- Changes in amino acid and glucose metabolism – in other words the way their body deals with proteins and sweet foods is altered.
- Changes in vitamin and mineral turnover.

ALUMINIUM AND ALZHEIMER'S

There has been much publicity about the link between aluminium and Alzheimer's disease. It originally arose because high levels of aluminium were found in the brains of some patients with Alzheimer's, and some studies suggested that Alzheimer's disease is more common in areas where there is a greater level of aluminium in the drinking water. Many of my patients worry that drinking tap water will cause them to develop Alzheimer's. There is no evidence to support this, as the aluminium level in drinking water varies from glass to glass and the value does not give an indication of the bioavailability of the aluminium; the ability of the body to absorb it. In many instances the aluminium is simply excreted without passing into the body's cells. I advise patients to carry on drinking water from the tap, or use an approved water filter if they don't like the taste. If you are worried about your water, contact your local water authority.

The only concern I have is with the use of aluminium cooking pans. There is some evidence to show that aluminium can dissolve from the pan and pass into certain foods. Although the evidence is not conclusive as to whether aluminium toxicity causes Alzheimer's, I would suggest that you use non-aluminium cooking pans.

Food considerations

As well as Alzheimer's disease and pre-senile dementia there are many other types and causes of dementia. Although these conditions bring nutritional factors of their own, the following section on managing dementia may give you some useful tips.

People with dementia are often underweight. There are a number of possible causes. Their food intake may be poor because they have forgotten to eat, or they cannot find foods they fancy because of changes in their sense of taste and smell. If they are physically infirm, this affects their ability to prepare and eat foods, and in the later stages of dementia they can develop problems chewing. Some medications can cause the mouth to become dry or give a strange taste. Changes in taste and the ability to recognize what they should be eating can be dramatic: in some cases patients eat totally inappropriate things, such as tissues. In the final stages of dementia the ability to swallow and the desire for food or fluids can disappear. In homes or in hospitals dementia patients can fall victim to lack of time and inflexibility in the menu. Feeding someone with dementia can take hours: they may refuse mouthfuls, sit in silence for minutes or get up and walk away.

All this can be extremely challenging for anyone looking after them, but there are many things you can do to improve the situation. It is important not only to tackle the psychological, social and physical challenges, but also to provide the body with the appropriate nutrients to support the nervous system.

STIMULATING THE APPETITE
There are a number of tactics to encourage a dementia patient to eat more of the right foods:
• Build up a selection of small meals and snacks, rather than the traditional three meals a day. This increases the likelihood that they will, in the course of a day, consume more nutrients.
• Don't overface them with food. Serve small but tasty dishes; if they cannot eat a large serving, you are reinforcing the sense of negative achievement. If they get through a small portion you can always serve seconds.

- Take some time to think about the presentation of the dish, as this is paramount in stimulating the senses and encouraging them to eat.
- Choose one-dish meals such as casseroles, hot pots, risottos and soufflés rather than piles of meat with different vegetables. Sometimes it can be difficult to cope with more than one thing. There are plenty of one-dish meals which provide proteins, carbohydrate and essential vitamins and minerals.
- Augment favourite foods with something which makes them a little more nutritious. Even if they don't manage many mouthfuls, the nutrient and calorie value of each mouthful is increased. For example, make mashed potatoes extra creamy by adding a spoonful of double cream, sour cream or grated cheese. Serve fruit with cream, ice cream, thick Greek-style yoghurt or custard.
- Keep the taste buds on their toes; plan to have plenty of variety during the day in terms of colour, taste, temperature and texture. However, it is important not to confuse the taste buds within one meal. Dishes such as soup with croûtons or chocolate mousse with a crisp biscuit can be confusing; serve the mousse on its own, and offer the biscuit later. Crisp textures 'hidden' in smooth foods can cause choking, especially if the dementia affects the ability to swallow.
- Have little bowls of nibbles around the house. They stimulate the appetite, tempt the eye and in turn the taste buds. If the patients find cheese straws, dried raisins and apricots, or filled dates at their fingertips, you will be surprised how they will graze their way through quite a lot without realizing it!
- Have slices of fruit, arranged in a small bowl, covered or chilled in the fridge for them to pick at. Do the same with raw vegetables such as sticks of carrot or celery with a dip of mayonnaise or soy sauce in a small ramekin dish. Some may find raw vegetables hard to eat; if so you could have small slices of pitta or ciabatta bread with the dips.

MAKE A LITTLE EFFORT TO PLAN

One of the most demanding aspects about looking after someone with dementia is the time it takes to feed them. Carers find it very disheartening to spend hours trying to make an appetizing dish only to have it refused. They take it as a rejection not only of their cooking but also of their love.

The best way to go about cooking for and feeding someone with dementia is to make a special effort to plan. Depending on their mental and physical state you should try to include them in the planning; on some days they fancy one thing in particular. Food will often seem more appetizing if they are able to join in with simple activities such as going to the shops to buy some fruit, looking at unusual vegetables, or even choosing a ready-prepared chilled meal. Try not to disempower them by choosing all their meals, unless they are too ill to participate. If they are unable to leave the home, bring home a selection of things that have caught your eye and discuss what they would like to eat.

If they live alone and can manage to cook, but need some help organizing their food store or deciding which meals to prepare, I suggest you make a large batch of a dish such as a casserole or flan and stock up their fridge and freezer with individually wrapped portions. Keep them supplied with easily eaten foods which don't need tin openers or scissors to crack the packaging. You can also make cakes and biscuits for morning and afternoon snacks.

The best time of day for eating is usually in the morning up until lunchtime, as cognitive abilities are generally better at these times. Confusion and agitation tend to increase as the day goes by.

It also helps if you refrain from having distractions such as television on during meals, as this can confuse them and distract them from eating.

DON'T OVERFACE THEM WITH CUTLERY

Sometimes people don't bother with eating because they find it difficult to deal with cutlery. If this is the case, choose finger foods such as little quiches, open sandwiches, flat breads and crisps with cheese and yoghurt dips. Serve deep-fried potato skins to scoop up a casserole.

I suggest you set just the cutlery needed to eat one course at a time, as too many things on the table can confuse dementia patients.

I think geriatric bibs are unnecessary and a little degrading. A napkin, even if it is disposable, placed over the clothing is much more civilized. You can buy beautiful plastic tablecloths to protect the table. Remember not to overfill cups and glasses as this increases the risk of spillage.

FOOD SAFETY

Remember to respect food hygiene advice (see the chapter on Food safety). In the homes of people who live alone it is a common occurrence to find food out of date and stale. Check the stock of food regularly as the last thing you want is for anyone to end up with food poisoning.

REFUSAL TO EAT

People suffering from dementia often refuse to eat. They can be so insistent that they refuse to open their mouths or sit down at the table. This can be a result of depression or a physiological response to the brain damage. Some drugs can also kill the appetite. Grasp every little opportunity for them to eat.

If they don't want to eat proper meals, try them with some nutritious drinks such as homemade milk shakes made with puréed fruit (bananas, strawberries and raspberries are good), which can be enriched with ice cream or yoghurt. I have given some recipes for fruit drinks such as strawberry and passionfruit punch on page 342. Hot chocolate (see page 90) is good for keeping up their calcium intake. Homemade soups (see recipes, pages 306–309) are easy to eat or drink from a mug.

The odd day of not eating much will not cause them any harm, the likelihood being that they will make up for it on the following day. However if you find that they are going for a few days without eating, you must seek medical advice.

The effects of medication

Discuss the times of taking medication with their doctor; sometimes taking medication before or after food can make a big difference to their appetite, nutrient absorption and taste buds. If they say they have a strange taste in their mouth, it may be that a change in medication could improve the situation.

- Strongly flavoured foods such as red meat sometimes taste metallic. In this instance, choose protein dishes based on cheese, fish, eggs, poultry or pulses.
- You may find that tea and coffee taste unpleasant. The positive side of this is that reducing the intake of tea and coffee helps with the absorption of important vitamins and minerals. However, removing tea and coffee leaves a gap in the day which traditionally provides an opportunity to eat a snack. Look for alternatives such as herbal or fruit teas, orange blossom tea or ginger tea (see page 343). Or try a glass of boiled water with a slice of lemon or lime; it cleanses the palate and provides the comfort of sipping a hot drink.
- An uncomfortably dry mouth can be caused by drugs that affect the natural process of salivation. Not surprisingly, it tends to be dry foods that aggravate a dry mouth and make it sore, so avoid grills, roasts and fries as well as very hot or spicy foods. Instead, try casseroles or fish with a sauce.

    Have on hand plenty of cool, refreshing drinks such as freshly squeezed fruit juices and drink these throughout the day.

SWALLOWING DIFFICULTIES

Difficulty in swallowing (dysphagia) is common in the later stages of dementia. Some may simply have difficulty managing solid things such as pieces of meat or crusty bread, whereas others may only be able to take liquid foods. Whichever form it takes, you can usually find a tasty option to enliven your meals.

- Try to choose foods which are naturally soft and easy to swallow, such as soufflés, omelettes, mousses. Cook interesting recipes and encourage the patient to eat with you, rather than isolating them with a dish of 'slop'.
- If they can only face liquids, remember that soups come in many flavours and textures. See the recipes on pages 306–309.
- Encourage them to take small sips of a drink while they eat, as this can help ease the food down.

ALCOHOL?

Check with their doctor first, because some medications do not mix well with alcohol. If the doctor approves, a pre-meal tipple can help increase the appetite and stimulate the taste buds.

    Something you may discover by trial and error is that alcohol adversely affects some dementia sufferers, causing them to become agitated or depressed. If they want a drink before a meal, which in some households forms part of the ritual of eating, but you don't want them to have alcohol, serve a sparkling mixer or fruit juice in a special glass as a refreshing alternative to alcohol.

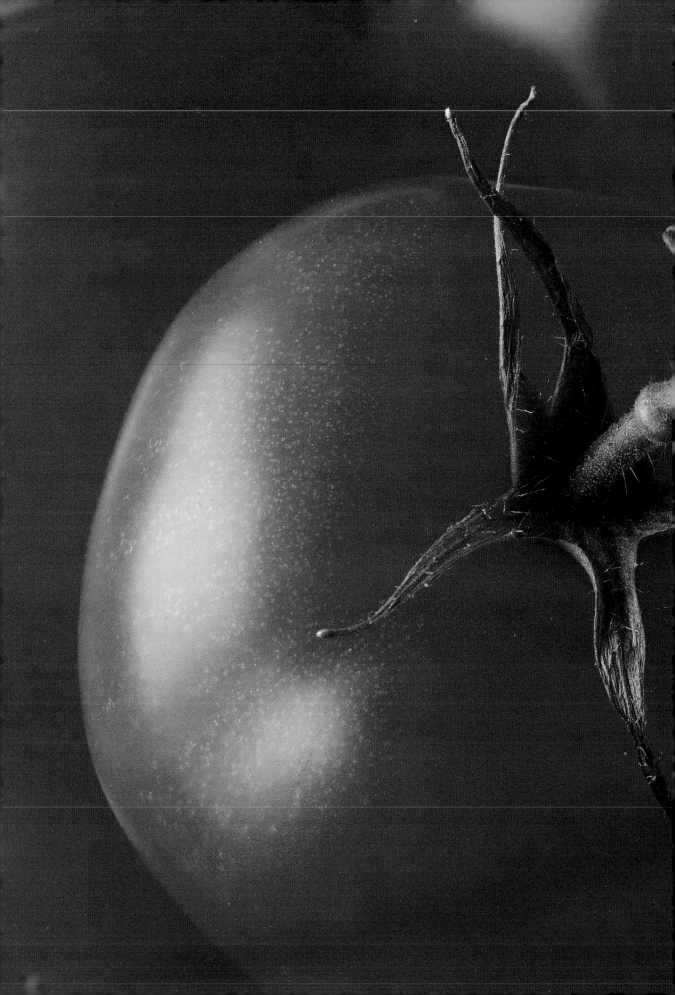

Cancer

Cancer affects us all, either directly, or indirectly as we become involved through caring for a relative or offering sympathy to a friend. One in three people develops cancer and one in four people dies of cancer in the United Kingdom. It is a sensitive illness to discuss, evoking fear and other difficult emotions. However, as with most things that worry us, the more the topic is out in the open, the more the fear of it dissipates. The more opportunities we have to discuss how to fight cancer, the better prepared we will be. Throughout this book you will pick up the message that there is a definite correlation between what you eat, how you eat, your general state of health and your ability to resist disease; cancer is no exception.

All the evidence shows that the earlier in life we start eating and living healthy lives, the smaller the risk of developing cancer. According to the World Cancer Research Fund, 30 to 40 per cent of cancer incidence worldwide is preventable by eating a healthy diet, maintaining a healthy weight and exercising regularly. Food always has a role to play, either as a preventive measure or as a therapy which boosts the immune system and provides the body with the nutrients it needs not only to fight the cancer cells but also to support cancer treatments.

There are many delicious combinations of foods that will boost your nutritional status and your immune system. Most importantly, you need to keep the issue of food in its right place. Eating should not become a task; you should enjoy putting together meals that contain the nutrients that will help your body. Don't set apart the person with cancer. It shouldn't be necessary to serve them something completely different at the meal table – banish liquidized meals and supplement drinks. Recipes can be found and adapted that will satisfy all the nutritional and physical requirements and still enable you to enjoy your food.

One of my patients had cancer of the oesophagus, the feeding tube that leads from the mouth to the stomach. The treatments made his throat exceedingly sore and swallowing difficult. He had been advised that he could get all the nutrients he needed from manufactured supplemented drinks, which in essence was correct. But what a way to spend your life, drinking milk shakes. We managed to put together meals containing dishes such as chicken and almond soup, soufflé omelette with a wild mushroom sauce and crème caramel. With these dishes he was able to join in with normal meals and command some self-respect – something that frequently disappears when you have a serious illness and have to rely on others to care for you.

Lifestyle changes

Food is a powerful weapon in the fight against cancer, but it can only perform its special magic in the right environment. Above all, respect your body.

TRY TO STOP SMOKING

You will be doing yourself a big favour. Not only will giving up smoking decrease your risk of cancer and heart disease, it will also improve your skin and energy levels. Avoid passive smoking as much as you can. Parents should be vigilant about avoiding their children's exposure to passive smoking.

TAKE REGULAR AEROBIC EXERCISE

Ideally you should take a brisk, lengthy walk every day and exercise vigorously for a total of one hour a week. Exercise is not only a valuable stress reliever, but it has also been shown to help the body produce anti-cancer substances and generally help the body stay healthy and strong. Exercise decreases the risk of developing cancer of the colon and possibly cancer of the breast and lung. If you are unable to exercise vigorously, just try to get out into the fresh air as much as possible and mobilize your body. Every little activity helps.

KEEP YOUR WEIGHT WITHIN THE IDEAL RANGE

Several studies suggest that overweight people are at greater risk of developing cancer, particularly of their reproductive system: the uterus, endometrium, and possibly the breast in postmenopausal women, and the prostate in men. The prognosis is also less positive in people who carry excess weight.

WASH FRESH FRUIT AND VEGETABLES BEFORE EATING

Fertilizers, pesticides and chemicals from industrial and vehicle pollution can build up in the body and become carcinogenic. However, it has to be said that on current evidence if you eat a varied and balanced diet the likelihood of you taking in sufficient levels of chemicals to cause cancer directly is small. Eat organic produce if possible (see page 63).

CHECK YOUR BODY REGULARLY

Monitor any changes and note any lumps, particularly in the breasts or the testes. The majority of lumps found in the breasts are non-cancerous, but it is a good habit to check the breast and surrounding area once a month, after your period. One of the main reasons why cancer of the prostate can be particularly virulent is that men are generally not as diligent as women at examining their body for abnormal lumps and bumps, so the tumour can be there for a long time before it is detected. If detected and treated early the prognosis in the majority of cases is good. Men should examine their testes and surrounding area once a month. Men over the age of fifty should see their doctor annually for a prostate check, which includes a PSA antigen blood test.

The anti-cancer diet

Food's interaction with cancer can be seen in two ways. First, food can be a major preventer: it can help keep your immune system strong and your body more capable of fending off damage from its environment. Strong professional opinion throughout the world supports the role of nutrition in helping to prevent major diseases such as cancer.

Secondly, food can be used to help treat certain cancers, either directly through boosting the immune system or indirectly by helping to relieve symptoms of the cancer or the cancer therapy. Food, finally, can provide a positive, refreshing interlude in a life dominated by illness and treatments.

The cancer-resisting plan is based on a well balanced diet, described in the section on Understanding your nutritional needs. Some points are particularly relevant for the prevention of cancer, so let's look at these in more detail.

THINK FIBRE

This means eating plenty of fresh vegetables, fruits, pulses, wholegrain cereals and wholegrain bread, brown rice and wholewheat pasta. A diet rich in fibre can decrease the risk of cancer of the mouth, pharynx, lungs (evidence is strongest for green leafy vegetables) and stomach (particularly raw vegetables, green vegetables and the allium, or onion, family). Diets rich in carrots, tomatoes and citrus fruits decrease the risk of cancer of the colon and rectum.

One of the main reasons why everyone is recommended to eat at least five helpings of fresh fruits and vegetables a day is that they are not only rich in fibre, they also contain important antioxidant vitamins and minerals.

THINK ANTIOXIDANTS

There has been a great deal of research linking antioxidant vitamins and minerals with the prevention and treatment of cancer. I believe that as a first goal you should look to boosting the amount of natural antioxidants in your diet, eating them in a way that allows your body to metabolize them efficiently. If you take a supplement it should be under the guidance of a doctor or dietitian, but in 99 per cent of cases supplements shouldn't be necessary. The antioxidants found naturally in foods seem to be used better by the body than those in supplements. In addition, it is quite easy to take an excess of certain vitamins and minerals from supplements, particularly if you take a combination of them. It is usually impossible to overdose on any particular antioxidant from natural foods – the bulk of the food and monotony of chomping through piles of carrots, for instance, usually stops people from overdoing it.

The main antioxidant vitamins are beta-carotene (converted to vitamin A by the body), vitamin C and vitamin E. The best food sources of all three are fresh fruits and vegetables; in addition, vitamin E is provided by nuts, seeds, vegetable oils and wholegrain cereals (for further sources, see pages 37–41). Remember that vitamin C is lost through storage and cooking, so the fresher your fruits and

Brazil nuts are a magnificent source of selenium. Two Brazil nuts a day provide you with more than your daily requirement of selenium. Almonds, cashews, pecans and walnuts are also rich in selenium.

vegetables and the quicker you cook them (better still, eat them raw) the more benefit your body will receive.

One of the main antioxidant minerals is selenium. Research has linked low levels of selenium in the body with an increased risk of cancer, which means that if you eat a diet rich in selenium you have a lower risk of developing cancer; in addition, if you have cancer, you have a greater chance of fighting it. A well balanced diet will give you more than enough selenium. Good sources of selenium include fish of all sorts, chicken, rabbit, liver and kidney, wholegrain products, nuts and mushrooms.

THINK VEGETABLES AND SALADS

The benefits of vegetables do not stop with fibre, vitamins and minerals; they also contain individual substances that can help protect the body against cancer and other diseases. The best way to include the recommended five daily helpings of vegetables and fruit in your diet is to eat them as part of your meals: in soups, as main ingredients or accompaniments, in puddings – don't leave them until you are too full to enjoy them.

- Green vegetables such as lettuce, spinach and broccoli are rich in nitrates, which are converted in the body into a potent antibacterial chemical. This is one of the body's natural lines of defence against food poisoning. In addition, the 'disinfectant' effect of this on bacteria in the stomach is thought to help protect the stomach against cancer by killing the bacterium *Helicobacter,* which is now believed to cause many cases of the disease.
- Folic acid can help in an anti-cancer diet because it is needed for the production of deoxyribonucleic acid (DNA), the molecule that controls aspects of cell growth and division. Boosting your intake of folic acid rich foods, which include asparagus, spring greens, fresh peas and broccoli, will help your body resist cancer and other diseases. See page 39 for other sources of folic acid.
- Watercress can help smokers fight cancer. It does this by neutralizing one of the most dangerous chemicals in tobacco, NNK, by causing the body to release Phenethyl isothiocyanate (PEITC). You will receive most PEITC when you eat raw watercress, so try it in salads, such as watercress and smoked mackerel salad, or as a sandwich filling with salmon and cream cheese. Far more effective, of course, is to give up smoking.
- Tomatoes also have a role to play in cancer prevention. Harvard University researchers report that men who eat at least ten servings of tomato-based foods a week are up to 45 per cent less likely to develop cancer of the prostate. The 'secret ingredient' here is lycopene. Low levels of lycopene, a substance found in tomatoes, have been associated with an increased risk of prostate cancer. Ten servings may sound a little daunting, but is not too difficult if you think of grilled tomatoes, sliced tomatoes in sandwiches, tomato sauces, soups and salads.

Stay good

THINK ALLIUMS

The Allium family includes garlic, onions, shallots, leeks and chives. This family, particularly garlic *(Allium sativum)*, contains a complex mixture of chemicals displaying immunity-boosting, anti-cancer, anti-viral, antibacterial, anti-blood clotting, cholesterol-reducing, decongestive and digestive properties. There is much evidence to support the theory that eating these foods helps to reduce the incidence of cancers of the colon, liver and breast. Unfortunately, many people undergoing cancer treatments, in particular chemotherapy, find the smell or taste of garlic offensive and nauseating. If this is the case don't worry about not including garlic in your cooking; use onions, leeks and shallots if you like, and bear in mind that there are many cancer-preventing foods, so keep up your intake of fruits and vegetables.

THINK PULSES

Pulses are strong anti-cancer foods. To look at them they don't immediately conjure up creative thoughts, but there are lots of things that can be done with the wide variety of pulses available. Many restaurant menus feature either fish or roasted meats served on a bed of Puy lentils, or soups made with pulses, such as Moroccan chickpea soup. Although the basic taste of pulses, tofu and other soya bean products can be quite bland, you can use fresh herbs, garlic and spices such as cumin, coriander and ginger, to turn these foods into delicious meals. See my recipes for minty chickpea soup, lentil, chicken and ginger soup, bean and rosemary soup (pages 308–309). Pulses can also be used to 'stretch' meats: make chicken 'burgers' with leftover roast chicken, mashed chickpeas, chopped onions and garlic; add lentils to a shepherd's pie.

THINK VARIETY

Try to eat a diet that has a variety of different proteins. We need protein to help keep our muscles and immune systems strong.

Meat has come in for some bad publicity, having been implicated in food hygiene scares, and excessive amounts of red meat have been linked to an increased risk of some cancers – particularly of the colon, rectum and possibly the breast and kidney. However, a small amount of red meat, in the region of 85 g/3 oz a day, two or three times a week, provides a number of useful vitamins and minerals and is perfectly healthy, assuming that it is good quality, lean meat.

There are many other protein-rich foods that can be eaten on non-meat days: fish and shellfish, poultry and game, pulses, tofu and eggs.

Children are sometimes reluctant to eat protein, as they may dislike chewing meat or worry about bones in fish. Try disguising meat and fish in pies with tomato or cheesy sauces, or make your own burgers, fish cakes, or rissoles.

There is another advantage to eating plenty of fish. Oily fish, such as mackerel, herrings, tuna, sardines and salmon, are rich in omega 3 and omega 6 fatty acids. These fats are thought to have a powerful 'cancer-slowing' action.

**Five things to do
with pulses**

- *Enjoy baked beans on toast – with a dash of Worcestershire sauce or a pinch of curry powder*
- *Mix lentils with fried onions and tomato purée*
- *Incorporate pulses into pies or corned beef hash*
- *Make salads of mixed beans or chickpeas with tuna, chopped tomatoes, cucumber, spring onions and a vinaigrette dressing*
- *Throw some chickpeas into a tomato soup and add some freshly chopped mint*

WATCH THE BARBECUE

There is evidence to suggest that if you eat a lot of chargrilled and barbecued foods you increase your risk of developing cancer. The foods are thought to react to direct contact with the flame. Although restaurants may chargrill foods over a fierce flame, a popular alternative for the home cook is to use a ridged chargrilling pan. It is heated to a high temperature and the food is placed on the hot pan, sealing it and marking it with the distinctive 'grill lines'.

KEEP FATS LOW

Animal fats consumed in large quantities have been implicated in the development of various cancers, including those of the breast, prostate, lung and colon. Breast cancer seems to be more prevalent in women who have a diet high in animal fats and low in fibre.

Some low-fat spreads contain high levels of a particular type of fat, known as trans-fatty acids; if eaten in large quantities these increase the risk of certain cancers. I always recommend that you use a natural fat such as butter or olive oil, but use only small amounts.

Choose foods that are naturally low in fat and limit the consumption of obviously fatty foods such as fried dishes and those coated in copious amounts of creamy, cheesy and oily sauces. Enjoy butter, cream and good quality cheese but remember to keep quantities small. Do not be tempted to eat only fat-free products; this is both unnecessary and virtually impossible to do without becoming obsessive. Fat free and fat reduced products are also likely to be high in sugar and artificial additives. Remember that children in particular need some fat in their diet.

DON'T BE TOO SWEET

Most of us have become accustomed to a much higher level of 'sweetness' than is natural and healthy. The more sweet foods you eat, the more your body will demand to avoid swings in energy level and moods, so try not to encourage a 'sweet tooth' in your children, as this will set a pattern for adulthood. Remember that many manufactured foods have sugar added in one form or another (see page 69), and even those that claim 'no added sugar' or 'sugar free' often contain artificial sweeteners. Artificial sweeteners have been implicated, but not proven to be, a factor in the development of certain cancers. For most people the risk is very slight, but if artificially sweetened drinks, sweet snacks and convenience foods feature heavily in your diet, try to wean yourself off sugary foods and drinks – if you do this gradually you will find it quite easy.

It is much healthier to take advantage of naturally occurring sugars, such as glucose, sucrose or fructose (fruit sugar) rather than artificial ones. Think of fruit as the primary sweetener for desserts or snacks. Fruits can be puréed to mix with yoghurt or spread on breads; dried fruits such as sultanas and dates sweeten cakes and tarter fruits such as apples.

Cutting the crusts off soft cheeses such as Brie or Camembert reduces the fat content by half. For hard cheeses, use a cheese slicer so that you enjoy thin slices rather than big chunks.

JUST A PINCH OF SALT

There is evidence to support the theory that high intakes of salty foods increase the risk of stomach cancer. You don't need to remove delicious salty cheeses, olives, cured meats and fish from your diet altogether, but neither should you be eating them every day. Before adding salt when you are cooking, stop and think how much you really need. One way to cut down on salt is to look to herbs, spices and other flavourings, such as a dash of wine in casseroles, to enhance the flavour of your foods.

WATER, THE ESSENCE OF LIFE

Adults should aim to drink two to two and a half litres/four to five pints of water every day. Children should be encouraged to drink plenty of water and healthy fruit drinks. Water helps your body glean all the beneficial anti-cancer nutrients such as antioxidants from the food you eat and also helps your body produce urine, through which it excretes unwanted toxic substances.

CUT DOWN ON CAFFEINE

Keep your intake of caffeine-containing drinks low. Large doses of caffeine not only deplete your body of essential water but they also inhibit the absorption of vitamins and minerals from the gut. Stick to a maximum of two to three cups in total of caffeine-containing drinks, such as tea, coffee, cola or hot chocolate. Instead, explore the many herbal and fruit teas that are naturally caffeine-free, and see page 343 for some delicious ideas. Elderly people should be encouraged to try alternative hot drinks, rather than the endless cups of tea they sometimes drink out of habit. Tempt your child to drink fruity, non-caffeine drinks rather than any of the cola or 'sports' drinks that are often astonishingly high in caffeine.

'MINE'S A GLASS OF RED WINE, PLEASE!'

Studies are emerging that suggest that red wine in moderation, a couple of glasses a day, can not only reduce the incidence of heart disease, but also of cancer. Red wine contains a host of antioxidant substances (such as anthocyanins, tannins, resveratrol, rutin, catechin, quercetin) that are present to different degrees in different grape varieties. Flavenoids (such as resveratrol) are antioxidants found within the grape skins; they are thought to inhibit the development of cancer. Some of the studies have been very specific about linking certain grape varieties with certain cancers. For example, wines made from Pinot Noir grapes in the damper regions of France seem to help prevent cancer of the digestive tract.

Check with your doctor before you drink any alcohol, to make sure that any medications you are taking will not interact adversely and that there is no other contraindication in your health.

For those of you who don't like red wine, some flavenoids are also found in fresh grapes, mulberries and peanuts.

AVOID NUTRITIONAL SUPPLEMENTS

There is little evidence to persuade me that your body needs supplements if you eat a well balanced diet. In fact, the body's natural balance can be disturbed if you take even one supplement, let alone the handfuls of pills people swallow every day. Some people think that it is better to take something to be safe than sorry. I don't agree. You should realize that vitamin, mineral and other nutrient supplements can easily cause the body to become unbalanced, which can bring its own problems and symptoms of toxicity.

The only exception is when people have health problems that prohibit them from eating certain foods, which could cause them to become deficient in a particular nutrient. In this case a supplement would be beneficial; it will probably be suggested by your doctor or dietitian.

LOOK AFTER YOUR GUT BACTERIA

The bowel is home to a colony of 'gut flora' that play a number of roles in keeping your body healthy; one of these roles is the production of anti-cancer substances. To replenish your gut bacteria I recommend that you include some healthy bacteria in your diet by eating a small pot of live yoghurt, especially the kind made with acidophilus and bifidus, every day.

A word of warning. People who have a sensitive immune system or gut, including those with irritable bowel syndrome, Crohn's disease or arthritis, should seek advice before taking these flora as they have the potential to irritate the gut and immune system. If you can't eat yoghurt you could ask a dietitian to suggest another source.

Specific targets

There is not any one food that has been shown to cause cancer directly: it is more a question of not having the right balance of foods in your diet. People who eat lots of fast foods on the hoof, without a fresh fruit or vegetable in sight, are the prime targets. Having said this, I must point out that some people unfortunately develop cancer despite eating a well balanced diet, because of the role of genetics and environmental factors. But food is something we can act on – all you need to know is how to choose the best foods and how to eat them in a way that gives your body the best chance, particularly if you are concerned about a certain type of cancer that may be linked to your family's genes.

BOWEL CANCER

It is thought that a healthy diet could cut the incidence of colon cancer by three-quarters. A high-fat diet that includes large amounts of fried foods, lots of dairy products, fatty cuts of meat, pies, pastries and very few vegetables and fruits is the worst sort of diet. The best way to keep your fat intake low is to eat just a small amount of the natural products such as cheese and butter along with plenty of fibre.

There is also evidence supporting exercise's role in reducing the incidence of cancer of the colon and rectum. Try to exercise vigorously for at least an hour every week and keep yourself active – even if it is only a brisk walk every day.

You should also keep your alcohol intake within the healthy guidelines: 21 units a week for women and 28 units for men (a unit means a glass of wine, half a pint of beer or a single measure of spirits).

STOMACH CANCER

There has been some convincing research that shows that people who consume a lot of salty and smoked foods have an increased risk of developing stomach cancer, especially if they don't eat many fresh fruits and vegetables. Make sure you include plenty of vegetables and fruits in your diet. Remember that too many salty foods can also increase your risk of high blood pressure, so limit your intake of pickles, olives, salt beef, pickled herrings, kippers and smoked salmon.

The most common non-food cause of cancer of the stomach is the bacterium *Helicobacter pylori*. Foods, particularly green leafy vegetables such as spinach and broccoli, have been shown to help the body kill this bacterium.

MOUTH, THROAT AND LIVER CANCER

There is a strong link between these cancers and excessive alcohol intakes. Stick to the recommended 28 units a week for men and 21 units for women, hopefully including some red wine (see page 241). Smokers should be particularly careful not to drink too much alcohol as the combination of excessive drinking and smoking greatly increases your risk of throat and mouth cancer.

BREAST CANCER

According to the cancer charities and research organizations, eating a healthy diet could halve the incidence of breast cancer. Yet again it is the level of fat and fibre which seem to be the core areas where we need to concentrate our efforts, but not only in our adult years – evidence also suggests that the earlier in life we start eating healthily the greater our chance of avoiding breast cancer. A high saturated/animal fat intake seems to cause hormone levels, particularly of oestrogen, to change within the female body, which increases the risk of breast cancer. There also appears to be a link between low fibre intakes and breast cancer. So boosting your fibre intake and keeping your saturated fat intake low, as part of a normal healthy diet, is the best advice. Keeping your alcohol intake within the recommended limits and weight within the ideal range after the menopause also help to decrease the risk of breast cancer.

PROSTATE CANCER

Cancer of the prostate is threatening to become even more prevalent than breast cancer, although with both diseases the prognosis is relatively good if it is diagnosed and treated early (see page 236).

As discussed on page 238, some exciting research is under way regarding tomatoes. Try to have at least ten tomato-based foods a week. You could have pasta with tomato sauce, grilled tomatoes for breakfast or as a vegetable dish, tomato soups (see recipes, page 306) and sliced tomatoes in sandwiches (think about the other ingredients as well – tomatoes are not a magical food that cancels out the negative effect of, say, a high-fat pâté).

The Pittsburgh Cancer Institute has found that vitamin D inhibits prostate cancer in animals, which gives us the hope that it may in future be useful both as a preventive anti-cancer vitamin and as a treatment for prostate cancer. Vitamin D is formed by the action of sunlight on the skin and is found in oily fish (herrings, kippers, mackerel, salmon, tuna and sardines), eggs and full-fat dairy products such as milk, butter and cheese. This may cause some men to throw their arms up in exasperation, as full-fat dairy products are widely condemned as cholesterol-forming and to be avoided because of the risk of heart disease. Yes, these foods when eaten in excess can form cholesterol in the blood, but it is possible to find a happy medium by boosting your fibre intake. Fibre helps the body excrete unwanted cholesterol (see page 255), so men can include these vitamin D rich foods in a healthy diet, as long as they eat plenty of fibre.

As well as including tomatoes and other fruits and vegetables, and natural carbohydrate foods (see page 25), try to keep your intake of meats and animal fats low, don't smoke or drink too much, and keep yourself active.

After a diagnosis

The response to a cancer diagnosis largely depends on how much you had been expecting the news. It may come as a terrible shock, but some people feel unwell for months and once they know why, there can be a strange feeling of relief that they know what they are dealing with and that they have a team of health care professionals behind them. They can then start building up a plan of attack.

Food can be an essential part of your plan; it provides your body with the ammunition to fight the cancer cells, prevents others from appearing and also provides you with the inner strength to tolerate cancer therapies. If you find that your appetite goes, don't worry, just manage what you can, remembering that the sooner you can get back to eating, the stronger chance you will have of beating cancer.

Some people find the easiest way to kickstart their anti-cancer lifestyle is to cleanse the body with a 24-hour fruit and vegetable diet with lots of water. Although this can be a strong psychological tool because you feel as if you are clearing the cancer-causing toxins from your body, it doesn't actually boost your immune system in any way.

There is no proof that any of the macrobiotic diets or radical diets do any real good. In fact, one problem with diets based primarily around vegetables and non-animal foods is that, although plant foods contain a lot of fibre and other substances that can help the body to fight cancer, the bulk of a vegetable

Juggling tastes and
textures to titillate the
tastebuds

- *Two different cheeses, some grapes and a crisp oatcake*
- *Warm soup followed by a platter of cold cuts and homemade chutney*
- *Grilled lamb cutlet and grilled tomato, sprinkled with fresh basil or dill, served with a cool, crisp salad*
- *Chocolate milk shake made with real chocolate (see page 00), with ice cream or clotted cream on top*
- *Fruit fool, ice cream or mousse with a thin, crisp biscuit*

and fruit diet can get in the way of your body receiving the nutrients it needs. Fibre reduces the absorption of proteins and other essential foodstuffs. So when you are feeling under the weather and not up to eating much, a small vegetable or fruit meal won't give you as much sustenance as a small meal that contains some animal proteins. You should try to make sure that your body receives not only plants, but also a regular amount of meat, poultry, fish, cheese and eggs.

Don't take risks with food hygiene. A bout of food poisoning is the last thing you need when your immune system is low. Read the section on Food safety (page 77) for more information. Discourage young people from eating food from roadside stalls such as hot dog stands, as these carry a higher than average food poisoning risk. Suggest other places where they can meet their friends .

Attacking the problems head on

No two people with cancer will feel the same. For some people nausea is the worst aspect, for others alterations in the way food tastes makes them very depressed. However you feel there are things you can do to ease your symptoms; food can be very empowering. The following problems are the most common, but if the advice does not seem to help you, consult your doctor and dietitian, as nine times out of ten there is something which can help.

LACK OF APPETITE

Lack of appetite can hit you when you have the initial shock of diagnosis, but you may also find throughout your battle with cancer that there are days when you simply cannot face food. The odd day of not eating much will not cause any harm, because the likelihood is that you will make up for it the following day. However, if you find that you are going for a few days without feeling like eating, you must seek medical advice.

- The first thing is not to panic or put pressure on yourself. Just try something small and light – anything, even if it is just a nutritious drink such as a milk shake or simply a biscuit, is better than nothing. Maybe an hour or so later you may be able to manage another small something.
- Grab every opportunity to eat. The time between feeling slightly peckish and actually preparing something can kill the impulse, so keep your fridge stocked with cheeses, fruit compote and dips for vegetables. Have little bowls of nibbles around the house or on your desk. Nuts (being careful if you have young children around), chocolate (preferably good quality chocolate or homemade truffles), crisps, cheese straws (recipe on page 316), or crystallized fruits are a few suggestions; for more snack ideas, see page 66.
- I would urge you to choose organic produce whenever possible. If you are eating only a small amount, it is important to have the most nutritious foods you can find. An organic tomato, for example, will be higher in vitamins and have a far better flavour than a non-organic tomato that is full of water and potentially high levels of pesticides.

- The best way to juggle what your body needs with your mood is to feed yourself really well on the days when you feel up to it; this leaves you with a little flexibility and a 'cushion' for those days when you don't feel like eating much.
- Alcohol can increase the appetite and stimulate the taste buds, so an aperitif before the meal or a glass of wine with your food could be just what you need. Do check with your doctor to make sure there are no reasons why you cannot take alcohol. However, heavy drinking can make the appetite can disappear – it is a question of balance and moderation.
- Fresh air can also stimulate the appetite. In summer, picnics are a good idea. If possible try to take a walk outside before a meal; if you are not well enough you could sit on a veranda or by an open window.

LACK OF INTEREST IN FOOD

Sometimes you can stare at the cupboards and be unable to think what on earth you can eat. Going to different shops and delis, flicking through recipes in magazines or watching one of the many TV shows dedicated to food can get your imagination going. If you are preparing meals for someone else who has cancer, discuss the different things you see in the shops and ideas as to how you can prepare them. Sometimes a brief but enticing description can tempt someone to try eating.

- Buying something different can spark your appetite – try some new cheeses or fish, unusual fruits and vegetables, breads flavoured with herbs, seeds or olives.
- Making a little effort with the simpler things, such as adding freshly chopped herbs to scrambled eggs, or slicing some grilled tomato on top of cheese on toast, can make you feel more like eating them.
- Juggling the colours, textures, temperatures, tastes and tantalizing smells of foods sends signals to the part of the brain which will become excited about eating. One of the gripes I have with the carton drinks formulated for cancer patients is that not only do they have a chemical taste, but they all taste very similar and don't stimulate either the mouth or the imagination. They have their place in keeping up nutrient intake, but most people would feel much better for enhancing and adapting foods they would normally choose, for example by adding cream to a vegetable soup or fruit compote.

THE NEED TO PLAN AHEAD

Stocking your cupboards, freezer and fridge, and planning a few simple basic meals for the week, can make a big difference to the amount you eat.

- When you are feeling well make a list of the things that you normally like and which are easy to prepare, so that on bad days you can quickly throw something together.
- Have a plentiful supply of high-energy foods, such as cheese, milk, creamy yoghurt, cream, natural sugar and honey at the ready so that you can easily make a small but concentrated food, such as cheese on toast or Greek yoghurt

with honey and banana. You can also use these foods to enhance the nutritional value of each mouthful, for example by adding some cream to mashed potato, or serving some bread and cheese along with a rich soup; this can really help when you can only manage a few mouthfuls of food.

- Buy a selection of breads and rolls, store them in the freezer and take them out when you fancy them. Warming them in the oven brings out delicious aromas and flavours and can be more appealing than a slice of cold bread.

CHANGING TASTE BUDS

If you are undergoing cytotoxic therapy such as chemo- or radiotherapy, your food preferences can change. You may have fancied something in the past but now your body sends out completely different signals. I see some patients who have always loved plain food develop a real taste for spicier dishes.

- Coffee and tea can begin to taste unpleasant; this is generally beneficial, because they can hinder the absorption of vitamins and minerals. Nevertheless, you will want an alternative hot drink. One of my favourites is mint tea, made simply by pouring hot water on to fresh mint leaves and infusing them for a few minutes. Ginger tea is very refreshing (see page 343 for this and other ideas).
- If a particular food such as wholemeal bread starts to taste bitter or too rough, think of similar foods as replacements; in this case another type of bread, or pasta or potatoes. Don't just stop eating the food, as this could cause your diet to become unbalanced or deficient in certain nutrients.

'I AM ALWAYS FULL'

A heavy, full feeling can arise even when you have had nothing at all to eat. It is frequently associated with radiotherapy to the stomach or following surgery to have part of the stomach removed.

- Make a point of sitting down to eat, laying a place and taking time to eat your main meals. When you rush food, you tend to take in air, which contributes to bloatedness and stress.
- Resist drinking while you are eating. Drinks fill your stomach with fluid rather than valuable nutrients. If you find it hard to swallow food without a drink, take small mouthfuls and choose moist or sauced food. Wait half an hour after you have eaten before you have a drink; by then the stomach will have more space available.
- Rather than three large meals, break up the day with a series of appetizing snacks, which are small but concentrated in nourishment.

DRY MOUTH

People who are taking strong anti-cancer drugs frequently suffer from dry mouth. It happens because the cocktail of strong drugs cannot differentiate between good and bad cells, so it kills many cells as well as the cancerous ones.

Here's a tip I picked up in Australia: serve jugs of water with fresh mint, pineapple chunks and slices of orange. It looks great, and the fruits add lovely flavours to the water.

The mouth, hair and stomach are prime targets. The rapidly proliferating cells in the mouth and stomach are particularly likely to be affected by chemotherapy, and this affects the natural process of salivation.

- Have on hand plenty of refreshing tangy juices, and drink these throughout the day. Homemade lemonade, mango juice, or freshly squeezed orange and grapefruit juice can be kept in a jug in the fridge and are a real pleasure to drink. Serve with a leaf or two of fresh mint and you'll be surprised at the delicious flavour. Sorbets are also good when you have a dry mouth.
- For main courses, prepare dishes with plenty of sauce, such as casseroles. Dry foods, and hot, spicy foods, tend to aggravate a dry mouth, so avoid grills, roasts and fries.
- Although a little alcoholic drink can increase the appetite, it reduces the production of saliva in the mouth, which can in turn aggravate swallowing. Choose a non-alcoholic drink with your meal.

SWALLOWING DIFFICULTIES

Difficulty in swallowing (dysphagia) is common in people with mouth or throat cancer. Sometimes a chilled drink will help the action of swallowing, and of course it is best to choose foods that are naturally soft, such as soufflés, omelettes, soups, mousses and vegetable purées. Although some health professionals recommend liquidizing all meals, this is not necessary and generally not very appealing. It's important not to isolate yourself with sub-standard food.

STOMACH AND BOWEL UPSET

Many cancer patients seem to suffer from constipation; I have given advice about this on page 149. If diarrhoea is the problem, try to stick to dishes that are not too high in vegetable fibre, as fibre can be too rough for the stomach and bowel to tolerate. You also need to avoid fatty foods. If you are trying to put on weight and need to boost your calorie consumption, stagger your fat intake throughout the day, so that your body can tolerate the fat more easily. Have six small meals containing some fat, rather than having non-fatty foods all day and then eating fish and chips in the evening, for example.

- Avoid a lot of dairy products in one go, because sometimes the concentration of lactose (milk sugar) can upset the stomach. Instead, use dairy products combined with other ingredients in a recipe.
- Ginger, camomile and mint teas are good digestive settlers.

SENSITIVE STOMACH

The stomach seems to fare badly when you are taking chemotherapy drugs or having radiotherapy on the stomach. This happens because cancer treatments attack cells that rapidly divide; cancer cells behave in this way, but unfortunately so do stomach cells, so the treatments bombard it. In addition, the strong pain-killers that are prescribed to help ease your discomfort can sometimes make your stomach even more sensitive. To minimize the negative effects of painkillers, it is best not to take them on an empty stomach.

- Choose plain rather than highly spiced food.
- Try to eat a little something every three to four hours, to give your stomach a coating. It could just be a biscuit or a slice of bread with a little cheese or cold meat.
- Avoid the temptation to drink milk. Although this gives you an initial cooling effect, it makes your stomach secrete more acid in the long run. Try ginger drinks or camomile or mint tea, which are much more settling. (For more information, see the section on indigestion, page 155.)

SICKNESS AND NAUSEA

Although food is the last thing you want to think about when you are feeling sick, sometimes just managing a little something, however small, can help ease the nausea. This is because the food soaks up some of the stomach acids that can aggravate nausea. It also stops your blood sugar level from going too low, which can in itself cause you to feel sick. There are a few simple steps you can take to ease nausea and sickness.

- If you have someone to help you cook, let them do it for you when you are not feeling well. Cooking smells can sometimes put you off your food.
- While food is being prepared, go for a little walk if you are up to it. Not only will the fresh air perk up your appetite, but it will also reduce the stale feeling of sickness. If you are not well enough, simply sit outside for a little, or by an open window. Fill your lungs with fresh air, and you will feel more lively and keen for your meal.
- If you are eating alone, settle for cold dishes. Often these are more appealing when you are feeling sick. Try something light but flavourful, such as ciabatta bread with Parma ham, or a tomato, mozzarella and avocado salad.
- Keep stores of favourite things in your freezer, so that you can get them out when you do not feel up to much else.
- Ginger is one of the most settling flavours. Some people find sucking on a piece of crystallized ginger relieves nausea. Keeping some ginger drinks in the fridge is a good idea. See my recipes for ginger punch (page 50) and ginger tea (page 343), or you can buy ginger cordial, which mixes with still or sparkling water.

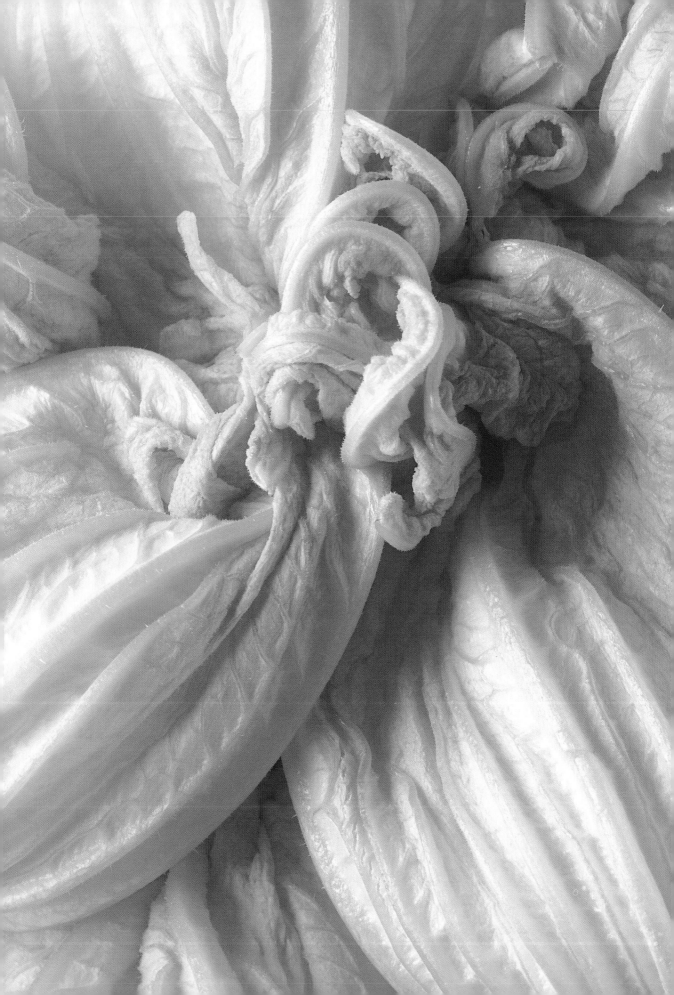

High blood cholesterol

There is a lot of confusion about cholesterol. Most people know that it is linked to heart disease and fat – but that's about the extent of their knowledge. Cholesterol is a whitish, fatty, wax-like substance (a lipid) that is both produced in the body and found in foods. Excess cholesterol in the bloodstream can clog and narrow the arteries, increasing the risk of heart attack, stroke and kidney disease. Hyperlipidaemia is the technical name for the presence of abnormally high levels of lipids (cholesterol and triglycerides) within the blood. A high level of blood fats is a risk factor in heart disease, which kills 83,000 men and 70,000 women in Great Britain every year, but the positive news is that evidence strongly suggests that improving the blood fat profile helps reduce the risk of heart disease.

As many as two in every three men, and increasingly more women, have unhealthy levels of blood fats. Symptoms include yellowish nodules of fat in the skin beneath the eyes, elbows, knees and in the tendons, or in some cases a whitish ring around the eye. The majority are unaware of these symptoms – opticians may be the first ones to notice. People may discover that they have hyperlipidaemia when they undergo a routine blood test.

Astonishingly we are now finding children as young as eight or nine with raised lipid levels and even the first signs of atherosclerosis, furring of the arteries. This is a trend we need to stop. Encouraging your child to eat and live healthily is most important.

CHOLESTEROL

Cholesterol is produced by the body, primarily in the liver. It is also present in certain foods. The cholesterol we eat is known as dietary cholesterol, and has little relationship with the cholesterol in the blood. Cholesterol is not all bad news. It plays an essential part in the production of sex hormones, is involved in the synthesis of vitamin D and is also needed for the production of the myelin sheath, the protective substance which surrounds the nerves.

Cholesterol only creates a problem when you have too much of it in your body; then, it can promote the production of a fatty plaque, which can clog up your arteries. If this happens the blood flow is interrupted, which in a main heart vessel can cause a heart attack, or in the blood vessel leading to your brain, a stroke. Blocked arteries also cause circulation problems; numbness and pain in your hands and feet.

The cholesterol made within the body needs to be broken down into a usable form and delivered to the cells which need it. The liver repackages cholesterol as low-density lipoprotein (LDL). As LDL flows through the blood, it latches on to receptor sites on the cells which need the cholesterol. When the cells have had enough cholesterol, they stop producing the receptor sites. When this happens, the unused LDL stays in the blood and can irritate the blood vessel lining, which in turn causes a fatty plaque to form.

Other factors can irritate the cells in the lining of the blood vessels and make them more susceptible to developing a plaque. The nicotine from cigarettes, and abnormally high sugar levels, such as are found in uncontrolled diabetics, are two such factors. Fundamentally, however, the plaque would not be able to form if there was no LDL around. If you have too much LDL in your blood, this is usually referred to as having 'bad' cholesterol.

The 'good' type of cholesterol is high-density lipoprotein (HDL). HDL carries the excess LDL cholesterol from your blood back to your intestine, where it is excreted.

TRIGLYCERIDES

These are another type of blood fat, produced in the body in response to alcohol, hormones and sugar. Although they are different from cholesterol, they too have been linked with heart disease – and pancreatic cancer – so it is important to keep them within the ideal range.

REFERENCE AND SUGGESTED 'HEALTHY' RANGES FOR PLASMA LIPIDS IN ADULTS UNDER 60 YEARS

	Reference range mmol/l	Suggested range mmol/l
Total cholesterol	3.5–7.8	<5.2
Low density lipoprotein (LDL) cholesterol	2.3–6.1	<4.0
High density lipoprotein (HDL) cholesterol	0.8–1.7	>1.15
Triglycerides	0.7–1.8	0.7–1.7

mmol/l = millimoles per litre

Taken from Manual of Dietetic Practice, second edition, 1994. Edited for The British Dietetic Association by Briony Thomas.

Blackwell Scientific Publications

The figures in the table are given to help you interpret a doctor's test of your blood fats (plasma lipids). The reference range is calculated from the mean of an apparently healthy population. Age and sex differences need to be considered:
• Blood fats may increase with age, consequently a cholesterol value in the reference range of 7.0 mmol/l would be much more noteworthy in a person of 25 years than one of 55 years.
• Triglycerides are generally higher in men than women; HDL levels are higher in women than men.

Up until a woman enters her menopausal years, the female hormone oestrogen alters the metabolism of cholesterol and helps to keep LDL levels low. After the menopause, when oestrogen levels drop considerably, the effect is lost, which explains why women's risk of heart disease and strokes increases at this point. Nowadays more and more women are sidestepping the menopausal years by taking hormone replacements for various reasons. Hormone replacement therapy can lower LDL and increase beneficial HDL levels, but so far this has been demonstrated only among women who take a pure oestrogen-based hormone replacement, which is prescribed only to women who have had their womb removed.

Other hormonal medication, such as the contraceptive pill, can increase LDL and lower HDL levels, which is one of the reasons why doctors need to make regular checks on women taking the pill.

For men there does not appear to be any hormone-related change in their life risk of developing heart disease.

TESTING YOUR BLOOD FATS

As I have already said, many people are unaware that they have a blood fat problem. In this case, ignorance is not bliss; high blood fats present a serious risk of heart disease, but the risk can be reduced through modifications to your diet and lifestyle. Your doctor can give you a blood test, or you can buy accurate self-testing kits at pharmacies. Since the food you eat can raise your blood fat levels, doctors recommend that you take a 'fasting' sample; this is best done first thing in the morning, because you must not eat anything for eight to ten hours before the test. Look at the results in conjunction with the previous paragraph to see whether, or to what extent, you need to alter your eating habits.

WHY DOES IT MATTER?

To reduce the risk of heart disease you need to make sure your LDL and triglyceride levels are low and your HDL level is high, to excrete as much LDL as possible. Every case of hyperlipidaemia is slightly different, but the best way to see your way through the jungle of advice is to understand how to build up a good blood profile.

If you have high blood fat levels, you can decrease them by 25 per cent by adopting a healthy diet. Your body produces 75 per cent of your blood fats, regardless of what you eat. However, the 25 per cent reduction can significantly reduce your risk of developing heart disease and therefore should be taken seriously. It is never too late to change your blood profile for the better.

If you don't have raised blood fats, this is the point at which you should pay most attention, as the longer you can stave them off the healthier your life should be. Equally, those of you with children should remember that hyperlipidaemia is not confined to adults; young people die of heart disease, so the sooner you begin to protect your child's blood vessels the better.

How to build up a good blood profile

There are several nutritional measures which can change your blood fat profile. Some people believe that eggs, shellfish and offal (liver, kidneys) should be banished from their diet and margarine should replace butter. This is not strictly correct. Although these foods contain cholesterol (as do all animal-derived foods, including cream, cheese, chicken and fish), they do not have a significant impact on blood cholesterol levels. The cholesterol from the foods we eat is broken down quite efficiently. Obviously, if you have a lot of these foods and few of the cholesterol-lowering foods, your blood cholesterol level may be a little high. But in the majority of people I see, this is not the situation.

So lobster, prawns, liver and eggs need not be banned from the table (they all contain plenty of other useful nutrients), they just need to be eaten in moderation and in a way that allows the body to metabolize the food efficiently. This normally means combining them with some fibre (see next page).

The major principles in building a healthy blood scenario are:
• to keep your intake of saturated fats low
• to keep the HDL level high enough to excrete the LDL
• to prevent excess LDL from depositing in your blood vessels
• to avoid exposure to any other heart disease risk factors.
You need to know which foods to eat more of and which are the foods to watch.

KEEP YOUR INTAKE OF SATURATED FATS LOW

The major influence on the level of LDL in the blood is not the intake of cholesterol-rich foods, but the intake of saturated fats. Sometimes these are found in the same foods – butter, cream, cheese – but prawns and offal, although high in cholesterol, are low in fat. Saturated animal fats stimulate the liver to produce more LDL, therefore keeping the intake of these foods low is the best way to keep your blood cholesterol level down. Choose lean meat rather than fatty cuts, and have small amounts of butter, cream and cheese because you enjoy the taste, not just out of habit.

I do not suggest that you avoid all cheese; not only is it delicious, it is also a good source of calcium and other nutrients. Interestingly, the creamier cheeses such as Brie and Camembert contain slightly less fat than the harder varieties. Also, if you cut off the white rind, you virtually halve the fat content.

Saturated fat is also found in some margarines, especially hard margarines. Even if you do not buy them as such, remember that they are used in many shop-bought cakes, biscuits and pastry products.

For cooking, stick to using a small amount of vegetable oils such as olive or sunflower.

One trap that some of my patients fall into is to think they can 'cure' their high cholesterol levels and then go back to their old ways. They go for weeks replacing butter with margarine, cheese with 'low fat' cheese substitutes, avoiding eggs, shellfish and offal, and feeling deprived and desperate for the day when the results come back from the lab saying that their cholesterol level has come down, so that they can get back to eating the 'real' foods they love. It is much better to adjust to a generally healthier lifestyle which can include butter, cheese, and other delicious foods, as long as they are eaten in moderation and in a way that helps the body deal with fats efficiently – with some fibre and water.

INCREASE YOUR INTAKE OF FIBRE

The best way to control the amount of LDL in the body is to change the balance between foods that produce LDL and those that allow the body to excrete LDL. Fibre helps your body in two ways. Firstly the fibre produces substances that help to clear the blood of LDL and secondly the presence of fibre in your meals acts as a buffer. Less fat is brought into contact with your blood vessels, which means that less fat is absorbed and more LDL is kept bound within the gut and then excreted.

A healthy, well balanced diet rich in high fibre foods such as wholegrain breads and cereals, pulses, vegetables and fruits enables the body to excrete more LDL. Eating the recommended five helpings of fresh vegetables and fruits and a selection of other high fibre foods every day really helps to bring your blood fat profile within the ideal range.

Oats are a particularly good form of fibre for reducing cholesterol, so begin your day with porridge or an oat cereal, have oatcakes as snacks and use oats in main meals such as fruit or vegetable crumbles. Oats are useful for people who have a limited tolerance of gluten; the gluten content is far lower than in wheat products such as bread and pasta. Oatcakes are a perfect partner for cheese: the oat fibre reduces the intake of saturated fat from the cheese and helps your body produce more HDL, which will enable LDL to be excreted.

INCREASE YOUR INTAKE OF HDL-PRODUCING FOODS

Two foods that have been the subject of much research are oily fish and garlic.

Oily fish such as herrings, mackerel, tuna and salmon contain beneficial types of fat called omega 3 and omega 6 fatty acids. These fatty acids encourage your body to produce HDL, which helps to remove LDL. Garlic also contains a substance which raises your HDL levels. Both garlic and oily fish contain other substances which reduce your risk of developing a blood clot or thrombosis. A clot is a collection of blood cells which can block a blood vessel in a similar way to a deposit of fatty plaque, so the more we can do to prevent this, the better.

Try to use garlic and oily fish in your weekly eating plan. Garlic could be included almost every day, and I recommend that you aim to have two or three fish-based meals every week. Many of the soups and savoury recipes in this book contain garlic, and for your 'fish suppers' you could try seared tuna on a bed of spinach (see page 323), or simple barbecued sardines or grilled herrings. If you worry about the aftertaste and smell of garlic, chewing a sprig of parsley or sucking a coffee bean are said to reduce the effects.

GOOD OLD ALCOHOL

Another foodstuff which has been shown to increase HDL cholesterol and there-fore reduce LDL levels, and also reduce the risk of thrombosis, is alcohol – in moderation. Alcohol in excess of the recommended maximum of 28 units for men and 21 units for women can increase not only the total amount of choles-terol and LDL, but also blood triglycerides, all of which increase the risk of heart disease. Excessive alcohol also increases the risk of cardiomyopathy (disease of the heart muscle) and liver damage.

Wine drinkers seem to enjoy better cardiovascular health than either beer drinkers or teetotallers, provided they have no more than two glasses of wine a day. The next best drink seems to be cloudy (sedimented or yeasty) beer, but all forms of alcohol are better for the blood fat levels than abstention.

Red wines are also rich in antioxidants (see below), substances that prevent LDL from depositing in the blood vessels. Recent studies suggest that a couple of glasses of red wine a day can reduce the risk of heart disease because of high levels of the antioxidants anthocyanin and tannin. See page 48 for more information. For those of you who don't like red wine, the darker beers contain more beneficial antioxidants than paler beers, but not as many as red wine.

Do check with your doctor before you drink any alcohol, in case any medica-tion you are taking is likely to interact adversely, or indeed there may be another contraindication in your health.

KEEP UP YOUR INTAKE OF ANTIOXIDANTS

There is little harm in fat circulating around the body, unless it starts to deposit. In order for fat to deposit, it needs to oxidize. Nutritionally we can stop this by eating plenty of foods containing antioxidants, as well as drinking a moderate amount of alcohol (see above).

The most powerful antioxidants found in food are beta-carotene (which the body converts to vitamin A), vitamin C and vitamin E. Good sources of these are discussed in more detail in the section on Understanding your nutritional needs, but basically if you eat at least five portions of fresh fruits or vegetables every day you should cover your needs. By a portion, I mean a piece of fruit such as a whole orange or kiwi fruit, a large helping of spinach, broccoli or carrots, or a bowl of vegetable soup. I suggest you have three pieces of antioxidant-rich fresh fruits and include a salad or vegetable portion at your two main meals. Besides green leafy vegetables and avocados (a particularly rich source), vitamin E is also found in nuts such as almonds and hazelnuts, seeds such as sunflower seeds – and therefore sunflower oil – and wholegrain cereals.

There has been so much interest surrounding antioxidants in connection with reducing heart disease and cancer that many people wonder whether they should be taking a supplement. I do not believe that this is necessary, as long as you are eating a well balanced diet with at least five portions of fresh fruits or vegetables every day, don't smoke and don't bombard your body with junk food.

Stay good

HOW GUT BACTERIA MAY HELP

Two bacteria found in the intestine, acidophilus and bifidus, are thought to produce substances which encourage the body to excrete more LDL and possibly raise HDL levels. Research is still in its early days, but I suggest you eat a small pot of live yoghurt containing these bacteria every day.

EAT SMALL MEALS OFTEN

Leaving your gut without any food for hours and hours and then putting a large meal into it is not healthy. This habit not only puts a strain on your digestion, it is also thought to raise your LDL levels.

Other risk factors

Besides the above nutritional measures you can take to improve your blood fat profile, there are other influences to consider. Some are hormonal (see page 253), but other factors seem to affect men as well as women: these include smoking, being over-fat, and lack of exercise. Diabetics are prone to suffer from heart disease, but hopefully as we come to understand more about controlling blood sugar levels (see the chapter on Diabetes) this will cease to be such a risk factor.

- Caffeine and nicotine both irritate the blood vessel linings, making them more likely to develop fatty plaques. Try to keep your caffeine intake down to no more than two or three cups of coffee, tea or cola a day, and stop smoking.
- Exercise, particularly aerobic exercise, helps to reduce blood fat levels and also helps reduce your risk of developing heart disease in other ways. Three times a week try to include a twenty-minute session of an aerobic exercise such as running, jogging, power walking or brisk walking, swimming or cycling. Always check with your doctor before you take up any form of exercise.
- In addition to the lipid-lowering effects of aerobic exercise, exercise is a good stress reliever. Stress can cause your liver to produce more fat, in particular LDL cholesterol. Since stress is also a risk factor in many other diseases, you should take steps to reduce the stress levels in your life.
- Excess weight, or more specifically excess fat, especially around the middle, is bad news for your heart in two ways. Firstly, obesity tends to reduce the levels of the 'good' HDL cholesterol in your blood, and secondly it leads to an increased risk of high blood pressure (see next chapter). It is the fat which fills the stomach area and puts pressure on the major blood vessels to the heart that causes most concern. This tends to be more common in men than women.

  Cutting down on your intake of saturated fats and increasing the amount of vegetables, fruit and high fibre foods will encourage healthy weight loss. If you need more advice, see the chapter on Achieving your ideal weight. Don't be tempted to crash diet, as this can place undue strain on your heart.

High cholesterol is a risk factor, not a disease. If your lifestyle is healthy and your lipid levels remain slightly above the ideal, don't worry too much.

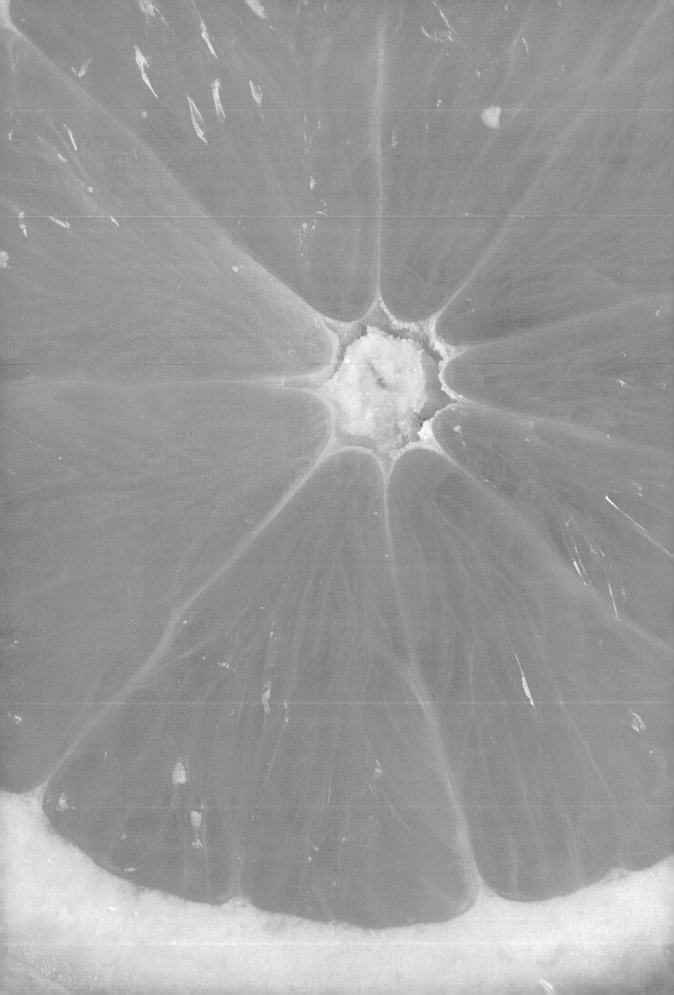

High blood pressure

High blood pressure, or hypertension, is a well documented risk factor in heart attacks, strokes and angina. Most people with high blood pressure have no symptoms, but it is commonly observed during company and routine medical checks. The development of high blood pressure is one of the first signs that the body is not coping with some aspect of life; it could be excess weight, smoking, stress, lack of exercise, poor eating habits.

While many people are told that they have high blood pressure, few know what it means and how food and lifestyle changes can help them correct it. Blood pressure is the force exerted by the flow of blood through your blood vessels. Blood pressure readings are expressed as one number over another. The upper (systolic) measurement reflects the force when the heart is pumping blood around the body; the lower (diastolic) reading is the pressure which exists in the blood vessels when they are relaxed between heart beats. Normal blood pressure readings are in the region of 120/80. The latter figure, representing diastolic pressure, is the important one in terms of establishing whether you have hypertension. Those with a diastolic pressure between 90 and 105 are considered to be mildly hypertensive; 105 to 120 represents moderate hypertension; severe hypertension (high blood pressure) is when the pressure is above 120.

Hypertension can be caused by heart or kidney problems, but in nine out of ten cases there is no known cause. Hypertension tends to run in families, and blood pressure usually increases as we get older. If there are underlying problems you may need to take medication, but for the majority of people, who suffer from simple hypertension, you can help yourself by a few modifications to your lifestyle: reducing stress; taking exercise; quitting smoking; looking at the way you eat; and choosing foods and drinks that help rather than hinder your body.

Why worry about high blood pressure?

If hypertension is ignored it can lead to problems such as heart disease, strokes or kidney problems. Some people need to take medication to help control their blood pressure, but most doctors suggest exploring all of the non-drug remedies first. Remember that all drugs have side effects; in the case of antihypertensives these may include weight gain, chronic tiredness, feeling low, and in some cases lack of libido and impotence. It is much better to see what you can do within your diet and lifestyle to help bring your blood pressure down.

How to correct hypertension

The most common contributory factors to hypertension are excess weight, stress, and high blood fat levels. Smoking is a strong risk factor in the development of hypertension and of course in many forms of heart disease and cancers. If you smoke try to give up.

TRY TO KEEP YOUR WEIGHT WITHIN THE IDEAL RANGE

In particular, excess fat around the middle of the body presses on the important blood vessels leading to and from the heart and hence aggravates blood pressure. Women with 'pear-shaped' figures – with more weight round the hips – have less of a problem than 'apple-shaped' women and men, who commonly tend to stack the weight around their middles. If you are carrying excess fat in this area you may well find that if you reduce it your blood pressure will improve and may even cease to become a problem. Some people become obsessed with their body weight, hopping on the scales every day. This is unnecessary, and is not really telling you anything you cannot see for yourself in a mirror. The scales may put you within your ideal weight range, but fat around the middle will still aggravate hypertension. Be honest with yourself and if necessary read the chapter on Achieving your ideal weight. Do not 'crash diet', as this can put your body under stress. Never take drugs to help you lose weight as they can cause dramatic rises in blood pressure.

TRY TO REDUCE STRESS

Build time into your daily schedule to allow yourself to relax. There are many excellent courses, tapes and books designed to help you reduce stress, so hunt them out. Some people learn to meditate or experiment with aromatherapy, others play a musical instrument, paint, or take yoga classes.

TAKE REGULAR EXERCISE

One of the easiest ways to reduce stress and also improve your general feeling of well-being is taking physical exercise. Try to get into the habit of doing some regular aerobic exercise throughout the week. Good aerobic exercise includes brisk walking, swimming, running, cycling and roller blading. (Exercise such as weightlifting and squash is not as effective in bringing blood pressure down, although you may think you thrash out stress on the court. These exercises that use short bursts of power tend to increase blood pressure; gentler, longer-lasting exercises are the ones to go for.) Always check with your doctor before you embark on any exercise programme, as he or she will be able to advise you as to the type and level at which you should train. Some people fall into the trap of trying to force exercise to fit into their schedule. Workers rush from the office to work out at lunch time and then rush back to the office feeling shattered. Treating fitness as a military exercise creates stress and will not help lower your blood pressure. Neither will pushing your body to the limits on the running machine. You would be much better off exercising in a more relaxed manner, perhaps only managing twice a week in the gym and taking a brisk lunchtime walk or roller blading in the park on the other days.

How food can help

Many of the points made in the previous chapter about how to improve the balance of the different types of fat in your blood are relevant here. If excess fat is deposited in the blood vessels, it reduces the space through which blood can flow and causes the pressure within the blood vessels to rise. If you have a high cholesterol level, do everything you can to keep it as low as possible. Keep your intake of animal fats such as butter, cream and cheese low, and boost your intake of fibre and water.

Some exciting research has recently shown that a diet rich in fresh fruits and vegetables can significantly reduce blood pressure. This is independent of their cholesterol-lowering effects, but may be linked to both their antioxidant content and their potassium content. Everyone should try to eat at least five portions of fresh fruits or vegetables every day.

First of all, make sure your diet is well balanced: besides plenty of fresh fruits and vegetables, you need plenty of high fibre starchy foods and water, smaller but regular amounts of lean proteins and dairy products, with minimal amounts of fat, sugar and caffeine (coffee, tea and cola drinks). Consider organizing a family health day (see page 81), as this will give you the time to take stock of your life and encourage you to instigate the necessary changes in your diet. In addition to a generally healthy lifestyle, a few specific areas of your diet may be particularly effective in reducing blood pressure.

A PINCH OF SALT

As well as watching your fat intake you need to make sure that you are not consuming too much salt. Salt (sodium chloride) can increase fluid retention and blood pressure. Sodium naturally exists in small amounts in many foods, including vegetables and fruits, but it is found in far greater quantities in prepared foods. Salt acts as a preservative, helping to keep food free of harmful bacteria, and also enhances flavour.

Rather than avoiding all processed foods, you can reach a sensible compromise by including small quantities of them in your weekly eating plan alongside plenty of fresh foods. Keep very salty foods down to a minimum. Your tongue and taste buds will usually tell you which these are, but they include olives, salted nuts, pickles, and cured and tinned fish and meats such as kippers and Parma ham. (Occasionally your taste buds can be fooled: cornflakes have a greater salt concentration than the Atlantic Ocean!)

Another step in reducing your salt intake is to get out of the habit of adding unnecessary salt in cooking. Try to wean yourself off this habit, as the more salt you have, the more your body thinks it needs before it recognizes the salt taste.

Look for the natural flavours of fresh fish, meat and vegetables first, then think about enhancing them rather than masking them with copious amounts of salt. Experiment with other flavours, such as herbs and spices, or marinate foods in wine before cooking. Mix vegetables and fruits to create different tastes. Always taste food before adding salt at the table. If you cut down your sodium intake, your blood pressure should improve.

BOOST YOUR POTASSIUM INTAKE

The best way to reduce the sodium level within your body is to increase the amount of potassium. These two minerals work together like a pair of scales – you should aim to get the balance right. By boosting your intake of potassium-rich foods your body should be able to maintain a healthy sodium level. It is usually people who overindulge in salty foods and don't eat a generally healthy diet who run into problems with salt-induced hypertension. You should not take any form of potassium supplement unless prescribed by your doctor. They are potentially very dangerous.

Potassium is found in abundance in most fresh (not canned) fruits and vegetables. The following are especially rich sources:

Fruit: apricots, bananas, blackcurrants, dates, grapes, grapefruit, kiwi fruit, cantaloupe melons, oranges, passionfruit, paw paw (papaya), peaches and plums, being even higher in the dried versions such as prunes, apricots, sultanas and raisins.

Vegetables: avocados, broad beans, peas, potatoes, tomatoes, squash such as courgettes and pumpkins. Cook vegetables without salt, and taste them before you add salt.

INCLUDE SOME DAIRY PRODUCTS IN YOUR DAILY DIET

Milk and natural yoghurt are rich in potassium, and, along with other dairy products, are also the major source of calcium in the Western diet. Calcium has been found to be helpful in correcting high blood pressure. Of course, some dairy products (cheese, butter, cream) are high in saturated fats, so you should not go overboard with them or you risk an increase in blood fat levels, but dairy products in moderation can help improve blood pressure. You can easily obtain sufficient calcium if you incorporate skimmed and semi-skimmed milk in drinks and naturally lower fat dairy foods such as yoghurt and fromage frais in your everyday cooking. If you don't like dairy products, or for more information on calcium, see page 42.

GARLIC

Several studies suggest that garlic contains substances which help reduce high blood pressure. Get into the habit of including garlic regularly in savoury dishes, sauces and dressings.

OILY FISH

Mackerel, fresh herrings, sardines, pilchards, salmon, trout and tuna are all rich in omega 3 fatty acids, beneficial oils that help prevent cholesterol from depositing in your blood vessels. Eating a meal based on oily fish two or three times a week can help control your blood pressure.

ANTIOXIDANTS

Antioxidants help reduce blood pressure as well as helping to prevent blood fats from depositing in your blood vessels. A healthy, well balanced eating plan will include foods rich in natural antioxidants (especially beta-carotene and vitamins C and E), found chiefly in fresh fruits and vegetables. Try to have five pieces of fruit or helpings of vegetables every day.

Don't forget that there are also antioxidants in red wine (see page 48). One or two glasses a day can be beneficial, unless there is another reason why you are unable to take red wine.

There is no need to take antioxidant supplements. Not only are they unnecessary, they can cause the balance of nutrients within your body to become unbalanced.

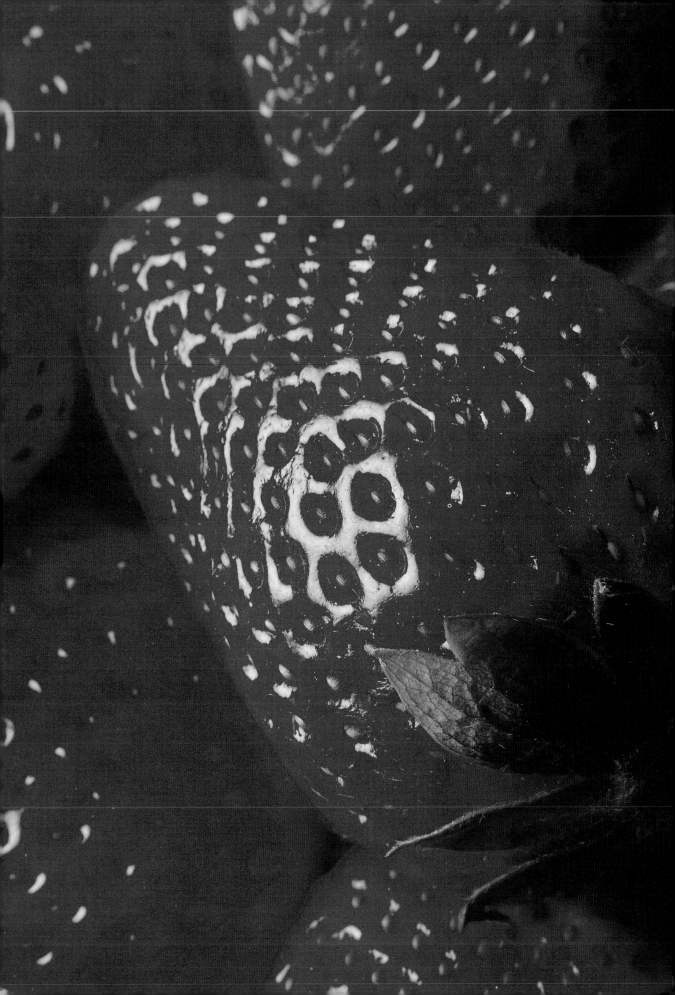

Diabetes

Today, diabetes mellitus, the most common form of diabetes, is easily managed; professional sports people cope, and even young children go about their day-to-day lives without any fuss. It's just a question of understanding how your body can compensate for its inability to control blood sugar levels. Experiences and lifestyle challenges differ, depending on age and the severity of diabetes, but the more normal you consider the situation, the less over-protective you are of your child or a diabetic partner, friend or relative, the more likely you all are to lead a happy and healthy life.

What is diabetes?

Diabetes mellitus takes three forms, distinguished by their treatment protocols. Some diabetics can control their diabetes simply by monitoring their diet; others need tablets to stimulate the body to produce more insulin; some diabetics require insulin injections.

The condition is characterized by an increased amount of sugar in the blood. This happens because there is a lack of insulin, the hormone the body needs to process sugar effectively. After you have eaten foods containing sugar, your blood sugar level rises, whereupon the pancreas releases insulin to help the cells absorb and use the sugar. The blood sugar level should then return to normal. With diabetes there is not enough insulin in the body to help the cells absorb the sugar. The sugar is present, but the body cannot use it.

This happens for two main reasons. In some people the pancreas is incapable of producing any insulin, as is most commonly found in children and young adults. In this case they need to have insulin injections. This type of diabetes is called insulin-dependent diabetes mellitus (IDDM). In other people the pancreas can produce some insulin, but not enough for the body's needs. This type, non insulin-dependent diabetes mellitus (NIDDM), is more common in older people, especially those who are overweight. Either the pancreas gets tired or the cells, particularly fat cells, seem unable to take up the sugar. Some diabetics in this category can control their blood sugar levels by losing excess weight (in particular, fat), as this takes the strain off the pancreas and improves the body's ability to utilize the small amounts of insulin produced. In some cases the pancreas is capable but seems unable to produce the insulin when it is needed; it needs a kick start from tablets.

Abnormally high quantities of sugar in the blood can cause potentially serious problems. In the long term, if the sugar levels continually run high, a state called hyperglycaemia, several tissues in the body start to suffer, especially the eyes, kidney and blood vessels leading to the arms and legs. But once the sugar level is corrected and controlled, diabetics lead normal, healthy lives.

One of the first symptoms noted by diabetics is an excessive, unquenchable thirst, often associated with frequent passing of urine (the most effective way for the body to get rid of excess sugar is by passing urine). This can be coupled with fatigue, headaches and nausea. Children appear listless and tetchy. Some people feel unusually hungry, because even though your body has excess sugar in the blood, it cannot utilize it without insulin.

Many people do not recognize the symptoms of diabetes and go to the doctor reporting a different complaint. For example, men go to the GP believing they have a prostate problem, only to find that they are diabetic. Other people are diagnosed as diabetic by accident; a routine blood test can reveal a raised blood sugar level. Every year around 60,000 people in the UK are diagnosed with diabetes; 1,500 of these are children. Some children are diagnosed at birth, others develop diabetes a little later, or even in their late teens.

Treatment

Many factors determine the type of treatment that will be effective. It is usually the case that the younger you are when you develop diabetes, the more likely you are to need insulin. Older people are often able to control their condition with a few adjustments to their diet and lifestyle.

Diabetics' lives have changed profoundly over the past decade. Tablets can now stimulate the pancreas to produce more insulin, and synthetic and animal insulins have become so efficient that they can act both on a short- and long-term basis, which gives those of you who need insulin injections a greater flexibility with eating and lifestyle. Injections are now administered by pen-like needles which are so fine they can be popped into the body through clothes, making them almost fuss-free.

Equally, gone are the days when it was almost a foregone conclusion that you would have to eat at set times, measure all carbohydrates, and banish all sweet foods, including fruit, from your diet. With young children it is sometimes necessary to measure foods to begin with, so they can get an idea of how much food they need to take and at which times. For others, it may be necessary to stick to some sort of schedule until the insulin and diet balance is achieved.

Some doctors find that the best way to control a diabetic diet is to measure the blood sugar levels. However, not all diabetics need to do this; it is usually suggested only for insulin dependent diabetics and uncontrolled diabetics whom the doctors want to stabilize. Tablet takers may be asked to monitor their blood sugar levels from time to by testing their urine for sugar. Insulin dependent diabetics are often encouraged to monitor their blood sugar level regularly by taking small samples of blood from a pinprick to the thumb. Accurate and easily available devices offer precise blood sugar level measurements and so assist in making adjustments to the insulin or diet. This should always be overseen by your doctor and dietitian.

Diet and diabetes

In terms of what diabetics need to eat, the principles are the same as for a non-diabetic person: a healthy, balanced diet that includes a regular intake of high fibre foods, plenty of water, some fresh vegetables and fruit, some lean proteins and dairy products, and a small amount of fat. The only differences are that you need to be extra diligent about balancing your diet with your medication, if you take it, and that you need to be more regular in your eating habits. While non-diabetic people can go for days before a bad diet catches up with them, diabetics don't have this flexibility.

A diabetic diet is a healthy diet. There are foods such as chocolate gateaux in which you shouldn't overindulge – but neither should non-diabetics. As long as you are aware of the effect the food will have on your body and act appropriately, you should be able to enjoy birthday parties, restaurant meals and all 'foodie' occasions.

There is no need to include special diabetic products in a diabetic diet. Not only do many of them taste very unlike their non-diabetic equivalents, they often contain unnecessary substances that have no part in a healthy diet. For example, many diabetic products contain sugar substitutes such as sorbitol and manitol, which can have a laxative effect The calorie content is sometimes higher than the non-diabetic, 'normal' equivalent, which can lead to weight gain – the last thing you need.

There are two major targets to achieve with your diet:
• to achieve and maintain control of your blood sugar level
• to regulate your body weight within the ideal range (see page 109).
The key points of a healthy diabetic eating plan are as follows:

HIGH FIBRE CARBOHYDRATES
Your body needs sugar for energy, and when you are diabetic, it's a question of regulating the amount. The best way of maintaining a steady release of sugar into your blood is from high fibre carbohydrates, such as wholemeal bread, wholewheat and oat cereals, brown rice, potatoes. The fibre in these foods slows down the release of sugar into the blood. This makes it easier to keep the blood sugar level within the desirable range.

Try to keep to roughly the same amount of carbohydrate in each of your meals. With the help of your doctor and dietitian, work out how much carbohydrate you need to maintain good blood sugar and energy levels and maintain your weight at a comfortable level. The majority of people will find they need roughly the same amount they would choose had they not been told they were diabetic. The advantage of high fibre carbohydrates is their satiety value – they make you feel appropriately full and contented, which can help you judge when you have eaten enough.

Don't think that high fibre foods are all heavy, dry and boring. These days you can buy delicious wholegrain and seeded breads with nuts, sun-dried tomatoes, herbs and spices. Look for the dark German rye breads, or Irish wholemeal soda breads. Serve strawberries or poached pears with your porridge, or try homemade apricot muesli (see page 304). I have also given plenty of recipes for high fibre desserts.

Having said this, various groups of diabetics need to moderate their consumption of high fibre carbohydrates. For example, children – and diabetic people with other medical conditions such as cancer – need a combination of high fibre and low fibre foods. If they just eat high fibre carbohydrates, they may not receive enough energy and essential vitamins and minerals from their food. People with digestive complains such as irritable bowel syndrome or Crohn's disease may have a problem balancing a diabetic high-fibre diet with their other medical requirements. Seek the advice of your doctor or dietitian.

If you need to include some lower fibre carbohydrate in your diet, you should regulate the portion size of the lower fibre carbohydrate and boost the fibre content of the meal with vegetables, pulses or fruits. There are no more calories or carbohydrates in white bread or rice than in the wholegrain versions, it's just that they release their sugar into the bloodstream more quickly; you are aiming to slow down that release by including some non-cereal fibre in the meal.

FRUIT AND VEGETABLES
As with any healthy diet, try to have five portions of fresh vegetables or fruits every day – not only does their fibre content help to regulate your blood sugar levels, they are also high in health-giving vitamins and minerals.

Some people mistakenly believe that fruit is too high in sugar for diabetics to enjoy. Although fruits do contain some sugar, mainly fructose, the fibre within the fruit helps to slow down the release of the sugar and therefore poses few problems for diabetics. It's good to get into the habit of having a portion after and in between meals. A portion would be a whole pear, orange, apple, a large plum, half a paw paw (papaya), about ten grapes or fresh strawberries or raspberries. The 'sweeter' fruits such as pineapples, mangoes, Galia or Charentais melons, bananas and figs have a little more sugar than apples and oranges, so I would suggest that you just have one of these a day. As well as puddings or toppings for breakfast cereals, serve melon or figs with Parma ham as a first course, or make fruit shakes: strawberry and passionfruit or raspberry and orange are just two delicious ideas. Tinned or frozen fruits are fine, as long as they are stored in their natural juice rather than sugary syrups.

Aim to have at least two helpings of vegetables during the day. This could be a main course salad, a bowl of vegetable soup, or salad in your sandwich at lunch time and then a vegetable main course or a good-sized selection of vegetables with your evening meal. Frozen or tinned vegetables can be fine on occasion; they often contain as many if not more vitamins and minerals as fresh. (Do not count potatoes as part of your helpings of vegetables – they should be treated as carbohydrates.)

FATS

Diabetics are more prone to developing heart disease because their blood contains more sugar than in non-diabetics, causing the blood cells to become 'sticky' and more likely to pick up circulating fats that can obstruct the blood vessels. It is therefore important to keep your intake of saturated fats down to a minimum; the same advice is given to non-diabetics. Avoid large amounts of cheese, butter and cream, as well as hydrogenated oils (found in bought pastry, cakes, biscuits and many other manufactured products). Instead, use just a small amount of vegetable oils such as olive oil and choose lean proteins: fish, poultry, game and lean cuts of meat.

DAIRY PRODUCTS

Dairy products are a valuable source of calcium, which is particularly important for women and children. Calcium is needed when you are growing, for healthy teeth and bones, and also when you are going through the menopause and have an increased risk of developing osteoporosis. Men rarely develop osteoporosis, but anyone taking medication that interferes with the balance of calcium in the body, such as strong steroids, should pay attention to their calcium intake. The elderly or bedbound, and people who don't do much exercise, should also take care to include some dairy products in their diet – exercise helps to build and maintain strong bones. Generally the advice is the same as for non-diabetics (see page 42): try to include a certain amount of semi-skimmed, skimmed or calcium-enriched soya milk in your daily eating plan, together with a small pot of 'live' yoghurt containing acidophilus and bifidus cultures. Fromage frais and cottage cheeses are lowest in fat; small amounts of other cheeses are fine for most people.

Dairy products don't adversely affect blood sugar levels, unless they are sugary products such as ice cream or sweetened yoghurts.

ALCOHOL

If you have diabetes, there is no reason why you shouldn't continue to drink alcohol, unless your doctor has told you not to. The only difference is that once you are a diabetic you need to modify the way that you drink, and drink only in moderation. Drinking to excess can make the control of diabetes problematic because of the way it affects your blood sugar levels. In addition, the symptoms of a hypoglycaemic attack (see page 272) are very similar to those experienced when you have had too much alcohol to drink, so your friends may not distinguish one from the other. This is potentially life-threatening.

It is essential to accompany alcohol with some food, especially if you take insulin. Choosing wine with a meal is fine, but drinking on an empty stomach – the pint after work or six o'clock whisky – should be avoided. This is because alcohol causes your blood sugar level to drop, by inhibiting the breakdown of sugar from the glycogen stores within the liver. Don't be fooled into thinking this is advantageous, because the level drops in an uncontrolled, unhealthy way.

All alcoholic drinks are metabolized in a similar way, so choose one you like and drink a small amount of it. The ones to watch are, firstly, sweet wines such as Sauternes. These contain a lot of sugar, so are best left for very special occasions and only when you have eaten plenty of high fibre foods. Spirits combined with mixers should be kept to a minimum; ideally you should choose diet mixers as these contain less sugar. Low-sugar (Pils) beers were created for diabetics, but this was long before current thinking on the management of diabetes. These beers tend to be high in alcohol, so avoid them for this reason.

WATER

As with other people, adults should drink at least two and a half litres/four to five pints of water a day. This amount of water helps excess sugar to be excreted from your body, helps to keep your kidneys and other organs healthy, and allows the fibre in your diet to regulate your blood sugar, as discussed above.

SWEETS AND SUGARY FOODS

Sweet foods are high in a type of sugar which very rapidly enters into the bloodstream. If they are eaten on an empty stomach, they can cause your blood sugar to rise very high. By sweet foods I mean the obvious candidates such as cakes, biscuits, sweets, liquorice and chocolate, honey and sugar-coated cereals, ice creams, canned drinks, squashes and fruit juices. Try to wean yourself off sweetening tea or coffee with sugar or honey.

However, sugary foods can be enjoyed on occasion, as long as you have them in small amounts, within meal times, making sure some fibre is present to cushion the effects of the sugar. For example, instead of having a large chocolate bar in the middle of the afternoon, wait until your evening meal and have a small amount of a good quality, high cocoa bean chocolate after the main course. Choose cakes and biscuits made with wholemeal flour or oats (see the Taste Good section for recipes for fruity malt loaf, apple flapjacks and brownies), or fruit-based desserts such as wholemeal or oat crumbles, fruit kebabs or fig and orange boats (see recipes) – which all contain some fibre. Instead of sweet ice creams, consider fresh fruit sorbets made with less sugar.

Be aware that even when a boiled sweet or other candy contains no sucrose or glucose, just fructose, in a low fibre setting the fructose will increase your blood sugar level in the same way as the other types of sugar. They are all best avoided.

Lifestyle concerns

VEGETARIANS AND VEGANS

Vegetarianism or veganism can be easily integrated with diabetes as long as you follow a healthy, balanced eating pattern. Because a vegetarian diet can be bulky, diabetic children need to have their diets carefully planned so that they still receive enough energy as well as other fibre-containing foods.

MILK INTOLERANCE

People with milk intolerance should be aware that some soya milks have added sugar, frequently labelled sucrose, so choose an unsweetened one.

PREGNANCY

If you're a healthy woman there is no reason for diabetes to stand in the way of a very happy and healthy pregnancy. The better controlled you are prior to conceiving the better, as this helps prevent any unnecessary complications cropping up during the pregnancy. You may need to change the pattern of your meals and snacks while you are pregnant as your hormone levels change, which can make you feel sick, starving at unusual times of the day and prone to strange cravings. If you know your body and diabetes well enough you should be able to work around these, but if in doubt ask your dietitian or doctor for their advice. Bear in mind that when you're pregnant, the baby will take and use some of your sugar; this should help you to realize the importance of eating regularly and keeping an eye on your sugar and medication levels.

EXERCISE

As with non-diabetic people, you should include some aerobic exercise in your daily routine. Exercise helps keep the body tissues supplied with oxygen, the muscles toned, the heart healthy and the mind content. The only thing to remember is that exercise lowers your blood sugar level, as the muscles use glucose as a form of fuel. You therefore need to make sure that you have enough carbohydrate to keep your sugar level normal. Insulin-dependent diabetics should have a sugary snack before any strenuous exercise.

It is important to stress to diabetic children that they can and should partake in sports. Point out famous sports people who are diabetic, to reassure them that the two are compatible. Provide them with a sugary snack to eat before they have a sports event at school and make sure that their teacher is fully aware that they are diabetic, so that they give them plenty of time to have a snack before doing any sport. The teacher should also know how to spot the signs of hypoglycaemia, just in case the sport is more energetic than expected.

Some older people seem to find that delaying the taking of insulin can help athletic performance, but you should discuss this with your doctor before you change your routine. This is only advisable for people whose diabetes is well controlled and who are mature enough to juggle the insulin and their bodies.

For non insulin-dependent diabetics, exercise should not pose any problems and indeed can bring down excess body weight, which can help your body regulate the sugar levels more efficiently.

ILLNESS

When you are ill, your metabolism slightly changes. The body naturally produces more glucose so blood sugar levels tend to rise. It is therefore vital if you're an insulin-dependent diabetic that your insulin is taken, regardless of whether or not you eat anything. Even if you don't fancy eating something solid, you should have a regular intake of carbohydrates, such as glasses of milk, fruit juice, soup, ice cream or yoghurt.

When you have a temperature your body loses a lot of water through sweating, so it is extremely important to drink plenty of clear water. If you have a young baby with diabetes I suggest you contact your GP and dietitian when they are unwell so that you can discuss the issue of their blood sugar control.

Hypos and hypers

Blood sugar levels change all the time, according to what you have eaten and what you have been doing to use up the sugar, such as exercise. If your sugar level goes too low because there is too much insulin in the body and too little sugar, you may suffer from hypoglycaemia (also called 'a hypo'). If there is too little insulin and too much sugar, the condition is referred to as hyperglycaemia. Both of these scenarios can on the whole be avoided by eating properly and taking medication if necessary. If you are unfortunate enough to experience them, they can be easily rectified.

HYPOGLYCAEMIA

'Hypos' are episodes when your blood sugar drops too low. Symptoms include dizziness, headaches, extreme hunger, blurred vision, odd behaviour such as crying, sweating, pins and needles, trembling, paleness and inability to speak.

The symptoms can come on extremely quickly, sometimes in a matter of minutes, but the condition is easy to correct. It can arise for various reasons: most often, if you haven't eaten enough carbohydrates; if you've left too long a gap between your injection of insulin and eating; or if you have done some energetic sport that has used more of the body's sugar reserves than you'd anticipated.

Once you've worked out how your body responds to exercise and how much carbohydrate you need to get through the day, hypos shouldn't occur. The best way of avoiding them is to be aware of what is happening in your body, for example if you are feeling slightly sweaty or dizzy, and don't push your body to the limit. Remember to have a mid-afternoon snack if this is what you normally do; don't think your body can hang on until you have journeyed back from the office, it won't. Always play safe.

Stay good

Your doctor will explain what to do when you have a hypoglycaemic attack, but the first thing is to have something sweet as quickly as possible. To stop a little 'hypo' from escalating into a big one, always carry a sugary snack around with you. This is especially important for children, and their carers should be notified as to where it is. Good portable snacks include bananas, biscuits, pieces of cake or chocolate, bottles or cartons of fruit juice, milk or milk shakes, or full-calorie fizzy drinks. Diet drinks won't help as they don't contain the right sort of sugar. Follow your sugary snack with a nourishing meal, containing some high fibre carbohydrate, as soon as possible.

You should contact your doctor immediately if you don't feel any better. If you're treating a friend whose blood sugar has dropped so low that she has lost consciousness, you should:

- turn her on to her left side
- make sure that her airway is clear by tilting the chin up slightly
- check that the tongue hasn't rolled back, as this could obstruct the throat
- then call the doctor or ambulance.

Never give anyone who is not fully conscious anything to eat or drink.

If you are having frequent hypos and you've checked that you are taking the correct dosage of medication and eating properly, consult your doctor. Non-insulin dependent diabetics should not have hypos. See your doctor for advice, as your symptoms may indicate something else.

Always inform your diabetic child's friends, parents, playgroup organizers and school teachers. Make sure that they know the basic things to do. Asking them to be diligent and flexible when it comes to your child's eating habits can save a lot of unnecessary worry.

HYPERGLYCAEMIA

The opposite to a 'hypo' is a hyperglycaemic attack. Hypers are commonly experienced when you have not taken enough insulin; you have eaten something too high in sugar; or you haven't done the sport or activity you planned. Mild 'hypers', which you detect by testing your urine or taking a blood sample, can be easily corrected by avoiding very sugary foods and taking the correct amount of insulin on time. Sometimes diabetics can have severe hyperglycaemic attacks, if for example they are ill or unable to take their insulin. The symptoms are similar to those experienced before diagnosis, including extreme thirst, lethargy, weight loss and frequent urination. It is important to realize that these symptoms are different to 'hypo' symptoms – you must seek medical advice immediately and not treat it yourself by taking a hypo-correcting sugary food. This will make your sugar level go even higher.

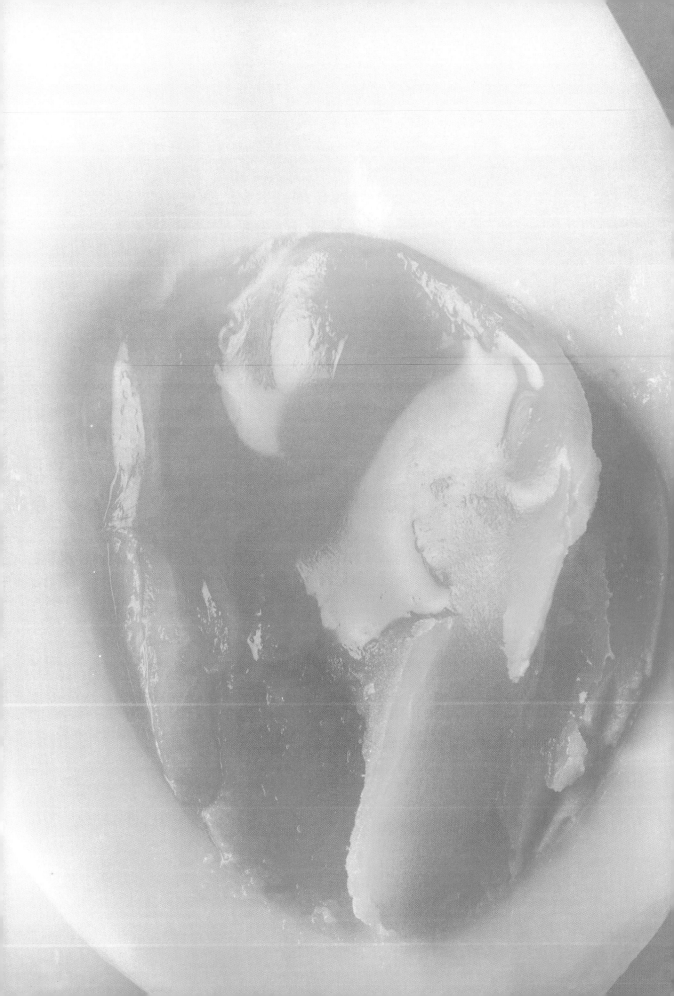

Anaemia

Anaemia affects many people at some time in their lives. It is most common in people who smoke, in women who have heavy periods, people who have an eating disorder such as anorexia, elderly people with poor appetites, people who suffer from intestinal bleeding, and those with malabsorption conditions such as Crohn's and coeliac disease. It is defined as a reduction below the norm of the blood concentration of a protein called haemoglobin, which enables the red blood cells to carry oxygen around the body.

There are many different sorts of anaemia, including folate deficiency and pernicious anaemia, but the most common form is iron deficiency anaemia. It is believed to affect between fifteen and twenty per cent of women in their child-bearing years and between six and nine per cent of elderly people. It is also becoming increasingly common in young children.

One of the reasons why the incidence of iron deficiency anaemia is on the increase is that people are eating less red meat, which is one of the richest sources of iron. Their motivations are varied. Some people are frightened about the health risks associated with the consumption of red meat, such as the increased risk of heart disease and certain kinds of cancer. Some people find that eating red meat aggravates their irritable bowel symptoms, another condition that is becoming more prevalent. Others are apprehensive about the risk of 'mad cow disease' or BSE; the way that meat is produced and the conditions in which animals are reared are also a growing concern.

The symptoms of anaemia include tiredness, irritability, loss of appetite, pallor and a general feeling of being 'run down'. Severe iron deficiency anaemia can lead to breathlessness, headaches and an inability to complete even simple tasks. One of the most common causes of hair loss in women is lack of iron in their diet.

If you have any of these symptoms, it is wise to go to your doctor in order that he or she can check the cause. It is important to establish which sort of anaemia you have before you embark on any self-help programme – don't just diagnose yourself or your child. Iron deficiency anaemia is relatively easy to correct through changing the foods you eat and your general lifestyle, but the other sorts of anaemia are a little trickier. Iron deficiency anaemia can usually be attributed to one of four factors.

YOU HAVE AN INCREASED DEMAND FOR IRON

The body may at certain times start to require a little more iron than it previously needed. In childhood the body rapidly uses iron as it builds the body, which is why you need to make sure your child has an iron-rich diet. Your demand for iron is drastically increased during pregnancy and breastfeeding, when extra iron is needed to satisfy both the baby's growth requirements and the blood loss you experience at childbirth.

The body also needs increased iron if you are being physically active, for example training for a serious athletic event, when your muscles, heart and lungs are put under greater strain.

LOSS OF BLOOD

For many women this occurs when they are experiencing heavy or lengthy menstrual periods. Other causes include intestinal bleeding, such as a burst ulcer or piles. The strong anti-inflammatory drugs prescribed for conditions such as rheumatoid arthritis can erode areas of the stomach lining, which also causes internal bleeding.

FOODS AND DRINKS THAT INHIBIT THE ABSORPTION OF IRON

The chief culprits are tannins and caffeine, found chiefly in coffee, tea and cola-based soft drinks. Chocolate contains oxalates, which also inhibit iron absorption.

INSUFFICIENT VITAMIN C

Vitamin C helps your body absorb the iron within the food. If you lack vitamin C the iron will stay in the gut and won't be absorbed. People who either don't eat many fruits or vegetables that contain vitamin C, or who smoke, are particularly susceptible to developing iron deficiency anaemia. People often make the mistake of boosting their iron intake but forgetting about vitamin C.

Dietary solutions

For the majority of people, iron deficiency anaemia is a question of negative iron and vitamin C balances; you retain less than you lose through menstruation or through internal bleeding or you fail to absorb efficiently the iron from your diet. These negative balances mean that you do not have enough iron to form sufficient haemoglobin to carry the oxygen needed for energy creation and tissue formation.

The usual response of people who are diagnosed anaemic is to buy a supplement, but it is much healthier to look at your diet and explore the reasons why it has occurred, and work through the practical ways in which you can use foods to correct and prevent it from re-appearing. Supplements have their place, but only when other issues have been explored. It is important once you have embarked on an anaemia-correcting eating plan to keep in touch with your doctor.

- *Steam and dress with a
  little butter and freshly
  grated nutmeg*
- *Eat the raw young leaves
  with charcuterie, with olive
  oil drizzled on top*
- *Steam or sweat in oil or
  butter. Beat two eggs with
  a little milk or cream, salt
  and pepper. Stir in the
  spinach and cook as an
  omelette*
- *Tear the leaves into freshly
  cooked pasta, along with
  chargrilled leeks*
- *Use young raw leaves
  in a salad with avocado,
  watercress, pine nuts and
  crisp grilled bacon*

ANAEMIA IN INFANCY

Babies born at full term have laid down stores of iron that will last them for four to six months. Pre-term babies, however, have not always had the chance to acquire sufficient stores of iron and because of this can easily become anaemic. For this reason pre-term babies are usually given extra iron and folic acid and may in certain cases be given top-ups of fresh donor blood. Breast milk contains very little iron, so if you have not weaned your baby on to formula by the age of six months, it is important to talk to your doctor about the possibility of either iron supplements or providing sources of iron through baby's first foods.

BOOST YOUR IRON INTAKE

There are two sorts of iron in food. Haem iron, found in animal foods such as lean red meat, liver and other offal, is easily absorbed by the body. Non-haem iron is derived mainly from non-animal foods, such as dark green vegetables (spinach, broccoli, Savoy cabbage, curly kale, watercress), pulses and nuts (see page 44 for other sources of iron). The exception to the animal link with haem iron is eggs, which are considered in the same way as vegetable sources.

Non-haem iron foods contain substances that hinder the absorption of iron, meaning that your body cannot absorb the iron from these sources as efficiently as it can from foods containing haem iron. You therefore need to eat a lot more of them to derive sufficient iron.

As with all nutrients, iron relies on a healthy gut to absorb it. Some people with digestive problems such as irritable bowel syndrome, chronic constipation, Crohn's disease or ulcerative colitis, can have slightly disrupted iron absorption. If you have a specific bowel problem see your dietitian or doctor for advice; a change in your diet could trigger the condition to relapse.

Generally, however, to prevent or correct anaemia I suggest you eat a rich source of iron two or three times a week. If you are not inspired by a chop or a steak, what about spaghetti bolognaise, beef Stroganoff, grilled calves' liver, lamb, venison and other game meats such as grouse and pheasant? These are all rich in iron. Pregnant women should avoid offal, as its vitamin A content is very high, which can lead to problems during pregnancy. Children may say they don't like the texture of meat – 'it's too chewy' – but can be coaxed to eat it in lasagne, homemade hamburgers or shepherd's pie. Meat dishes can be frozen, as long as you have begun with fresh meat, and not frozen.

In addition to red meat you should eat plenty of non-haem sources of iron most days – a substantial portion of green leafy vegetables, or eggs, or a lentil, bean or nut-based main course. A surprising source of non-haem iron is black treacle, which can be deliciously made into parkin or ginger biscuits – perfect mid-afternoon iron boosts! Dried fruits such as apricots and figs also contain good levels of iron; include them in muesli for breakfast and fruit compotes for snacks and desserts. If you are a vegetarian or just don't like red meat, it is essential that you eat some of these foods every day.

BOOST YOUR VITAMIN C INTAKE

In addition to looking at the iron content of foods, it is also important to address the vitamin C issue. You need to concentrate on having plenty of oranges, grapefruits, kiwi fruits, cranberries and other berries, and potatoes. Dark green leafy vegetables contain vitamin C as well as iron.

Aim to have a source of vitamin C with every meal, perhaps a glass of freshly squeezed juice or a fresh fruit salad to finish. (The only exception here is for people with high blood fat levels, who should wait until lunchtime before they drink fresh fruit juice, as fresh juice on an empty stomach in the morning can increase production of blood fats. If you cannot eat citrus fruits (perhaps because of an allergy) you should include some green vegetables with each of your main meals: this could be in the form of a soup, a salad or a lightly cooked vegetable accompaniment.

Freshly squeezed juices are the best. Some cartons of drink labelled 'fresh' will have very little vitamin C left by the time you drink them, because the vitamin C content diminishes with time. Others can be quite high in vitamin C because artificial vitamin C (ascorbic acid) is added. Although some fruit squashes contain added vitamin C, their sugar contents are so high that they can cause extreme mood swings, tooth decay and excess weight.

There is very little difference between the vitamin C content in raw versus cooked foods, as long as you don't overcook them. Experiment with vegetables stir-fried, steamed, baked, or boiled for a very short time, so they retain a lot of their crisp texture. There can also be a lot of vitamin C in frozen and tinned fruits and vegetables, but organic or home-grown produce is the ideal.

CHOOSE ALCOHOLIC DRINKS WITH CARE

One of the great myths is that stout contains a lot of iron. A more accurate statement would be that it contains a small amount of iron, not enough to have magical, health-giving properties, and not enough to make you drink it if you don't particularly like it. Champagne is relatively high in iron because of the limestone soil in the Champagne region of France. Wines grown in the limestone areas of southern Britain are rich in iron for the same reasons. Some red wines are even higher in iron, containing virtually twenty times as much iron as champagne. I am not suggesting you down pints of champagne, but a glass or two of champagne or red wine can do wonders for your iron levels.

AVOID FOODS AND DRINKS THAT INHIBIT THE ABSORPTION OF IRON

The worst offenders are coffee, tea and cola-based drinks. Also remember that chocolate contains caffeine and other substances that hinder iron, so don't over-indulge, especially if you are feeling tired. A healthier energy boost would be a fruit shake, a bowl of fruit compote or a piece of fresh fruit. Keep your tea, coffee and cola drinks intake down to a maximum of two or three cups a day and allow at least one hour between drinking tea or coffee before or after a meal. This elapse of time should allow your gut to absorb the iron from the food more efficiently. Other hot drinks to try include herbal or fruit teas, mugs of warm milk, hot water with slices of lemon, or the drinks suggested on page 343.

KEEP THE BULK DOWN

While you are trying to boost your iron and vitamin C intakes, try to keep the amount of cereal fibre such as wholegrain cereals and wholegrain bread low. This is because oxalates and phylates, two substances that naturally occur within these high fibre foods, can inhibit the absorption of iron. This is especially important for growing children and people with small appetites, as the last thing you want is fill them up with fibre and stop their body from absorbing the iron. I don't mean that you should cut fibre out completely, but try not to hide the red meat or vegetable source of iron in mounds of cereal fibre.

IRON SUPPLEMENTS

If you are unable to eat as much iron as you need, perhaps because your iron status is too low to be corrected by diet alone, you may need to take a supplement. I recommend that you discuss the issue with your doctor or dietitian.

There are plenty of supplements on the market; some contain just iron, others contain iron with vitamin C and/or folate. It is generally a good idea to choose a supplement that incorporates vitamin C. The majority of women should be fine on a supplement that provides 15 mg iron along with 500 – 1000 mg vitamin C; men need 9 mg iron a day. Children need 7 mg a day up to the age of six, 9 mg a day until ten and then they join the adult requirement. Herbal iron supplements contain an easily absorbed source of iron.

Some iron supplements can cause indigestion, diarrhoea or constipation. Avoid taking them on an empty stomach as this can make the problem worse. If you experience any of these symptoms, use the information in the chapter on Digestion. If nothing seems to do the trick, ask your doctor or pharmacist about changing the supplement. Some supplements are better tolerated than others.

Lifestyle considerations

In order to help your body replenish its store of iron and produce healthy blood cells, it is also important to make changes in your day-to-day life. I commonly see people who receive a diagnosis of iron deficiency anaemia, take an iron supplement and expect their body to recover overnight. It cannot happen this way. Your body needs time to recover, and I usually estimate three to four weeks to make any substantial improvements.

Get plenty of rest and try to reduce the amount of stress you are under. If your lifestyle normally demands a lot of physical exertion, you should try to cut this down. While a little gentle exercise helps keep the mood high and the heart going, strenuous exercise will make you feel lousy, because you won't have sufficient oxygen to feed your muscles. If you have anaemia, you need to slow down.

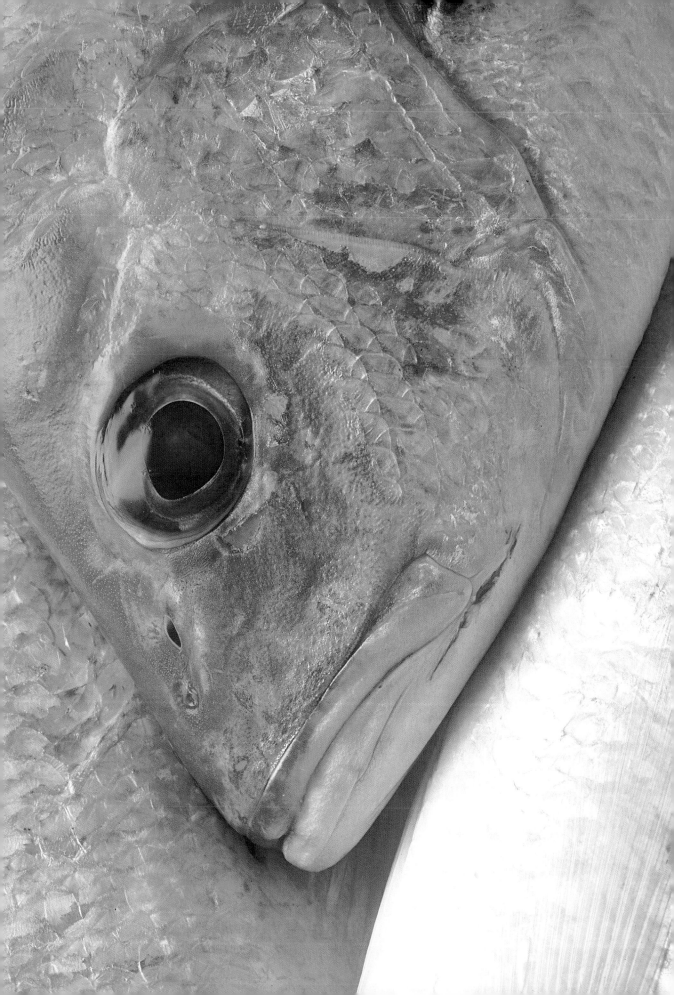

Arthritis and gout

While heart disease and cancer are the biggest killers in the Western world, arthritis remains a major cause of disability. The term arthritis means inflammation of a joint. Painful, swollen, contorted joints can be a severe handicap, especially when these are the joints of the hand or wrist. Arthritis is not confined to the elderly; there are several types that affect people of all ages, from the juvenile arthritis known as Still's disease, sometimes found in babies just a few months old, to alkylosing spondilytis, osteoarthritis, psoriatic, rheumatoid and crystal arthritis, also known as gout, which often begins when men are between forty and fifty.

Correct nutrition can bring tremendous relief to many arthritis sufferers, but it must be undertaken with care, as the different types of arthritis require different nutritional management. It will also take time – anything from a few days to weeks – to calm your body down from any food-related inflammation, and you should allow a couple of months to glean the full benefit from the foods you eat. You may be used to seeing quicker results from medication, but keep reminding yourself that in the long run your whole body will benefit.

Of course, some people cannot cope without medication, but the side effects of some of the powerful drugs used to treat arthritis range from chronic loss of appetite and mild indigestion to more serious gastric or intestinal irritation, even bleeding and subsequent anaemia.

In this chapter I shall concentrate on rheumatoid arthritis, osteoarthritis and gout, as these are most common in Western society, but will begin with some general advice. The guidelines are much the same as for any healthy person; they play an important role in both the treatment of arthritis and the prevention of complications.

First of all, follow a healthy eating plan. By this I mean that you should eat as wide a variety as possible of fresh foods: vegetables and pulses, fruit, cereal products (bread, rice, pasta etc.), dairy products, eggs, fish, poultry, meat. Vitamin and mineral intakes in arthritis sufferers are often low. This is partly because it can be difficult to shop, cook and care for yourself, and there may be days when you don't feel like eating much. Medication also has a number of side effects: some drugs take your appetite away or make you crave sweet foods, which don't tend to be high in vitamins and minerals. Others interfere with the metabolism of vitamins and minerals, or increase the amount of protein, calcium and zinc the body excretes. Lack of these essential nutrients can cause your body to become more susceptible to colds, infections and other health problems. You should have small meals at least three times a day, rather than skipping meals or having one large, blow-out meal, especially late at night. A regular eating pattern will give your body a steady intake of nutrients.

Water is necessary to keep your body functioning efficiently and enable it to glean nutrients from the food you eat. Aim to drink two and a half litres/four to five pints a day. The following points apply to most arthritis sufferers:

- Keep your caffeine and tannin intakes low. Coffee, tea, hot chocolate and cola-based drinks contain caffeine and tannin, which inhibit the absorption of vitamins and minerals from the gut. Caffeine can also make the gut more sensitive to the irritating effects of anti-inflammatory medication and can increase fluid retention, both of which can cause disability and pain. Ideally keep your intake down to two or three cups a day. Try herb and fruit teas and see page 343 for caffeine-free alternatives.

- Watch your weight. Excess weight puts stress on the joints, causing pain and discomfort. Remember it's much easier to stop weight piling on than to try to lose it later. Unfortunately it is very easy for arthritis sufferers to put on weight, especially if they are prescribed steroids to reduce the inflammatory process. The balance between calorie intake and expenditure goes against you when it is painful to move around and exercise. You also have to contend with the emotional aspect of being in pain and unable to do anything about it. We would all admit to comfort eating at times, and people with arthritis have more reason than most to turn to food for solace. When you are in pain it is tempting to grab something quick and easy – there are plenty of healthy foods which fit this description. See page 66 for some nutritious snacks.

- Try to keep organized. Most people with arthritis go through good and not-so-good periods. Use the periods when you are feeling better to stock up your cupboards and fridge and cook meals which can be frozen in small portions, so that when your joints are extra painful you have plenty of healthy food to fall back on.

- Any doctor or physiotherapist will agree on the merits of regular exercise. It is important to keep your joints moving, so that in the long run they will be more flexible and less painful and disabling. You need to include stretching and strengthening exercises as well as cardiovascular aerobic exercises.

There is a fine balance to achieve, though; while you need to exercise the joints, you also need to give them time to recover and rest. If they are particularly inflamed and sore, see if things get better with a day or two's rest. Once things improve, build up gradually with some exercise.

- Feeling tense, stressed, or guilty about resting are arthritis-aggravating emotions. To help you relax, consider aromatherapy oils, such as comfrey, lavender, neroli, vetiver and benzoin. Comfrey is particularly good at reducing inflammation. These oils can be used in a burner, dropped into your bath, or diluted in a carrier oil (such as grapeseed) and used in massage. It needn't be a whole body massage; a foot, hand or back massage can relieve an affected area.

- If you suspect that your arthritis is aggravated by additives and preservatives, I suggest you avoid ready-made, convenience and fast foods for a couple of weeks, instead eating simply cooked fresh foods. Replace your chilled or frozen, ready-to-cook dinners with pieces of chicken or fish which are just as easy to pop in the oven or under the grill. Instead of sweets or a bar of chocolate, treat yourself to some grapes, strawberries or other seasonal fruit.

    Taking this one step further, many of my patients feel much better when they eat organic produce and hence reduce their exposure to pesticides and other artificial food additives.
- Take your anti-inflammatories and painkillers with or after food. Many of the anti-inflammatories are particularly fierce on the stomach and intestine; taking them with food helps to minimize gastrointestinal discomfort. However, there are alternative ways of administering pain-relieving drugs, including suppositories, so discuss these options with your doctor.

Rheumatoid arthritis

Rheumatoid arthritis usually starts with swelling, pain or stiffness in the joints, especially the wrists, hands and feet, which is usually worse in the morning. With time the body becomes more and more riddled with pain. In the severest of cases the body can become so disabled that it picks up lung infections easily, which can lead to breathing problems and even pneumonia. The skin, liver and kidneys can also be badly affected. Rheumatoid arthritis plagues many elderly people to the extent that they become physically dependent on others, and this loss of independence, when their mind is still active, puts a strain on their relationships. In this situation food can be very empowering; choosing what to eat and how to manage your meals can have a positive effect on your life. You are making the decisions, instead of relying on doctors and carers.

   Diet is very important in the treatment of rheumatoid arthritis. In addition to the good eating habits outlined above there are several modifications which help some people reduce their symptoms:
- People with rheumatoid arthritis frequently find that a diet rich in oily fish significantly reduces inflammation and pain. Oily fish, such as mackerel, salmon, herrings and kippers, tuna, sardines and anchovies, are rich sources of omega 3 fatty acids. These fatty acids have a range of benefits; besides reducing inflammation they have been shown to protect against thrombosis and strengthen the immune system.

    Some people find oily fish a little heavy on the palate and digestion. The traditional way to cut the oiliness is to marry the fish with a sharp fresh flavour: a wedge of lemon or lime, ginger, horseradish, or a tangy fruit sauce such as gooseberry or rhubarb. Eating some fibre, such as wholemeal bread or a portion of spinach, can help your body deal with the fat.

    My patients seem to experience maximum benefit when they take these fatty acids in food, but if you really dislike oily fish you could take a supplement.

The optimum dosage would be 600 mg omega 3 fatty acid a day; check that your supplement has this level of omega 3 oil and not just any fish oil.

- If you are a vegetarian and cannot eat fish oils, evening primrose oil has a similar beneficial effect. It contains gamma linoleic acid (GLA), an omega 6 fatty acid which, like the omega 3 fatty acids, seems to reduce the inflammation process. The current recommended dosage of evening primrose oil is 2000–4000 mg a day, usually taken in 500 mg tablets. There does not appear to be any equivalent dietary source of GLA.

- One important point to remember when you are boosting your intake of omega 3 or omega 6 fatty acids is that you need to keep your animal fat intake low as part of a healthy eating plan. If you eat too much animal fat, such as butter, cream, cheese and fatty meat, the omega 3 fatty acids and GLA cannot work effectively, and therefore their potential healing power is lost. Many people are swallowing tablets with no chance of success.

- People suffering from rheumatoid arthritis may be the exceptions to my general advice that everyone should eat the equivalent of a daily small pot of yoghurt containing bifidus and acidophilus (bacteria that are beneficial to the digestive system). Sometimes these cultures can cause your symptoms to flare up. I suggest that you keep a food and symptom diary (see page 85) for a few weeks. Take a couple of spoonfuls of a yoghurt containing these cultures regularly, then avoid yoghurt for a few days, and note how your body responds. If you can tolerate them they will help your overall health. Yoghurts containing lactobacillus cultures should not upset you.

- Copper, zinc and nicotinamide supplements are sometimes advocated. Without further medical research, I wouldn't recommend taking any tablets containing these ingredients. A copper wrist band is a traditional arthritis remedy that cannot do any harm, so if you feel it helps, by all means wear one. It may be that a small amount of copper which seeps through the skin in some way reduces the inflammatory response.

FOOD INTOLERANCE

When you are in pain, it is tempting to try anything that might help, and you will hear of lots of remedies, many of them involving exclusion diets: no red meat or no citrus fruit for example. Before you cut anything out, take the time to ensure that your diet is well balanced; sometimes it is what you are not eating that can aggravate symptoms. It would be a pity to worry about avoiding foods if all you need to do is eat a healthy diet. I suggest you keep a food diary (page 85) to help you explore the relationship between food and your symptoms.

Scientists disagree as to whether food intolerances have any role in the cause and hence treatment of rheumatoid arthritis. While not scientifically supported, some specific dietary modifications can make you feel better. There are those that suggest excluding all meat, eating no cooked foods or grains, no citrus fruits, or drinking whole milk before meals, the respective theories being that meat (or wheat) causes arthritis, raw vegetables cleanse the body, citrus fruits create too much acid, milk helps to lubricate the joints. While these theories are not proven, it may be the case that the altered intake of nutrients beneficially affects the immune system, or the changes cause you to shed some excess weight. Even if it's just the placebo effect (i.e. if you believe that the diet is helping, the power of your mind helps you feel less pain and stiffness), it is always important to feel that you are doing something to help yourself.

In order for any food therapy to help rather than hinder your body, it needs to be carefully executed. A patient of mine was advised by a so-called nutritionist to cut out wheat, dairy products, meat, fish and of all things water from his diet. Without these sources of essential nutrients his body weight dropped danger- ously low and he became seriously weak. While the severity of this outcome is extreme, there are thousands of people eating inappropriately in the hope of curing their arthritis symptoms.

If you decide to explore food intolerances you should go about it in a controlled manner, keeping detailed notes of your food and symptoms. Some- times it is simply a matter of quantity: your body may be able to take a small amount of a specific food, but develops symptoms when you overstep the mark. Try reducing the quantity of a suspected food and see how your body responds. For instance if you suspect wheat, have just one meal based on wheat (bread, pasta) in a day. I suggest you allow a couple of weeks before you reach any conclusions, as the body needs a while to show any changes.

Some people need to eliminate the food completely to experience any relief. In this case, it is important to replace the food with an alternative source of nutrients. For instance, if you cut out bread, get your carbohydrates from rice or potatoes. If you cut out dairy products you need to find another source of calcium (see page 42); if you cut out red meat you need another source of iron (see page 44). Food can be the most amazing healer, but finding the right foods for your body takes time and care.

ANAEMIA

Anaemia is one of the most common secondary conditions affecting people who suffer from rheumatoid arthritis. This may arise as a result of a poor dietary intake of iron, folic acid or vitamin C. Those following exclusion diets can easily miss out on essential nutrients. Additionally, many of the anti-inflammatory and strong painkilling drugs interfere with the metabolism of vitamins and minerals, in particular the B group of vitamins, folic acid, vitamin C and vitamin E. Anaemia can also result from gastrointestinal bleeding, which can occur when you take a lot of non-steroidal painkillers. You can reduce the likelihood of intestinal bleeding by eating something before taking painkillers.

If you are feeling continually tired you should see your GP to ascertain the cause. If it is anaemia, there is a lot you can do to help yourself, mainly by choosing foods rich in iron. I suggest you read the chapter on Anaemia.

Osteoarthritis

Osteoarthritis is a degenerative condition which is more common as you get older – although I have patients as young as ten years old. Osteoarthritis develops as the cartilage around the joints – especially weight-bearing joints such as hips and knees – wears away and new bone material grows beneath the worn cartilage. With the growth of bone tissue the joint cannot move as smoothly as it is meant to and inflammation occurs. The joints become distorted, which leads to further pain, as muscles are strained and nerves get trapped.

CAN FOOD HELP?

Unlike rheumatoid arthritis, there is no special diet which greatly affects the progression and symptoms of osteoarthritis. However, some of my patients experience relief when they increase their intake of fish oils or evening primrose oil. A copper bracelet also seems to help some people. One unusual ingredient that is currently being investigated is the green-lipped mussel from New Zealand; results are suggesting that it may be able to relieve osteoarthritis.

EXCESS WEIGHT

The issue of weight is particularly relevant with this form of arthritis, since it commonly affects 'load-bearing' joints such as the knee and hip; if you are carrying excess weight you will place an enormous strain on these joints. Many surgeons advise that patients who need surgery to replace joints should reduce their body weight before undergoing surgery. Losing excess weight increases the success rate of the operation both short and long term. However, as I constantly reiterate, crash diets are not the answer; their effect is only temporary – the weight will soon come back, which will not help your new joint. You can continue to enjoy your food and still lose weight by approaching it sensibly. Read the chapter on Achieving your ideal weight.

DON'T SUFFER UNNECESSARILY

Your physiotherapist and/or occupational therapist can help make your life easier to manage. Ask for advice about exercises and modified or specially designed household utensils and machines.

Some patients don't like to make a fuss, but if you are suffering pain, don't be afraid to ask your doctor to review your medication. There are so many different types of painkilling drugs that there should be one that can relieve you of the majority of pain and discomfort.

Some patients find that a change of temperature can reduce the pain. Experiment with heat and cold: hot water bottles, warm baths, ice packs (or a bag of frozen peas) on the joints. You can also get special sound wave machines, called TENS machines, which help your body to produce natural painkilling substances. Ask your doctor or physiotherapist about these.

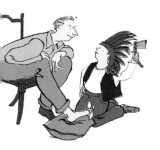

Gout

Gout, according to a friend of mine, is excruciatingly painful. 'It's as if someone is ramming a huge hot needle into your toe!' It generally affects men of middle age and older, although this particular friend is in his thirties, and women are not immune. Gout has traditionally been labelled as the disease of the heavy drinker and the rich, but not all sufferers fall into these categories. The cause is usually genetic, but occasionally gout is a side effect of certain diuretics.

Gout arises when crystals of uric acid deposit in the joints, causing them to become swollen and inflamed. It is most common in the toes, but also affects other joints. Gout is also known as crystal arthritis or hyperuricaemia.

Drug therapy using Allopurinol has largely replaced the need for dietary restriction in the treatment of gout, but as a second line of defence many men choose to restrict their intake of purines, the main dietary ingredient that causes the formation of uric acid crystals. Bear in mind that if you suffer an attack of gout it usually takes about five days for the body to rid itself of the dietary sources of uric acid. You should ensure you are drinking enough water to help your body excrete unwanted substances.

PURINES

Many men think that they need to avoid all types of red meat. This is not totally necessary; the richest sources of purines are game, offal and meat extracts (for example Oxo), and of course products made from them such as pâtés, sausages and pies. If you want to make gravy or soups, I suggest you use fresh stock rather than meat stock cubes. Meat such as beef, lamb and pork, as well as poultry, is lower in purines.

Some fish are rather rich in purines: anchovies, herring, mackerel, sardines, sprats and whitebait, as well as fish roes and shellfish such as crab and prawns. This leaves the whole range of white fish open for your enjoyment, from cod and plaice to turbot and Dover sole.

Smoked and pickled fish and meat are also high in purines, as are other salty foods, dried fruits, dried beans, peas and asparagus.

While it is good to steer clear of these items, there is no need to avoid them altogether. Instead, I suggest you look out for them, and avoid too many purine sources in one day. For example, by all means enjoy asparagus when it is in season, but follow it with chicken or white fish.

WINE

Red wine is traditionally associated with gout, since it can produce uric acid. However, you do not need to exclude all red wine. It is usually a question of quantity, as some men can tolerate more red wine than others. Some people find the lighter, Beaujolais-style wines suit them better than port, mature claret and burgundy. The best way of finding the wines you can drink without painful symptoms is to keep a food and drink diary (see page 85).

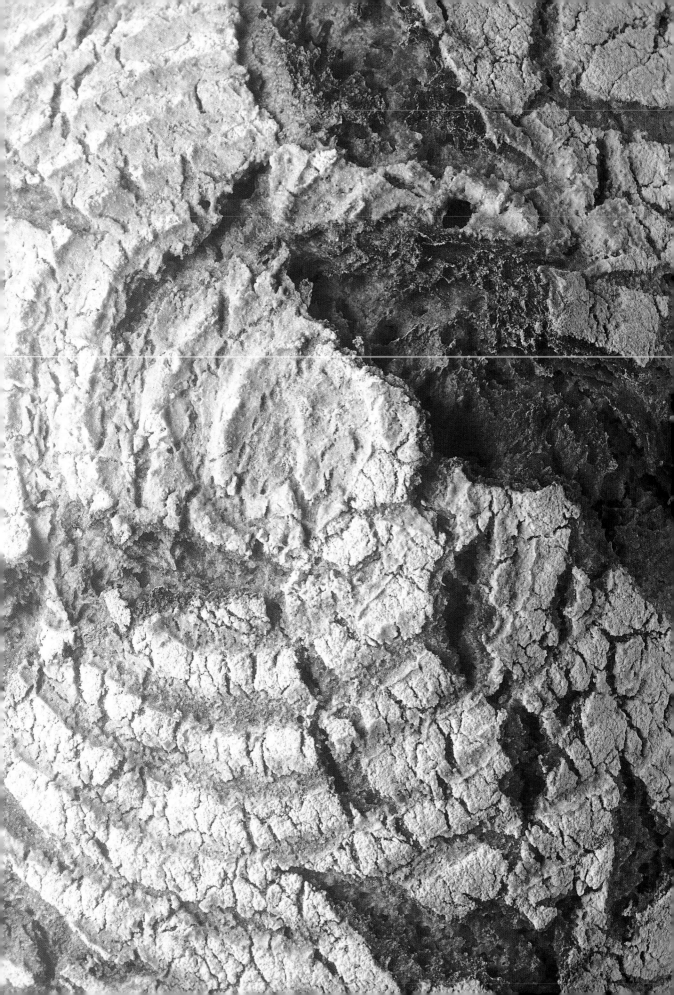

Gallstones; raised liver enzymes

The liver is the largest organ in the body, and one of the most important. It has many vital functions relating to the blood, and others relating to the digestion, absorption and storage of nutrients. The gall-bladder nestles below the liver and supports it in the digestion of fat; it acts as a reservoir for bile, the fat-digesting fluid produced by the liver. The gall-bladder stores the bile until it is discharged during digestion into the duodenum, the first part of the intestine. The majority of people don't realize they have a gall-bladder until they are hit with the excruciating pain that accompanies gallstones and inflammation of the gall-bladder. It has been estimated that ten per cent of the Western population suffer from gallstones.

Gallstones are pebble-like balls of cholesterol-rich crystals which form within the gall-bladder. There may be one walnut-sized gallstone or hundreds of them, smaller than grains of rice. Problems occur when they block the route of the bile to the intestine and irritate the lining of the gall-bladder, causing it to become inflamed (cholecystitis). If the bile's exit is blocked, its yellowish pigment will be returned to the blood via the liver, and the body can become jaundiced (the skin and whites of the eyes turn yellowy orange). Jaundice requires medical investigation and treatment, along with specific dietary advice from your doctor. Since the major function of bile is to help the body digest fat, the lack of bile causes fat malabsorption, which leads to other symptoms: bloating, nausea, diarrhoea and steatorrhoea (fatty, smelly stools).

Nutritionally, the best way to prevent and treat gall-bladder disease is to make sure that you eat plenty of high fibre foods, as these help your body rid itself of unwanted fat. Having said this, some people seem to have a genetic predisposition to developing gallstones, however healthy and well balanced their diet is.

Prevention of gallstones

Understanding your nutritional needs (see pages 25–47) explains the elements of a balanced, healthy diet. The general principles apply to anyone who wants to maintain good health and prevent disease.

While high fat, low fibre diets have been linked with the formation of gallstones, there is little evidence to say that you need to avoid fat completely. You need a certain amount of fat to provide and metabolize nutrients within your body. However, many people in Western society eat far too much fat. If you eat a lot of fried foods, takeaways, high-fat snacks such as crisps and chocolate, butter and cheese, I suggest you think seriously about your eating habits. Take things gradually: grill or bake rather than fry, plan a big healthy salad instead of a takeaway, make crisps and chocolate an occasional treat rather than an everyday snack.

Many people would also benefit from boosting their fibre intake. Fruits and vegetables, beans and lentils, wholegrain cereals, bread and rice should all feature in your daily or weekly eating plan. Make sure you drink plenty of water to help the fibre work efficiently in your body.

Some studies have suggested that coffee and tea can reduce the production of gallstones, but do not take this to mean that copious consumption will dissolve the stones; it will not. The disadvantages of excessive tea and coffee drinking far outweigh the benefits, so enjoy two to three cups a day, but no more.

Dealing with gall-bladder problems

Managing gall-bladder disease is all about discovering which foods upset you and which foods you can tolerate. To investigate how different foods affect your symptoms, try keeping a food diary (see page 85) for a couple of weeks. Some people think that fat will upset them, but when they keep a note of everything they eat they find that there is no correlation between fat and their symptoms.

The reason why fat can cause pain and nausea is that the presence of fat in the stomach stimulates the gall-bladder to contract and release bile. If there are stones in the gall-bladder or the gall-bladder ducts are inflamed, this contraction can bring about pain.

Many patients diagnosed with gall-bladder problems think they need to shop for low fat products. I do not generally recommend these because they don't really contribute to a healthy diet: they can be very high in sugar, artificial additives and preservatives, and the taste often leaves a lot to be desired. It is much better for you to stick to natural fats like olive oil and butter, but cut down on the amount you use.

The gall-bladder does not react any differently to saturated fats (found mainly in meat, butter and other dairy products) and unsaturated fats (found in vegetable fats such as olive oil, and in oily fish). However, if you have a raised cholesterol level (see the chapter on High blood cholesterol) you should consider choosing olive oil rather than butter.

Women with gallstones need to be particularly careful when cutting out dairy products, because these provide such a significant amount of calcium. Calcium is vital for maintaining healthy bones, and lack of it can increase the risk of osteoporosis, a condition common in women after the menopause. Younger women should be aware that they need to maintain bone density throughout their lives. The best way to approach this and prevent gall-bladder discomfort is to avoid having large lumps of cheese or glasses of full cream milk on an empty stomach.

Instead, incorporate small amounts of dairy products – semi-skimmed or skimmed milk, yoghurt, cheese – within meals. See page 42 for other calcium sources.

If you find from your food diary that fatty foods such as fried foods, cakes, or desserts laden with cream upset your system, simply avoid these foods. It is usually the large load of fat that causes problems. Instead, stagger your intake of fat throughout the day, and combine it with high fibre foods, for instance having butter on wholemeal bread or a light vinaigrette dressing on salads.

People sometimes forget that if you eat a lot the stomach may swell and press against the inflamed gall-bladder and cause pain. It may be nothing to do with the fat content of your meal, but simply the sheer volume of food in your stomach. Small meals often is the best eating style, as this not only limits the pressure on the gall-bladder, it also allows the body to digest the food most efficiently.

Of course, if you are carrying excess body weight, a gall-bladder problem may be the spur you need to lose weight by reducing the amount of fat and other concentrated sources of calories in your diet. But as with all weight loss programmes it is best to lose weight gradually and to find an eating style which doesn't make you feel deprived (see the chapter on Achieving your ideal weight).

The majority of my patients with gall-bladder problems find that, if they increase their intake of high fibre foods, this has a cushioning effect which stops the fat within the meal setting off any pain. Some patients notice that certain high fibre foods such as cauliflower and broccoli have a tendency to produce wind and bloating, which can set their gall-bladder pain off. This is nothing to do with the fat content of the diet. In this instance I suggest experimenting with different types of high fibre foods, drinking plenty of water and protecting the healthy bacteria in your gut (see page 47).

Some people find that excess tea and coffee can cause bloating, which can trigger pain, so limit yourself to two or three cups a day.

Removal of the gall-bladder
In the past the majority of people with gallstones had to have surgery to remove the gall-bladder, but now there are simpler, non-invasive treatments which can either dissolve the gallstones or smash them up with ultrasound. The symptoms usually disappear almost immediately, although the gall-bladder may remain inflamed for a few days after the procedure.

Some patients come to me having been told by their surgeon to lose excess weight before they can have the operation to remove the gall-bladder. It is tempting to go on a crash diet to lose the weight so you can be relieved of the pain, but it is better to try to lose it gradually by adjusting your eating habits, so that it stays off after the operation. You should be able to lose weight while managing your symptoms by adopting a higher fibre, lower fat diet, so that the overall efficiency of your treatment is good.

If you have your gall-bladder removed, you will need to address the fat content of your diet if you are to remain symptom-free. There is no reason why your body cannot digest fat, as it is the liver that produces the bile, not the gall-bladder. So when you have your gall-bladder removed the liver will still produce bile, but your body won't have a reservoir on which it can draw if you have a fatty meal. Most people find that keeping their intake of fat at a healthy level helps their digestive system to cope. Try to have small amounts of fat regularly, taken with high fibre foods, such as a slice of cheese on wholemeal bread with a bunch of grapes, rather than gorging on a plate of cheese on its own. This eating pattern will enable your liver to judge how much bile to produce. Don't go for long, relatively fat-free periods and then expect your liver to produce a large amount of bile to digest a fatty meal, as the liver takes time to respond.

People who have the stone dissolved or smashed by ultrasound shouldn't have any further problems digesting fat, but I suggest you keep a food diary (page 85) for a few weeks to check your overall nutritional balance.

Raised liver enzymes
Routine blood tests can occasionally show raised liver enzymes. The presence of abnormally raised enzymes in the blood suggests that the liver is working at a reduced capacity. This can occur for many reasons and your doctor will need to investigate further. The most common causes are infections such as those caused by the hepatitis virus (hepatitis A, B or C), or the side effects of certain drugs. In some cases a cancerous tumour will produce significantly high enzyme levels.

Often there is no underlying cause for the raised enzymes other than that the liver is not coping with your eating and drinking habits. In these cases, raised liver enzymes are a warning that you need to take your body seriously and start looking after it. Your doctor will be able to tell whether the Gamma GT level is raised, which usually suggests that you are drinking too much alcohol. However, some livers are just more sensitive than others. There are people who, despite leading a healthy lifestyle, always show raised liver enzymes. This may happen because of an earlier illness or as an unexplainable phenomena, which many doctors don't worry about unless the levels change significantly.

If you have been diagnosed as having raised liver enzyme levels and your doctor reassures you that all you need to do is start looking after your liver there are several nutritional issues you can address which will allow your liver to recover and stay healthy. This is definitely in your best interest, as liver failure is one of the most debilitating illnesses.

DISCUSS ALL MEDICATION WITH YOUR GP
Remember that everything you put into your body is metabolized by the liver. This includes nutritional supplements and homeopathic remedies, so don't take any medication, whether wholly natural or over-the-counter drugs, unless you have discussed them with your GP. It is important not to overload your liver with substances, be they food or drugs, that might compound the problem.

TAKE YOUR DOCTOR'S ADVICE ABOUT ALCOHOL

Your doctor may suggest that you abstain from alcohol until your liver enzymes return to normal. There are plenty of alcohol-free drinks, such as sparkling and fruit-flavoured waters, elderflower cordials, apple, cranberry and other fruit juices, that are quite delicious. Remember that you are saving your liver.

In other circumstances you may simply be advised to cut down your alcohol intake. Many people find that spirits – whisky, brandy, gin, vodka – hit the liver harder than wines, probably due to their high alcohol content. I advise that you stick to wine and don't drink on an empty stomach, as this causes a rush of alcohol into your system, which your liver has to work overtime to deal with. Drinking a small amount of wine with food is the best plan. Beware of dessert wines such as Sauternes and Tokaji, as these tend to be hard on the liver. Beers seem to be reasonably well tolerated, their main drawback being that you tend to drink them without food, which can cause your liver to complain.

CUT DOWN ON CAFFEINE

Caffeine irritates the liver, so cutting down on caffeine-containing drinks – tea, coffee, cola, hot chocolate – to no more than two cups a day will help your liver recover more quickly.

BE FOOD WISE

If you have raised liver enzymes but no other medical problem such as hepatitis, a well balanced, healthy diet, as discussed in the chapter on Understanding your nutritional needs, will enable your liver to recover as quickly as possible.

There is one area to which you should pay particular attention: fats. Fat is one of the hardest foods for the body to break down and metabolize, and it is often even more difficult for people with raised liver enzymes. They may suffer from indigestion, bloating, wind and a general feeling of heaviness when they eat fatty foods. It is therefore best to avoid fried foods, cream, butter-rich pastries and large pieces of cheese on their own. Keep food simple. Chargrilled fish, roast lean meats, steamed, baked or roasted vegetables can all be flavoured with herbs for plenty of variety; they don't need to be cooked with lashings of oil, butter or cream. Eat pasta with a tomato sauce rather than a creamy one, look to desserts based on fresh fruits.

If your body weight is on the low side and you are worried about cutting such a rich source of calories out of your diet, step up your intake of starchy foods (carbohydrates) such as pasta, rice, potatoes and bread, as well as pulses and lean proteins, to give your body the energy it needs.

Some people with raised liver enzymes get indigestion from certain foods such as bread or pasta. If you suspect a particular food, keep a diary of your food, drink and symptoms (page 85). If one item seems to be responsible, avoid it for a week or two, replacing it with an equally nutritious food, and see if there is any difference. I suggest you also read the chapter on Managing allergies.

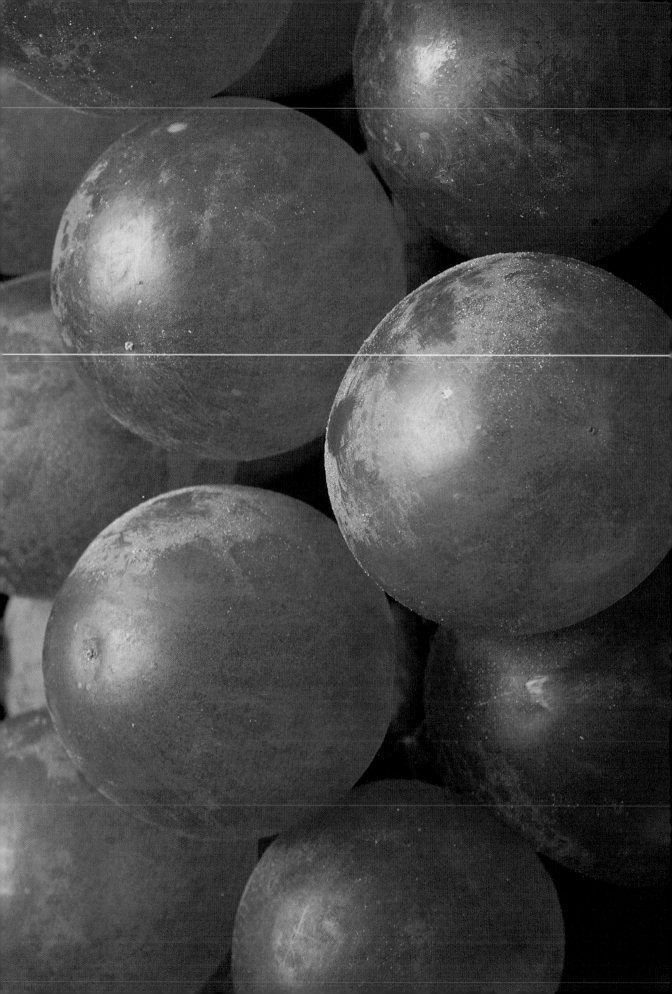

Parkinson's disease

Parkinson's disease affects approximately one per cent of people over the age of fifty, but it is also found in people in their twenties and thirties. It is a chronic, progressive disorder of the nervous system, resulting from the degeneration of certain brain cells. These brain cells produce a substance called dopamine, which is a neurotransmitter; in other words it helps the nerves communicate messages to one another. Without dopamine the nervous system falters.

The disease commonly starts with a tremor of one arm that occurs when the arm is at rest. As the disease progresses, movements gradually become more rigid, the face becomes frozen and there is progressive difficulty in performing simple tasks. Parkinson's disease affects not only the individual but also everyone around them, as the sufferer has to rely heavily on others for help. In Great Britain, there are only about two people with Parkinson's under each GP; many practitioners don't know the best ways of dealing with the disease. I would stress how important it is to be under the care of a neurologist who has an interest in Parkinson's disease; he or she will be able to put you in contact with a support network.

Drug treatment

Parkinson's disease is a distressing condition, but since the discovery of the drug Levodopa the prognosis has changed dramatically. Levodopa restores the deficiency of dopamine within the brain by providing the brain with the amino acid L-Dopa (L dihydroxy-phenylalanine) from which the neurotransmitter dopamine is derived.

How can food help?

While food cannot cure Parkinson's disease, what you eat can minimize the symptoms, help your body to feel stronger and generally improve both quality and quantity of life. When you are first diagnosed with Parkinson's you will need a little time to establish a good eating style; a diet that enables you to get the maximum benefit from the nutrients within your food and from Levodopa, if it is prescribed. Levodopa is taken by mouth and is absorbed most effectively through the upper part of the small intestine, the part encountered by food as it leaves the stomach. It is best taken on an empty stomach, as there are nutritional factors which in some people can interfere with the metabolism and ultimately the efficacy of the drug.

PROTEIN

In some people, certain amino acids (molecules within protein) interfere with the metabolism of Levodopa. If these protein-sensitive people eat protein foods and take Levodopa at the same time, the drug will not be able to work efficiently in the body.

One might think that the simplest thing to do would be to cut out protein, but this would lead to other malnutrition problems. Lack of protein itself can make your symptoms worse. Protein is essential in maintaining a healthy muscle system and is also needed to keep the body generally strong.

So it is a question of separating concentrated sources of protein from the dose of Levodopa, so that your body can glean the protein and respond well to the treatment. Your doctor and dietitian will be able to advise you as to the time you should leave between taking your medication and eating protein-rich foods such as meat, poultry, fish and eggs. (The slower absorption of protein from pulses – dried beans, peas and lentils – makes them less of a problem.) An hour before you eat seems to be commonly advised, but I cannot give an exact time, because everyone's metabolism is different, and indeed some people with Parkinson's are not at all affected by protein. They can eat a steak and take the Levodopa with no ill effect.

Other foods such as cereal-based carbohydrates (for example, pasta, rice, bread) and dairy products also contain protein, but in a less concentrated form, so these, and of course vegetables and fruits, will not interfere with the actions of Levodopa. So if you take Levodopa and want something to eat before your curfew time, these are the foods to choose. However, it is a good idea to try to separate medication from any type of food, unless your doctor advises otherwise.

Juggling your meals to include protein in the meals taken well after or before Levodopa, and carbohydrate-rich foods in the meals around Levodopa, is the way to balance a healthy diet.

I generally advise that you base breakfast and lunch on carbohydrates and save the protein until the evening, eating it an hour after you have taken your last dose of medication. Breakfasts could include toast, cereal, milk and fruit, for instance porridge with honey and banana, or rice pudding with poached pear. Lunches could be risotto, pasta with tomato sauce or roasted artichokes and onions and a little grated cheese, pitta bread stuffed with tabbouleh with a cucumber yoghurt dressing, or a simple sandwich. The evening meal could then consist of grilled lean meat or chicken, fish dishes like Caribbean casserole or chargrilled seabass with ginger, or venison with blackcurrants and redcurrants (see recipes, pages 322–327).

A BALANCED WAY OF EATING

As well as considering the protein aspect, you should also ensure that you eat a variety of fresh vegetables, fruits, and dairy products; in other words a well balanced diet.

Once you have established a good meal pattern, which allows your body to utilize the Levodopa efficiently and receive the correct balance of nutrients, it is important to stick to this sort of structure, in meal quantity, quality and timing. If you vary things too much, the action of Levodopa may be compromised. Having said this, it is important not to become obsessional. Always remember that food is to be enjoyed. As George Prentice said in 1860, 'What some call health, if purchased by perpetual anxiety about diet, isn't much better than tedious disease.'

TACKLING OTHER PROBLEMS

A vicious circle can develop: the disease can weaken and depress you, there is sometimes difficulty in swallowing, and it can be so physically difficult to prepare and eat meals that the desire to eat can disappear. Lack of nutrients leads to more depression, chronic fatigue, weight loss and reduced physical strength, all of which compound the problems of dealing with Parkinson's.

The best way to tackle these problems is to eat small meals often. Simple meals such as egg on toast or a rich soup are generally better managed than a whole roast lunch. Fruit fools, egg custard, soufflés and omelettes slip down easily if swallowing is difficult. It is still important to keep to a structured eating pattern and include protein foods at a set time every day. I suggest you read the chapter on the problems of ageing (page 225); although the symptoms and diseases are very different, the eating tips are useful.

Keeping a well-stocked refrigerator, freezer and cupboards full of simple-to-prepare foods such as cheese, sliced meats, individual portions of homemade soups and vegetable flans is a step in the right direction. Keep your cake tins stocked with nutritious bakes such as fruity malt loaf and apple flapjacks (page 331). Cakes also freeze well, so a batch of cakes can be stored for a month or two and eaten one at a time. Having small bowls of nuts, dried fruit and home-made biscuits such as raspberry bars (page 330) can help the Parkinson's sufferer seize a hungry moment, with little effort involved.

Multiple sclerosis

Multiple sclerosis, often referred to as MS, is a chronic progressive disease of the central nervous system. It affects more women than men on a ratio of about 3:2. According to the Multiple Sclerosis Society there are approximately 85,000 people with MS in the United Kingdom and 250,000 in the USA. The age at which MS strikes can vary from twelve to fifty years old, but the average age of diagnosis is late twenties to mid thirties. Once you have been diagnosed the next question is how will the disease progress? There is no predictable pattern; MS sufferers usually experience periods with few symptoms, called remission periods, then days, weeks or months later they will relapse. As the years go by the symptoms become more acute and/or new symptoms appear during a relapse. One of the hardest psychological aspects of MS is that you can feel so well during a remission, but just around the corner is a relapse, which can knock you for six.

Before discussing the ways in which food can be used to help you cope with MS, I would like to dispel some common misconceptions. Multiple sclerosis is not hereditary or infectious, nor is it a psychiatric disorder. MS is not a terminal condition in itself, but there are secondary complications which can result from the sometimes severe disability. It is these secondary conditions, such as chest or kidney infections, that can prove fatal.

Multiple sclerosis is caused by damage to the myelin sheath surrounding certain nerve fibres. How does this damage occur? Many believe that it is due to an aberration of the immune system. Generally, the immune system is our body's chief line of defence. It produces antibodies to fight against foreign matter, the bacteria and viruses that cause infections and illness. Sometimes, however, the immune system produces antibodies that destroy the healthy cells of the myelin sheath. When this becomes scarred, multiple sclerosis is diagnosed.

How will MS affect you?

The symptoms of MS are very variable, depending on the size and site of the neurological scarring. Common symptoms include altered sensations such as pins and needles, numbness, impaired speech or visual disorders. You may suffer from acute or chronic fatigue, muscular incoordination or spasms, tremor and partial paralysis. Some people forget things easily and find it difficult to concentrate. MS can also cause you to experience pain or become incontinent.

Not only are the symptoms distressing in themselves, they can also make the sufferer and their relatives and friends feel depressed. People find it hard to come to terms with the concept of being dependent on others, which sometimes makes them feel angry and resentful. There can also be a feeling of helplessness

in those around you; others cosset you and make you feel as if you can't do anything for yourself. Depression can set in and it can be hard to know how to get out of it.

As the years go by MS suffers will experience difficulties in living alone, so the practicalities of how they are going to be cared for and how they will afford help need to be addressed. Counsellors and social service professionals are out there to help you, your family and friends cope with MS, it's just a question of asking for help. In the first instance I suggest you contact the Multiple Sclerosis society (address on page 352).

What can be done to alter the progression of the disease?

While there is no proven way of preventing a relapse or deterioration, adopting a healthy lifestyle as far as is acceptable to the individual will maintain good general health. This includes getting plenty of rest and trying not to overexert yourself. It is tempting during a remission to try to act as if there is nothing wrong. A positive outlook is important, but overdoing it can exacerbate your symptoms. Try to establish a balance between proving something to yourself and others, and taking care of yourself, which will help you in the long run.

From a nutritional point of view, one of the most important things is to eat a healthy, well-balanced diet (see the chapter on Understanding your nutritional needs), with a good intake of polyunsaturated fatty acids, which I will discuss in more detail later.

It is also important to avoid other illness as far as possible. Read the chapter on Building a strong immune system, and tell friends to stay away when they are ill. They might be able to cope with a cold, but it can have a more serious effect on your system. Finally, the less stress you have in your life the better.

The role of unsaturated fats

The most talked-about link between food and MS is the theoretical link with fats. The first suggestion of a relationship between fats and MS came from studies of the incidence of this disease in different parts of the world. These studies suggested that the consumption of large quantities of animal fat was correlated with a prevalence of MS. It was pointed out that people consuming large amounts of animal fat were normally receiving a low intake of unsaturated fat. It was also found that people with MS, at some time during the course of their disease, had low levels of polyunsaturated fatty acids in their blood.

If we are to explore this issue further we need to understand a little about the different types of fat. The fats in most foods, whether animal or plant derived, are a combination of three main types of fatty acids: saturated, monounsaturated and polyunsaturated. Most animal fats, such as those found in meat, milk, yoghurt, cream, butter and cheese, have a high proportion of saturated fatty acids. Palm oil and coconut oil are also high in saturated fats. On the other hand, vegetable oils such as olive, sunflower and peanut (groundnut) have high

proportions of mono- and polyunsaturated fats. Oily fish are also proportionally higher in unsaturated than saturated fats.

The unsaturated fatty acids are essential fatty acids. That is, they are essential components of the diet required to support our growth and health. The three most important essential fatty acids are: linoleic, linolenic and arachidonic.

The essential fatty acids have two important functions in the body. Firstly, they are components of the membranes that surround the cells. The myelin sheath is part of such a membrane. (It is the myelin sheath that is scarred with multiple sclerosis.) Secondly, they are components of prostaglandins. Prostaglandins are hormone-like compounds found in all the body's tissues; among other things, they affect the nervous system and the immune defence system. One of the most important aspects of dealing with MS is making sure that the diet contains an adequate amount of essential fatty acids.

Trials have been carried out to test whether supplements of linoleic acid had any effect on the course of MS. One group of MS sufferers received a linoleic acid supplement in the form of sunflower seed oil capsules. Another group received a placebo (a dummy capsule). Neither group were aware of what they were taking. The results of these trials showed that the group receiving sunflower seed oil had less severe relapses of their MS and the relapses were of a shorter duration. The conclusion was drawn that a form of linoleic acid, taken as a supplement, MAY have some beneficial effect. I must point out that supplementing the diet with linoleic acid does not provide a cure for MS, it just appears to modify the course of the disease, reducing the severity, and perhaps the frequency, of relapses.

From a food point of view you should make sure that your diet includes plenty of essential, unsaturated fatty acids. These acids are present in most vegetable, seed and nut oils, such as olive, sunflower, corn, walnut – except coconut and palm oils, which are high in saturated fats. Dressing salads with olive or walnut oil, using vegetable oils for cooking, sesame oils with stir-fries, or drizzling rustic-style bread with warmed virgin olive oil instead of butter are all good ways of boosting your unsaturated fat intake. Fish such as salmon, tuna, herring, mackerel and sardines also contain essential fatty acids. Enjoy them grilled or barbecued, or see my recipes for seared tuna (page 323) and Scandinavian salad on (page 311).

Ideally you should include some essential fatty acids in your daily eating plan. If you doubt whether your intake is adequate, you can also purchase some of these oils in capsules, from health food stores and chemists.

Other dietary changes

I have little trust in some of the other diets that are sometimes recommended for multiple sclerosis sufferers. These include gluten-free and other 'food allergy' diets. Not only is there no evidence to support them, I worry that if people with MS start excluding things from their diet, they can easily become

malnourished, which can only make symptoms worse. However, if you feel you would like to investigate one of these routes, ask for professional help from an experienced dietitian, who will be able to ensure that your diet is well balanced. Some people feel better for excluding certain foods – and of course you may be the first person to start a trend of studies.

I am strongly against the raw/unprocessed food diets. There is a theory – but again no evidence – that these diets reduce the development of MS lesions. Of course in general health terms I encourage everyone to eat as many fresh foods and as few processed foods as possible, but I feel it is asking too much of people to avoid all canned, frozen and processed foods. Some of these can be extremely useful to have in the fridge, freezer and cupboard for occasions when you don't feel well enough to shop and cook much.

Many people ask me whether they should be taking any supplements or digestive aids such as aloe vera or enzymes? The answer is no, because there is no evidence supporting their use and I have seen cases of people taking too many supplements and suffering from toxic symptoms such as digestive upsets.

I can understand why sufferers look to supplements to help MS, but none of them have been proven to help, apart from those that boost your unsaturated fat intake. I always stress that the preferable first course of action is to derive the oils from food, rather than a supplement. Mother Nature cleverly delivers food as a 'package' of nutrients; meals featuring natural oils and fish are full of protein, vitamins and minerals, all of which will help your body feel and stay strong. A supplement can only give you the fatty acids.

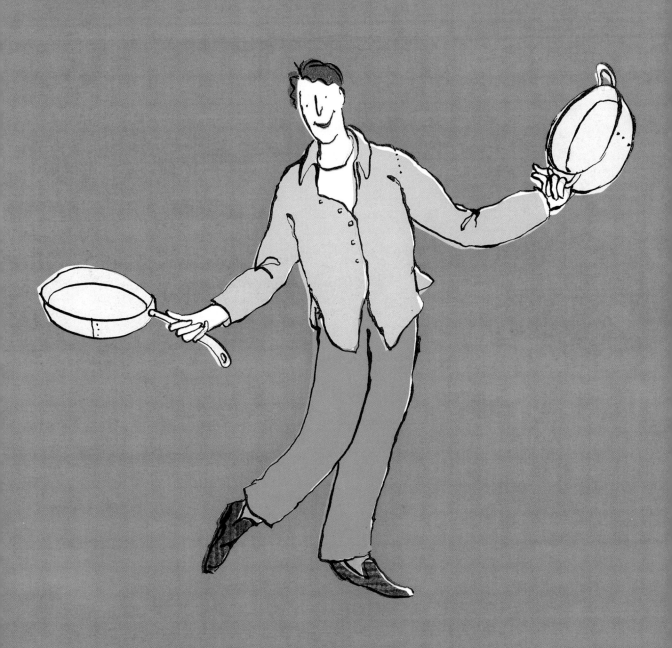

5

taste good

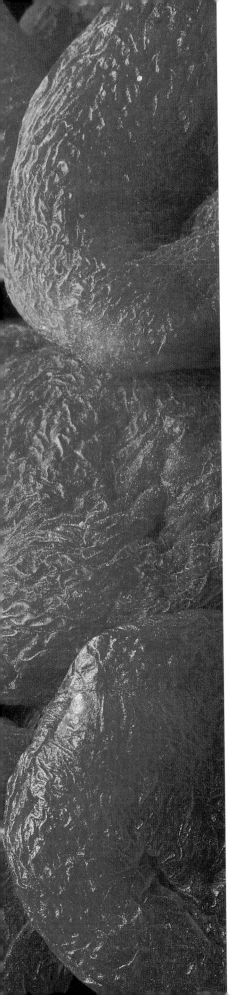

Porridge

Oats are rich in biotin, so a bowl of porridge is a perfect 'skin food'.

Remember to drink some water or freshly squeezed fruit juice at breakfast, to help your body deal efficiently with the nutrients and fibre from the food.

The size of the cup doesn't matter, it's just an easy way to get the right proportions of oats and water.

SERVES 1

1 cup porridge oats
2 cups water, milk or a mixture
    of the two
a pinch of salt or brown sugar

Place all the ingredients in a saucepan and bring to the boil, stirring all the time. Simmer for 5 minutes, stirring frequently, then serve at once.

You could add chopped banana, a handful of raisins or a spoonful of fruit compote.

Apricot muesli

Not only are oats good for the skin, they also help fend off cancers and heart disease and protect your body against ageing – what a way to start the day.

SERVES 4 – 6
50 g/2 oz wheat flakes
25 g/1 oz toasted bran
25 g/1 oz medium porridge oats
40 g/1½ oz dried banana flakes
25 g/1 oz ground, chopped
    or flaked hazelnuts
50 g/2 oz dried apricots, chopped
handful of coconut flakes

Mix all the ingredients together. Serve in small bowls with milk, natural yoghurt or fruit juice, and chopped fresh fruit.

Bagel with banana and peanut butter

You may think that peanut butter is too high in fat and sugar to be healthy. However, a good-quality peanut butter can give your body a little protein as well as energy in the mornings – and since it also contains fibre it helps to slow down the absorption of sugar into the body and therefore prevents sugar swings. For the same reason, the ideal bagels would be wholemeal, if you can get them.

If you or your child are allergic to peanuts you could substitute a thin layer of golden syrup.

SERVES 2
2 tablespoons good-quality crunchy
  peanut butter
2 bagels, sliced and warmed
1 large banana, sliced

Spread a spoonful of peanut butter on top of the bagel and arrange the banana slices on top. These should be made just before you are ready to eat them, as the bagel will become soggy and the banana will discolour.

Bananas on bread with maple syrup

Bananas are rich in potassium, which helps your body maintain a healthy blood pressure. They are also full of slow-release sugars, which makes them the perfect energy boost for the beginning of the day.

SERVES 4
4 thick slices of white bread
butter
2 bananas, thinly sliced
maple syrup

Thinly spread the bread with butter and layer the banana slices on top. Place under a hot grill until slightly browned. Trickle a little maple syrup on top and serve at once.

Orange and cinnamon breakfast bars

If time is short these biscuit bars will give your body a morning energy boost. They are also good as accompaniments to bowls of natural yoghurt and fresh fruit.

MAKES 6 LARGE BARS
125 g/4 oz plain wholemeal flour
½ teaspoon baking powder
½ teaspoon bicarbonate of soda
1 teaspoon ground cinnamon
125 g/4 oz unsalted butter, softened
125 g/4 oz soft brown sugar
1 egg, beaten lightly
1 tablespoon golden syrup
50 g/2 oz dried apricots, chopped
50 g/2 oz large raisins, chopped
50 g/2 oz dried figs, chopped
finely grated rind of 1 orange
175 g/6 oz coarse oatmeal

Preheat the oven to 180°C/350°F/ Gas 4. Grease and line an 18 cm/ 7 inch square baking tin with greaseproof paper.

Sift the flour, baking powder, bicarbonate of soda and cinnamon into a bowl.

Put the butter and sugar into a separate bowl and beat until light and fluffy. Beat in the egg a little at a time. If the mixture starts to curdle, beat in a tablespoon of the flour mixture. Add the golden syrup, dried fruits, orange rind and oatmeal, and mix until smooth. Mix in the flour mixture. Place in the lined tin and bake for approximately 15–20 minutes, until golden brown.

Remove from the oven and while still warm cut the mixture into fingers, but leave in the tin for 10 minutes to allow it to firm up slightly. Remove the biscuit fingers and leave on a wire rack to cool.

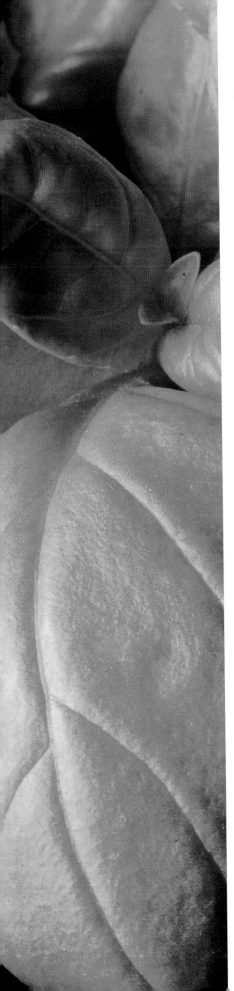

Tomato island soup

Tomatoes and lentils are two of the top ingredients in protecting your body against cancer.

SERVES 6

25 g/1 oz butter
1 onion, thinly sliced
2 garlic cloves, finely chopped
50 g/2 oz lean back bacon, chopped
1 potato, cut into small chunks
2 carrots, finely chopped
1 stick of celery, chopped
900 ml/1½ pints fresh vegetable
    or chicken stock
1 bay leaf
900 g/2 lb ripe tomatoes
4 tablespoons tomato purée
125 g/4 oz lentils
600 ml/1 pint milk
6 tinned plum tomatoes,
    drained of their juices
salt and pepper
natural yoghurt
6 sprigs of basil

Melt the butter in a large saucepan. Fry the onion and garlic until translucent. Add the bacon and fry until it starts to turn golden brown. Add the potato, carrots and celery and cook for a couple of minutes.

Add the stock, bay leaf, fresh tomatoes, tomato purée and lentils. Bring to the boil and simmer for 30 minutes, until the lentils are cooked.

Tip into a liquidizer and blend until smooth. Return to the heat and add the milk, drained plum tomatoes and salt and pepper to taste. Bring to the boil and simmer for a further 2–3 minutes, until piping hot. Serve with a plum tomato in each bowl, a swirl of yoghurt around the outside and a little freshly torn basil on top.

Summer tomato soup with basil purée

SERVES 6

2 tablespoons butter
1 large onion or 10 small leeks,
    finely chopped
1 bay leaf
5 sprigs of lemon thyme
700 g/1½ lb new potatoes,
    peeled and roughly chopped
1 teaspoon salt
4 tablespoons olive oil
450 g/1 lb ripe tomatoes, peeled,
    seeded and finely chopped
large bunch of basil leaves
champagne vinegar or red wine
    vinegar to taste
cracked black pepper

In a large saucepan, melt the butter with 125 ml/4 fl oz water and add the onion or leeks, bay leaf and thyme. Cook for 4–5 minutes, then add the potatoes and salt. Cover and stew for 5 minutes.

Add 1.2 litres/2 pints water and bring to the boil, then simmer, covered, until the potatoes are tender and falling apart. Pass the soup through a food mill and return to the pan (do not use a blender, which would make the soup gluey). Taste and add a little more salt if necessary.

Warm a tablespoon of olive oil in a frying pan, add the tomatoes, and cook until the juice has evaporated. Break up the tomatoes with a spoon and season to taste. Stir the tomatoes into the potatoes. If the soup is too thick, add a little more water.

Purée the remaining oil and the basil in a blender; season to taste with salt and vinegar. Serve the soup with a spoonful of basil purée in each bowl, sprinkled with pepper.

Parsnip and lemon soup

In this lovely lemony soup, the combination of fibre and slow-release sugars from the parsnips provides a long-lasting energy reserve.

SERVES 6

1½ unwaxed lemons
1 onion, finely chopped
1 tablespoon olive oil
4 large parsnips, peeled and chopped
1 Bramley apple, peeled and chopped
4 sticks of celery, chopped
1.2 litres/2 pints vegetable stock
150 g/5 oz natural yoghurt
dash of dry white wine

Cut the half lemon in half again and remove any pips.

In a large saucepan, fry the onion in the olive oil until golden brown. Add the parsnips, apple and celery and fry for 5–6 minutes until they turn golden. Add the stock and the two lemon quarters, bring to the boil, then simmer for 1 hour.

Meanwhile, pare the zest from the whole lemon and cut into thin strips; set aside. Cut the pared lemon in half and squeeze the juice. Purée the soup (including the lemon quarters) and return to the pan. Add the yoghurt, wine and lemon juice and heat gently to bring up to serving temperature, being careful not to boil it, as the yoghurt may curdle. Serve hot, garnished with strips of lemon zest.

Fresh pea soup with a mint 'cream'

Among other nutrients, peas provide magnesium, which helps the body metabolize energy. For the mint 'cream' you could use yoghurt or cream depending on whether you want a high or low fat soup. Add the mint mixture immediately before serving, as it will melt into the soup.

SERVES 6–8

50 g/2 oz butter
1 onion, thinly sliced
1 garlic clove, finely chopped
1.5 kg/3 lb peas, shelled (reserve the pods to make stock – see below)
salt and pepper
5 tablespoons thick natural yoghurt or thick cream
3 teaspoons finely chopped mint leaves

PEA-POD STOCK
175 g/6 oz pea pods, roughly chopped
10 lettuce leaves
1 carrot
1 stick of celery
1 bunch of spring onions
1 bay leaf

First make the stock: put all the ingredients into a large saucepan, add a good pinch of salt and 1.7 litres/3 pints of water. Bring to the boil, cover and simmer over a low heat for 1 hour. Strain and set aside.

Melt the butter in a large saucepan and add 125 ml/4 fl oz of the stock. Add the onion and garlic and stew over a low heat for 5–6 minutes, until the onion is soft and translucent.

Reserve a handful or two of peas and add the rest to the onion, with a good pinch of salt and enough stock to cover. Bring to the boil, then simmer until the peas are tender. Add the rest of the stock and purée until smooth. Return to the pan and season to taste with salt and pepper.

Cook the remaining peas in boiling water until tender. Drain and rinse in cold water. Add a pinch of salt to the yoghurt or cream and stir in the chopped mint. Serve the soup with a few whole peas and a spoonful of the mint 'cream' in each bowl.

Smoky potato soup

Potatoes help the body produce comforting, restful hormones – this is the perfect dish for warming lunches and slumbering suppers.

SERVES 6 – 8
50 g/2 oz butter
6 lean rashers of smoked bacon
3 leeks, white parts only, cut into
 5 mm/¼ inch rounds
1 teaspoon mustard
700 g/1½ lb red potatoes,
 scrubbed, quartered lengthways
 and thinly sliced
salt and pepper
thick natural yoghurt, fromage frais
 or single cream
1 tablespoon chopped fresh chives

Melt the butter in a large saucepan and fry the bacon and leeks until they turn a light golden brown. Add the mustard and 125 ml/4 fl oz water and simmer for 5 minutes.

Add the potatoes and cook for 10 minutes, stirring occasionally. Add 1.5 litres/2½ pints water and bring to the boil. Simmer until the potatoes are tender.

Tip into a liquidizer and blend until smooth; season to taste. Serve with a spoonful of yoghurt, fromage frais or cream in each bowl, and sprinkle with chives.

If you like, you could stir in some grated cheese, such as Emmental, Gruyère or mature Cheddar, so it melts into the soup. Add some wholewheat croûtons (see opposite) for texture.

Roasted pumpkin soup

Roasting the pumpkin before you make this soup really brings out the nutty taste. This soup is very creamy, perfect for calming the mind and body.

SERVES 4
900 g/2 lb pumpkin or other squash,
 peeled, seeded and chopped into
 large chunks
dash of olive oil
1 onion, finely chopped
1 garlic clove, finely chopped
½ tablespoon mild curry powder
600 ml/1 pint chicken or
 vegetable stock
salt and pepper
8 tablespoons thick natural yoghurt
 or cream
croûtons (see opposite)

Preheat the oven to 220°C/425°F/ Gas 7. Put the pumpkin on an oiled baking sheet and roast until the edges of the pumpkin turn golden brown and the flesh is soft to touch, about 25 minutes.

In a large saucepan, heat the olive oil and fry the onion and garlic until translucent. Add the curry powder and cook, stirring, for 1 minute.

Add the roasted pumpkin and stir for a couple of minutes. Add the stock, bring to the boil and simmer for 20 minutes.

Tip into a liquidizer, blend until smooth and season to taste. Add the yoghurt or cream and heat gently to bring the soup up to serving temperature. Serve with freshly ground black pepper and croûtons to provide a contrasting texture.

Minty chickpea soup

A trip to Morocco inspired this soup. The combination of nutty chickpeas – which ideally should be freshly boiled, although to be practical I have used canned chickpeas – with the mint and apple makes this the most delectable comfort soup; high in fibre and low in calories.

SERVES 6 – 8
1 tablespoon olive oil
1 onion, finely chopped
2 garlic cloves (optional)
2 parsnips, peeled and chopped
1 large Bramley apple, peeled,
 cored and chopped
2 teaspoons garam masala
900 ml/1½ pints fresh stock;
 either chicken or vegetable
2 x 400 g/14 oz cans of chickpeas
 (or 175 g/6 oz dried chickpeas,
 soaked overnight, then boiled
 for 1½ hours)
½ teaspoon celery salt
dash of white wine
150 g/5 oz natural yoghurt
1 tablespoon chopped fresh mint
salt and pepper

In a large saucepan, heat the oil and fry the onion and garlic until they are just turning golden. Add the parsnips and apple and fry for a further 5 minutes. Add the spice, warm for a minute and then add the stock and chickpeas. Bring to the boil and simmer for 25 minutes.

Tip into a liquidizer and blend until smooth. Return to the pan and add the celery salt, wine, yoghurt and mint. Taste and adjust the seasoning. Heat gently to bring up to serving temperature, being careful not to boil it, as the yoghurt may curdle. Serve hot.

Lentil, chicken and ginger soup

Lentils help the body to produce substances that ward off heart disease and cancer. In addition, because this soup is high in fibre it can cushion hormonal swings, aid digestion and improve skin.

SERVES 6

dash of olive oil

1 onion, finely chopped

1 garlic clove, finely chopped

2 teaspoons ground ginger

2 teaspoons garam masala

1.2 litres/2 pints fresh chicken stock

325 g/12 oz roast chicken meat, shredded

1 carrot, finely chopped

1 small parsnip, finely chopped

1 lemon, cut in half

225 g/8 oz Puy lentils

250 g/9 oz natural yoghurt

salt and pepper

Heat the oil in a large saucepan. Add the onion and garlic and fry until they begin to turn golden brown. Add the spice and stir for a minute. Add the stock and chicken meat, carrot, parsnip, lemon and lentils. Bring to the boil, then simmer for 25–30 minutes, until the lentils and vegetables are cooked.

Remove from the heat and remove the lemon. Tip the soup into a liquidizer and blend until smooth. Stir in the yoghurt, season to taste and heat gently to bring up to serving temperature, being careful not to boil it as the yoghurt may curdle. Serve hot.

Bean and rosemary soup

Beans are not only full of fibre, which helps keep a healthy digestive system, they also reduce the bad types of cholesterol in the blood and can cushion hormonal swings. For extra flavour, and if you don't mind increasing the fat content, you could add a dash of extra-virgin olive oil before serving.

This soup is delicious served with toasted Italian bread such as focaccia or ciabatta, spread with roasted garlic. You could also place the bread in the soup just before serving, which allows the bread to soak up all the lovely flavours.

SERVES 8

250 g/9 oz pearl barley, soaked in plenty of water, preferably overnight, but for at least 5 hours, until the barley is very swollen

2 litres/3½ pints chicken or vegetable stock

400 g/14 oz canned borlotti beans, drained

400 g/14 oz canned cannellini beans, drained

400 g/14 oz canned chickpeas, drained

dash of olive oil

75 g/3 oz pancetta, cubed

2 sprigs of rosemary, leaves stripped from the stem

3 garlic cloves, finely chopped

400 g/14 oz canned plum tomatoes

dash of dry white wine

salt and pepper

Drain the barley and place in a large saucepan. Add the stock, bring to the boil and simmer for 1 hour.

Add the beans and chickpeas and simmer for 20 minutes.

Meanwhile, heat the olive oil in another pan, add the pancetta, rosemary leaves and garlic and fry for a couple of minutes. Add the plum tomatoes and cook for 5 minutes. Add to the bean soup and cook for a further 40 minutes, until the flavours have married.

Add the wine and season to taste, adding plenty of freshly ground black pepper.

You may need to add a little extra water, but I like this soup thick and hearty. If you are serving it to someone who isn't able to eat whole beans you could liquidize it – in that case you probably will need to add more water.

Croûtons

Croûtons can make eating soup more fun for children – but that doesn't mean adults can't enjoy them too. They add a contrasting colour and texture to many soups, and if you use wholewheat or granary bread they also provide extra nourishment.

Use fresh thick slices of bread, cut into cubes. Place the cubes on a greased baking sheet and place either in a hot oven (200°C/400°F/Gas 6) or under the grill. Toast until brown on all sides, turning regularly.

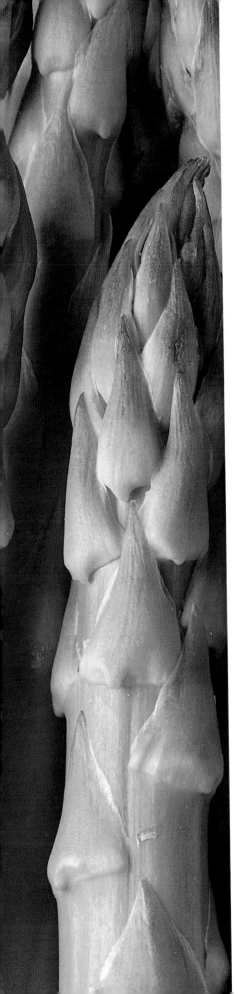

Purple sprouting broccoli and asparagus salad

SERVES 4

8 heads of purple sprouting broccoli
12 asparagus spears
2 spring onions, finely chopped
baby spinach leaves, washed
12 cherry tomatoes
1 tablespoon capers (optional)
chopped fresh dill

AVOCADO DRESSING

2 avocados
150 g/5 oz natural yoghurt
juice of ½ lemon
1 garlic clove, finely chopped
salt and pepper

Separate the broccoli into small sprigs and steam until just tender. Steam the asparagus until just tender. Combine the broccoli, asparagus and spring onions in a bowl.

For the avocado dressing, purée all the ingredients in a blender or food processor. Season to taste.

Mix the dressing with the broccoli and asparagus and serve on a bed of baby spinach, with the cherry tomatoes. Garnish with capers, if using, and fresh dill.

Orange blossom and carrot salad

This salad is deliciously simple, and gives a delicate flavour to health-giving carrots. It goes well with cold chicken, roast duck or freshly grilled mackerel.

Mix however much grated raw carrot you require with a few drops of orange blossom water. Leave in the refrigerator for 6 – 8 hours to allow the flavours to marry.

Spring vegetable tabbouleh

This tabbouleh is delicious on its own, but you could also include some roast chicken or cooked prawns. The combination of B vitamins present in wheat with the vitamin C rich asparagus and peas makes this a very moreish way to boost vitality.

SERVES 6

300 g/11 oz cracked wheat (bulgar)
600 ml/1 pint fresh chicken stock
200 g/7 oz French beans
100 g/3½ oz fresh peas
200 g/7 oz asparagus tips
200 g/7 oz cooked broad beans
4 spring onions, finely chopped
2 garlic cloves, finely chopped
4 tablespoons chopped fresh mint
8 tablespoons chopped fresh parsley
4 tablespoons virgin olive oil
juice of 1 lime
salt and freshly ground black pepper

TO SERVE

Cos lettuce leaves
cherry tomatoes, halved
a few mint leaves
1 lime, sliced

Soak the cracked wheat in the stock for about 30 minutes.

Meanwhile, steam or boil the French beans, peas and asparagus until just tender. Drain and refresh in cold water. Drain well.

Place in a large bowl and add the remaining ingredients. Drain any excess liquid from the cracked wheat and add to the bowl; season well.

Serve on the Cos lettuce leaves, garnished with tomatoes, mint leaves and slices of lime. If you like, drizzle with a little more olive oil just before serving.

Scandinavian salad

Sardines are rich in beneficial fish oils, which can help to improve blood fat levels and also reduce inflammation of the joints, skin and other body tissues. This recipe uses fresh sardines, but for a quick supper you could use tinned sardines, although the taste will not be as vivid.

SERVES 4
4 large ripe tomatoes, sliced in half
125 g/4 oz French beans
12 spears of asparagus
chopped fresh dill
few capers (optional)
4 small fresh sardines
bunch of rocket

VINAIGRETTE DRESSING
3 tablespoons olive oil
2 garlic cloves, finely chopped
1 teaspoon Dijon mustard
1 tablespoon lemon juice
salt and pepper

Cook the tomatoes under a very hot grill until they start to brown at the edges.

Meanwhile, boil or steam the beans and asparagus until just tender to the bite. Refresh in cold water to set the colour.

Place the tomatoes, beans and asparagus in a bowl, along with the dill and capers, if using.

Whisk together the ingredients for the dressing.

Grill the sardines, turning once.

Arrange the rocket leaves on four plates. Add the vegetables and spoon over the dressing. Add a grilled sardine to each plate. Garnish with fresh dill and serve immediately, with chunks of wholegrain bread.

Middle Eastern lentils with green salad

This recipe is bursting with Mediterranean flavours and packed with fibre. Begin by simmering the lentils; while they are cooking you can prepare the salad. I prefer green or brown lentils to the orange ones, but you could mix several colours together. For the salad, if you can get hold of the small cucumbers sold in Middle Eastern shops, so much the better, as they tend to have more flavour than larger cucumbers.

SERVES 4
225 g/8 oz lentils, soaked overnight
2 large onions, chopped
3 garlic cloves, chopped
½ tablespoon olive oil
85 g/3 oz wholegrain rice
1 teaspoon cumin seeds
1½ teaspoons salt
300 ml/½ pint fresh chicken
    or vegetable stock
2 spring onions, or 2 tablespoons
    chopped fresh parsley, to garnish

SALAD
1 Cos lettuce, or a bunch of baby
    spinach leaves
2 ripe tomatoes, seeded and diced
1 cucumber, peeled in strips,
    then sliced thinly
2 spring onions, chopped
1 red or green pepper, diced
1 avocado, sliced

DRESSING
2 tablespoons olive oil
1 garlic clove, crushed
2 tablespoons fresh lemon juice
    or wine vinegar
½ teaspoon paprika
¼ teaspoon mustard powder
¼ teaspoon salt
½ teaspoon sugar

Drain the lentils. Sauté the onions and garlic in olive oil until soft and golden. Add the rice, cumin and salt and continue to cook over a medium heat for 5 minutes. Stir in the drained lentils, add the stock, bring to the boil and cover. Simmer over a low heat for about 50 minutes, stirring from time to time to prevent sticking. You may find that the lentils need more liquid while they are cooking; if so, either add some more stock or just add water.

While the lentils are cooking, prepare the salad vegetables and place in a bowl. Mix together all the ingredients for the dressing, but do not dress the salad until you are ready to eat.

If the lentils are ready before you finish preparing the salad they can be kept warm in an ovenproof dish, covered with a lid.

When the lentils are ready, toss the salad with the dressing. Place spoonfuls of lentils on each plate and serve with the salad. Garnish the lentils with a little chopped spring onion or a sprinkling of chopped fresh parsley.

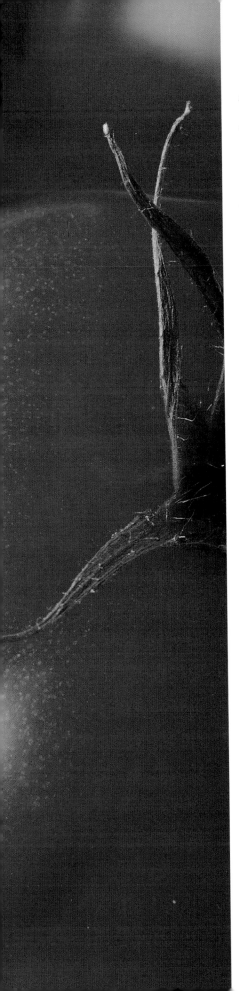

Tomato and tarragon dressing

Tomatoes are rich in beta-carotene and lycopene, two anti-cancer nutrients.

4 ripe, well-flavoured tomatoes, roughly chopped (alternatively use tinned plum tomatoes)
2 garlic cloves, roughly chopped
3 tablespoons red wine vinegar
½ teaspoon wholegrain mustard
salt and pepper
1 tablespoon olive oil
1 tablespoon chopped fresh tarragon

Put the tomatoes, garlic, vinegar, mustard, salt and pepper into a liquidizer and blend until the dressing is reduced to a pulp, but still retains some texture.

Add the olive oil very slowly, as if you were making mayonnaise. Add the tarragon and blend again. Adjust the seasoning to taste.

Vinaigrette

Use this and the other sauces and dressings on these pages to vary your daily vegetables and salads.

250 ml/8 fl oz olive oil
4 tablespoons wine vinegar, lemon juice or lime juice
1 teaspoon salt
freshly ground black pepper

Place all the ingredients in a jar with a lid and shake vigorously until it becomes thick and emulsified.

You can vary the taste by using different oils, such as walnut, sesame or sunflower oil. Experiment by adding finely chopped fresh herbs such as dill, mint, basil or parsley.

Tarragon walnut dressing

Yoghurt oozes calcium, a crucial bone-building and maintaining nutrient.
This is also good as a sauce for poached chicken.

250 g/9 oz natural yoghurt
50 g/2 oz walnuts, chopped
½ teaspoon mustard
2 tablespoons chopped fresh tarragon
1 garlic clove
salt and pepper

Put all the ingredients into a liquidizer and blend until smooth. Season to taste.

To make a slightly thicker dressing you could add a slice of fresh bread.

GARLIC AND DILL DRESSING
This is good with fish such as trout, sardines and mackerel.
Omit the walnuts and mustard. Replace the tarragon with 1 tablespoon chopped fresh dill.

PEANUT DRESSING
This is good with grilled, steamed or raw vegetables.
Stir 1 tablespoon crunchy peanut butter into 250 g/9 oz yoghurt. Season to taste.

HORSERADISH SAUCE
This is delicious with cold roast beef.
Mix 3 tablespoons freshly grated horseradish with 150 g/5 oz yoghurt. Season with a smidgen of mustard and a little salt and pepper.

Creamy lemon mayonnaise

You can use reduced-calorie mayonnaise if you like it, but I prefer the real thing, but then to use less of the dressing. This is delicious with cold roast chicken or poached fish, such as salmon.

150 ml/5 fl oz crème fraîche
150 g/5 oz mayonnaise
1 tablespoon fresh lemon juice
1 teaspoon mild French mustard
salt (optional) and freshly ground
　　black pepper

Stir all the ingredients together and season to taste with pepper, and salt if desired.

Salsa

Avocado is a rich source of the anti-oxidant vitamin E and is high in potassium. Salsa should be made at the last minute, as the avocado soon loses its green colour. Children may find the salsa a little hot; you could omit the chilli, but this would be a pity as it is the chilli that gives it its kick. Good for jaded appetites! Serve with baked or grilled vegetables, fish, or couscous.

1 small onion, chopped
1 small red chilli, chopped
12 ripe tomatoes, chopped
small handful of coriander leaves,
　　finely chopped
1 avocado, chopped
a dash of fresh lemon or lime juice
salt and pepper

Mix all the ingredients together, gently but evenly. Season to taste.

Rich tomato sauce

A simple, versatile sauce that can be served with fish or meat, pasta or vegetables. It can be stored in a covered container in the refrigerator for up to three days.

15 g/½ oz butter or a dash of virgin
　　olive oil
1 onion, thinly sliced
1 carrot, thinly sliced
1 garlic clove, crushed (optional)
900 g/2 lb tomatoes, skinned,
　　seeded and chopped
2 tablespoons chopped fresh basil
1 teaspoon sugar (optional)
salt and pepper

Melt the butter or heat the oil in a saucepan. Add the onion and carrot (and garlic, if using) and cook for about 5 minutes, until softened.

Add the tomatoes, basil and sugar (if needed to bring out the flavour of the tomatoes) and season to taste. Simmer for 15 minutes.

Inspirational sandwich fillings

Thinking of something exciting to put into sandwiches day after day can be a nuisance. Here are some ideas to get your taste buds tingling. They could also be used to fill jacket potatoes.

• Tuna, grated cucumber, Greek yoghurt, salt and freshly ground black pepper and chopped fresh coriander, on wholegrain rolls.

• Wafer-thin Parma or honey-roast ham, wholegrain mustard, gherkins and baby tomatoes, on light rye bread.

• Chopped roasted chicken in a mayonnaise or yoghurt dressing (see page 312) mixed with a little curry powder. Serve with watercress on stoneground bread.

• Grated Wensleydale cheese, sliced pickled onions and mango chutney, on walnut and onion bread.

• Vine-ripened tomatoes, sliced olives, mascarpone cheese and flat-leaf parsley, on sun-dried tomato or olive bread.

• Smoked salmon, avocado and grapefruit, on wholewheat bread.

• Lean Aberdeen Angus beef, horseradish and lambs lettuce on brown bread.

• Baby spinach and fresh herbs, topped with fromage frais or cottage cheese mixed with sultanas, dried apricots, walnuts, diced cucumber and quartered baby tomatoes, on crusty white roll.

Smoked chicken with grapes in wholemeal pitta

This gives you a good selection of nutrients: protein from the chicken, carbohydrates and fibre from the grapes and bread, and dairy products in the dressing. It is perfect for picnics or lunch boxes. Alternatively the topping can be stuffed into a jacket potato and served as a light supper dish.

SERVES 4
125 g/4 oz thinly cut smoked chicken
20 seedless grapes, quartered
4 baby wholemeal pittas

DILL DRESSING
1 tablespoon finely chopped fresh dill
3 tablespoons natural yoghurt
salt and pepper

Mix the chicken with the grapes and stuff into the pittas.

Mix all the dressing ingredients together and drizzle over the chicken. Serve at once.

Goats' cheese with celery and walnuts on granary bread

Goats' cheese is high in calcium and protein, making it a useful source of these nutrients for people who cannot tolerate cows' milk.

SERVES 4
softened butter
4 or 8 slices of granary bread
150 g/5 oz soft French goats' cheese, very soft
4 sticks of celery, finely chopped
25 g/1 oz walnuts, chopped
salt and pepper

Lightly butter the bread. Mix the goats' cheese with the celery and walnuts, season to taste and spread on the bread.

Parma ham with asparagus on cheese bread

Both Parma ham and cheese contain protein, making this a substantial protein-rich snack.

SERVES 4
250 g/9 oz asparagus
1 loaf of cheese bread,
    cut in thick slices
softened butter
100 g/3½ oz Parma ham
salt and pepper

Trim the woody bases of the asparagus, then steam or boil until tender. Drain and pat dry. Cut in half and keep warm.

Warm the bread slightly and lightly spread with butter. Place several pieces of asparagus on a piece of Parma ham and roll up. Arrange these on top of the bread, then sprinkle with salt and pepper.

Focaccia with chargrilled aubergines

A quick, satisfying supper, or a tasty alternative to a sandwich at lunchtime.

SERVES 4
1 aubergine, sliced
2 beef tomatoes, sliced
1 focaccia, sliced
black olives, pitted and halved

BASIL VINAIGRETTE
2 tablespoons finely chopped
    fresh basil
4 tablespoons extra virgin olive oil
2 tablespoons balsamic vinegar
salt and pepper

Preheat the grill. Cook the aubergine under the hot grill until browned, then leave to cool.

Mix together all the ingredients for the dressing and season to taste.

Place the aubergine and tomato slices on the bread. Sprinkle with the olives and dressing. Serve at once.

French bread pizza with cheese, chilli and salami

This is a quick supper, ideal for children. Shop-bought pizzas can be loaded with fat and additives; homemade pizza (see page 328) is superb; but this version, made with French bread, can be made in 15 minutes.

SERVES 4
½ teaspoon chopped fresh chilli
    or ½ teaspoon chilli powder
    (optional)
4 tablespoons tomato purée
1 baguette, cut in half and
    sliced horizontally
100 g/3½ oz Gruyère cheese, grated
100 g/3½ oz lean salami
10 black olives, pitted and halved

Preheat the oven to 190°C/375°F/ Gas 5.

Mix the chilli with the tomato purée and spread on the bread. Sprinkle the cheese on top, then the sliced salami and olives. Place on a baking sheet and bake for 10 minutes, until the cheese has melted. Serve at once, with a crisp salad.

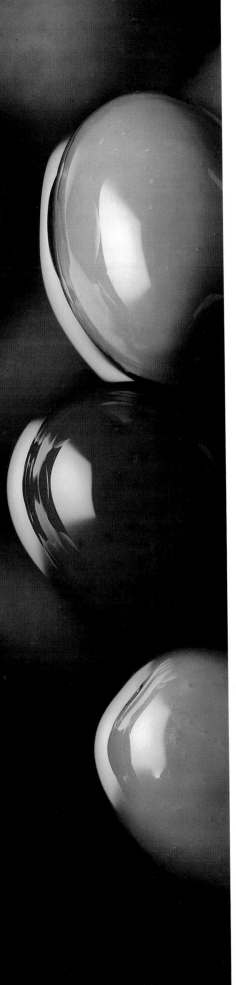

Tapenade

Tuna and anchovies both contain beneficial fish oils that are good for your blood, protect against heart disease and cancer, and help relieve arthritis. This is also a good appetite stimulant. It can be kept in the fridge for up to a week. Spread it on bruschetta or serve as a dip with sticks of raw vegetables.

SERVES 10–12
225 g/8 oz black olives
1 teaspoon lemon juice
50 g/2 oz canned tuna
8 anchovy fillets
85 g/3 oz capers
1 garlic clove
2 tablespoons olive oil
freshly ground black pepper

Put all the ingredients, apart from the olive oil and pepper, into a food processor and blend until smooth.

Add the olive oil gradually to make a thick paste.

Season to taste with a little black pepper and store in the refrigerator until needed.

Cheese straws

With a subtle cheese flavour, these pastry 'straws' are as light as air. They are good to serve with drinks before a meal as they are not too filling – and because they are homemade they will be far more satisfying to eat than shop-bought 'nibbles', not to mention free of undesirable additives.

MAKES ABOUT 40 CHEESE STRAWS
125 g/4 oz plain white
    or wholemeal flour
pinch of salt
pinch of cayenne pepper
50 g/2 oz butter, cut into pieces
50 g/2 oz mature Cheddar cheese,
    finely grated
1 egg yolk, beaten
1 teaspoon Dijon mustard

Sift the flour, salt and cayenne together into a mixing bowl. Add the butter and lightly rub together with your fingertips until the mixture resembles fine breadcrumbs. Stir in the grated cheese, then the egg yolk and mustard. Draw together with the fingertips to form a smooth dough, using a little cold water if the mixture is too dry. Chill in the refrigerator for at least 30 minutes.

Preheat the oven to 200°C/ 400°F/Gas 6.

Roll out the dough thinly on a floured board and cut into strips about 12 cm/5 inches long and 5 mm/¼ inch wide. Place on baking sheets and bake for 10–15 minutes or until golden. Remove from the oven, leave on the baking sheet to cool slightly, then transfer to a wire rack to cool completely. Store in an airtight tin.

Avocados with peppers and olives

This dish needs to be made at the last minute, as the avocados go brown very quickly. It is a good way to eat a generous helping of vegetables.

SERVES 4

2 small avocados
juice of 1 lime
1 red pepper, finely chopped
1 green pepper, finely chopped
2 carrots, finely diced
½ cucumber, finely chopped
2 ripe tomatoes, finely chopped
1 onion, finely chopped
10 black olives, finely chopped
½ teaspoon salt
freshly ground black pepper
Tabasco or other hot sauce to taste

Cut the avocados in half lengthways very carefully, discard the stones and carefully scoop out the flesh. Reserve the shells. Chop the flesh finely and place in a bowl. Add half the lime juice and toss gently.

Mix the chopped vegetables, olives, remaining lime juice, salt and pepper and a dash of Tabasco. Add the avocado and toss lightly, taking care not to break up the avocados too much while tossing or the salad will look mushy.

Pile the salad back into the avocado shells, or serve it from the bowl and scoop up with taco shells or pitta breads; you could also serve it on a bed of rocket or spinach.

Marinated mussels

Mussels are a good source of zinc, to boost your immune system.

SERVES 6

about 2 kg/4–5 lb mussels
juice of 1 lemon
4 tablespoons virgin olive oil
½ teaspoon salt
¼ freshly ground black pepper
1 teaspoon sugar or honey
2 teaspoons chopped mixed fresh
   herbs such as parsley, coriander
   and most certainly basil
1 tablespoon chopped fresh parsley,
   to garnish

Scrub the mussels and rinse in cold water, discarding any with broken or open shells. Place in a large saucepan over a high heat for 3–4 minutes, shaking the pan occasionally, until the mussels open. Discarding any that remain closed, remove the mussels from their shells. Keep half the shells for serving.

Mix the lemon juice, oil, salt, pepper, sugar or honey and mixed herbs and very gently stir in the mussels, taking care not to break them up.

Marinate the mussels in a shallow dish in the refrigerator for up to 3 hours, until you are ready to serve them (the longer the better).

To serve, lay out the shells on a platter and place a mussel in each shell. Sprinkle the parsley over the top. Serve with lemon wedges and French bread to mop up the marinade.

Fonduta (Italian cheese fondue)

Although fondue is usually associated with Switzerland, northern Italy has its own traditional fondue. Fontina is a mild, semi-soft cheese, but if you can't get hold of Fontina you could use Cheddar, Gruyère or Emmental, or a combination of cheeses.

This fonduta is rich in calcium, but high in saturated fats. Serve it with wholemeal bread and raw or very lightly cooked vegetables such as asparagus, broccoli or cauliflower to dunk into it, to help your body deal with the fat.

If you are lucky enough to obtain some white truffles, this is the dish to use them with – just shave a few slices over the top – the taste is out of this world!

SERVES 4

400 g/14 oz Fontina cheese,
   cut into small pieces
600 ml/1 pint milk
85 g/3 oz butter
4 eggs
salt and pepper
chopped fresh chives or white truffles
   (optional)

Put the cheese and milk into a bowl and leave for at least an hour – traditionally the cheese is left in the milk for about 6 hours.

Put the cheese and milk into a double boiler over a low heat. Add the butter and eggs, season to taste and heat gently, stirring all the time. It is important to keep the mixture moving, otherwise the cheese burns on the bottom of the pan.

When the mixture has become a smooth, silky sauce, pour into a warmed serving dish and shave slices of truffle on top or sprinkle with chopped chives.

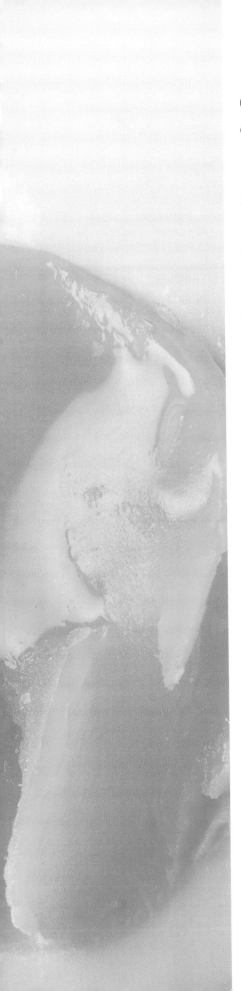

Chanterelle omelette

Omelettes are a nutritious fast food, high in protein, with a number of important vitamins and minerals. Pregnant women and elderly people should avoid omelettes because of the slight risk of salmonella poisoning which can come from uncooked eggs. Some people say that you could cook the omelette thoroughly, but it would be rather rubbery. Here are a few points to help you make a soft, delicious omelette.

- *Choose good-quality fresh eggs, ideally organic free-range eggs.*
- *Speed is the most important factor in making an omelette. You should be ready to eat the omelette before you start cooking, as it takes less than a minute to cook the egg mixture.*
- *Always have your filling prepared first, so that you can assemble the omelette at the last minute.*
- *Omelettes are best made for one (2–3 eggs) or two (4–5 eggs) people. Four people would need 8 eggs, and a 28 cm/11 inch diameter pan.*

SERVES 1
25 g/1 oz butter
about 125 g/4 oz fresh chanterelle
    mushrooms
salt and pepper
chopped fresh herbs such as tarragon
    or parsley (optional)
3 eggs

Heat half the butter in a small saucepan and fry the mushrooms for a couple of minutes. Add a little seasoning, and some herbs if you like. Remove the pan from the heat.

Meanwhile, break the eggs into a bowl and beat lightly with a fork.

Put an 18–20 cm/7–8 inch omelette pan over a high heat. Add the remaining butter and as soon as it begins to foam, add the beaten eggs and the cooked mushrooms and leave for about 10 seconds. Using the back of a spoon, stir the omelette lightly and then tip the omelette mixture on to a warmed plate and serve at once. The omelette should be creamy in the centre.

CHARGRILLED ONION AND SAUSAGE OMELETTE

Brush some canned artichoke hearts and quartered onions with olive oil and cook under a hot grill until they are deep brown around the edges. Grill a lean sausage, chop into slices and mix with the artichokes, onions and ½ teaspoon of mild mustard. Place on top of the cooked omelette and fold over.

SMOKED HADDOCK AND SPINACH OMELETTE

Poach a small piece of smoked haddock in a little milk, until the flesh flakes easily, about 5–8 minutes. Remove from the milk and flake into large pieces. Wash some spinach leaves thoroughly. When the omelette is nearly ready, put the fish and the raw spinach on top of the egg mixture in the pan. Grate a little nutmeg over the spinach, along with freshly ground black pepper. Fold the omelette in half, tucking the spinach into the centre. Cook for 1 minute, to allow the heat from the omelette to steam the spinach. Serve immediately.

Leek and asparagus flan

Leeks are members of the allium family, known to help prevent cancer; asparagus is a rich source of folic acid.

SERVES 6–8

275 g/10 oz white or wholemeal
    shortcrust pastry
50 g/2 oz butter
450 g/1 lb leeks, washed and sliced
    into 5 mm/¼ inch rings
12 asparagus spears
50 ml/2 fl oz dry white wine
½ teaspoon salt
2 eggs
150 ml/5 fl oz milk or single cream
2–3 tablespoons wholegrain mustard
85 g/3 oz Swiss cheese, grated
coarsely ground black pepper

Preheat the oven to 190°C/375°F/ Gas 5. Roll out the pastry and use to line a 22 cm/9 inch quiche tin. Line with baking parchment or greaseproof paper and baking beans and bake 'blind' for 8–10 minutes, until the pastry starts to lose its wetness and turn pale golden brown.

Melt the butter in a saucepan, add the leeks and any water that clings to them. Cook, stirring, for about 3 minutes, until they begin to look translucent. Add the asparagus, wine and salt, cover and simmer for about 15 minutes or until tender. Check after 7 minutes and add more wine or a little water if necessary.

Beat the eggs together, then stir in the milk or cream, mustard and cheese. When the leeks and asparagus are cooked, season with pepper and fold in the egg mixture. Pour the filling into the pastry case and bake until the top is golden brown, about 30 minutes.

Mediterranean vegetable and creamy custard flan

The combination of the vegetable topping – with beta-carotene rich peppers – a creamy, cheesy middle, and a walnut base make this flan delectable. It keeps well until the next day.

SERVES 6–8

1 small onion,
    peeled and thinly sliced
1 garlic clove, finely chopped
a little olive oil
1 small aubergine, sliced thinly
1 red and 1 yellow pepper,
    sliced thinly
1 courgette, sliced thinly
450 g/1 lb plum tomatoes
2 tablespoons tomato purée
225 g/8 oz mushrooms, sliced
dash of red wine
salt and pepper
2 eggs, beaten
100 ml/3½ fl oz milk
1 teaspoon wholegrain mustard
175 g/6 oz mature cheese
    (a mixture of Gruyère and
    Lancashire would be good)
bunch of fresh basil leaves
shavings of fresh Parmesan cheese

WALNUT BASE
150 g/5 oz wholemeal breadcrumbs
50 g/2 oz butter
25 g/1 oz walnuts, chopped
150 g/5 oz mature cheese, grated
1 garlic clove, finely chopped

Preheat the oven to 220°C/425°F/ Gas 7.

For the walnut base, put the breadcrumbs into a bowl and rub in the butter. Stir in the remaining ingredients and press into a 28 x 13 cm/11 x 5½ inch tin. Bake for 20 minutes, or until golden brown.

Reduce the oven temperature to 180°C/350°F/Gas 4.

Meanwhile, make the vegetable topping: gently fry the onion and garlic in olive oil until translucent. Add the aubergine, peppers and courgette and cook for 5 minutes.

Add the tomatoes, tomato purée, mushrooms and a dash of red wine. Bring to the boil, then reduce the heat and simmer for 25–35 minutes, until the vegetables are cooked and surrounded by a thick sauce. Season to taste and set aside.

Whisk together the eggs, milk, mustard, salt and pepper.

Put the cheese into the walnut case and pour over the egg mixture. Bake in the oven for 15 minutes, until the egg custard is starting to set. Take the flan out of the oven, tear some basil leaves into the tomato sauce and carefully spoon the vegetables on top of the flan. Return to the oven for 5–10 minutes, until the topping is bubbling.

To serve, tear some basil leaves over and shave Parmesan on top.

ARTICHOKE AND WALNUT FLAN
Drain 400 g/14 oz canned artichoke hearts and slice lengthways. Place on a lightly oiled baking sheet and drizzle over a little olive oil. Place under a hot grill until the edges of the artichokes are golden brown. Fry 50 g/2 oz lean bacon until well browned, then drain on kitchen paper to remove excess fat.

Put the artichoke hearts, bacon and cheese into the walnut case and pour over the egg mixture. Bake in a preheated oven at 180°C/350°F/Gas 4 for 20 minutes.

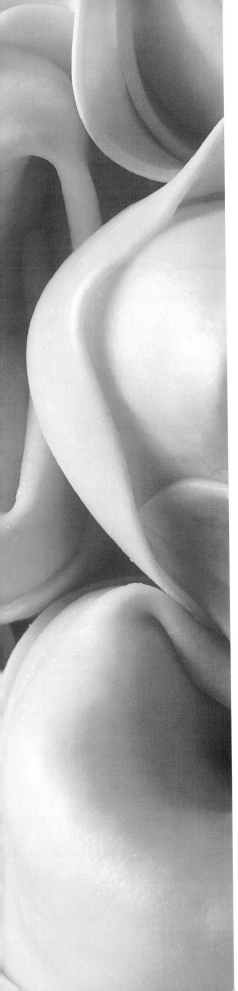

Pasta with grilled peppers, aubergine and roasted onions

SERVES 4

4 different coloured peppers
1 aubergine
8 small onions or shallots,
    peeled and root removed
virgin olive oil
50 g/2 oz black olives
2 garlic cloves
450 g/1 lb dried pasta
salt and pepper
bunch of fresh basil leaves
freshly grated Parmesan cheese

Slice the peppers in half lengthways and remove the seeds. Slice the aubergine into quarters. Arrange the onions or shallots, peppers and aubergine on an oiled grill pan. Drizzle with a little olive oil and place under a grill or in a very hot oven and cook until the pepper skins are black and the onions are golden brown. You may need to remove the onions before the peppers.

Once the peppers are blackened, place them in a plastic bag. Tie the top and leave to cool slightly. When the peppers are cool enough to handle, you will find that the skin is easy to peel away from the flesh. Discard the charred skins.

Scoop the aubergine flesh away from the skin and add to the peppers, together with the onions and olives.

In a large frying pan, heat a little olive oil and fry the garlic. Add the vegetables and cook for a couple of minutes. Keep warm while you cook the pasta. When the pasta is cooked until tender but still just firm to the bite, drain well and add to the vegetables. Season to taste and tear in the basil. Serve with Parmesan.

Spaghetti with Gruyère, rosemary and roasted onions

The starchy pasta encourages the body to relax – what better way to unwind at the end of the day? Carbohydrate is also useful for stocking up the glycogen stores prior to exercise.

SERVES 4

16 shallots or very small onions,
    peeled and root removed
olive oil
2 garlic cloves, finely chopped
450 g/1 lb dried spaghetti
bunch of fresh rosemary leaves,
    finely chopped
125 g/4 oz Gruyère cheese, grated
handful of black olives
1 teaspoon Dijon mustard
salt and pepper

Place the onions on an oiled grill tray, drizzle with a little olive oil and grill until they are tender and the outsides are golden brown; turn occasionally so they cook evenly.

If you like, you can fry the garlic in a little olive oil, although I generally prefer to add it uncooked at the next stage.

Cook the pasta until it is tender but still just firm to the bite, drain well and place in a large bowl. Add the onions, garlic, chopped rosemary, Gruyère, olives, mustard, salt and pepper. Return to the pan and quickly heat through to allow the cheese to melt. Serve immediately, garnished with a few sprigs of rosemary.

Pasta with sausage, grilled tomatoes and basil

Tomatoes are a good source of the anti-oxidant beta-carotene, which protects your body against disease and signs of ageing.

SERVES 4
900 g/2 lb fresh ripe tomatoes
olive oil
1 onion, finely chopped
2 garlic cloves, finely chopped
2 tablespoons tomato purée
dash of red wine
6 lean, good-quality sausages,
    grilled and cut into thick slices
450 g/1 lb dried pasta
bunch of fresh basil leaves
freshly grated Parmesan cheese

Slice the tomatoes in half, place on a grill tray and drizzle with a little olive oil. Place under a hot grill and grill until they are soft and slightly blackened around the edges.

Meanwhile, heat a little olive oil in a large saucepan and fry the onion and garlic until light golden brown. Add the grilled tomatoes, tomato purée and a dash of red wine. Cover with a lid and leave to simmer for 20–30 minutes.

Remove the lid and boil the sauce until it reduces and thickens, by allowing some of the water to escape as steam. Add the sausages and cook for a further 10 minutes, being careful not to stir too vigorously, otherwise the sausages will break up.

Meanwhile, cook the pasta in plenty of boiling water until it is tender but still just firm to the bite. Drain and add to the sauce. Tear in some fresh basil and serve with grated Parmesan.

Vine-ripened tomato risotto

This is great on its own, or you could serve it with ham hock or a flavoursome fish such as a grilled tuna steak. It is important that the tomatoes you use are ripe and tasty, otherwise the dish will be very bland.

SERVES 4–6
450 g/1 lb tomatoes on the vine
1.5 litres/2½ pints fresh chicken
    or vegetable stock
1 tablespoon butter
1 tablespoon virgin olive oil
2 rashers of lean back bacon
    (optional), chopped
1 onion, finely chopped
1 garlic clove, finely chopped
400 g/14 oz risotto (arborio) rice
125 ml/4 fl oz dry white wine
salt and pepper
large bunch of basil leaves
50 g/2 oz Parmesan cheese, shaved

Place the tomatoes in a bowl of boiling water for 2 minutes, then remove with a slotted spoon and place in a bowl of ice-cold water. Leave for 2 minutes, then lift out the tomatoes. You should find that the tomato skins fall away from the flesh. Discard the skins and slice the tomatoes in half. Scoop out the seeds and reserve the flesh.

Heat the stock in a saucepan and bring it to a gentle simmer.

In a large saucepan, melt the butter and oil over the heat. Add the bacon, onion and garlic and fry gently for 2–3 minutes until the onion is translucent and soft.

Add the rice and stir over the heat for 2–3 minutes. Add the wine and tomato flesh and cook for a further 2 minutes. Gradually add the stock, a little at a time, stirring constantly and making sure that the stock is absorbed before adding more. Repeat until all the stock has been used and the rice grains are swollen and tender, but retain just a little firmness in the centre (don't over-cook the rice otherwise it will go soggy). Season with salt and pepper to taste and, if you like, briskly stir in another tablespoon of butter. Take the pan off the heat and tear the basil leaves into the risotto. Serve at once, garnished with Parmesan.

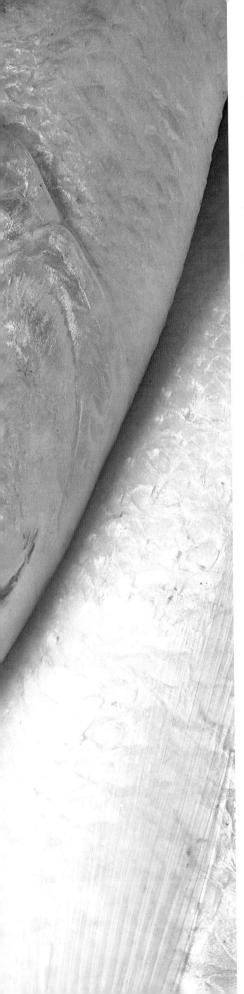

Prawn risotto

It is traditional to beat in a little butter just before serving a risotto – this gives it a wonderful flavour and creamy consistency. However, if you need to keep your fat intake down, this is optional.

SERVES 6
1.5 litres/2½ pints fresh fish
   or chicken stock
2 tablespoons olive oil
3 large garlic cloves, finely chopped
1 onion, finely chopped
6 tablespoons chopped fresh parsley
125 ml/4 fl oz dry white wine
400 g/14 oz arborio rice
salt and pepper
450 g/1 lb uncooked prawns,
   shelled and deveined
25 g/1 oz unsalted butter (optional)
slices of lime, to garnish

Heat the stock in a small saucepan and keep hot until needed.

Heat 1 tablespoon of the oil in a large saucepan, add the garlic and fry gently until it turns golden brown. Add the onion and 5 tablespoons of parsley and cook for few minutes.

Add the wine, bring to the boil and simmer for a few minutes.

Add the rice and stir over the heat for a few minutes. Gradually add the hot stock, about 125 ml/4 fl oz at a time, stirring constantly, making sure that the liquid has been absorbed before you add more stock.

After about 10 minutes, add salt and pepper and the prawns. Stir until the prawns turn pink. You may need to add a little more water, but make sure that the water is boiling.

Stir in the remaining parsley and the butter if you are using it, then serve at once, garnished with lime.

Chargrilled seabass with sesame and ginger

Seabass is a deliciously meaty fish which is a rich source of protein, without much fat – especially when cooked in this way, in a ridged chargrilling pan. If you don't have one you could cook the fish under a standard grill. The ginger dressing really lifts the flavour of the fish.

SERVES 4
4 small seabass, about 450 g/1 lb
   each, cleaned and scaled
a dash of olive oil
coarse sea salt and freshly ground
   black pepper

GINGER AND SESAME DRESSING
1 tablespoon finely chopped
   fresh ginger
4 tablespoons dark soy sauce
4 tablespoons sesame oil
4 tablespoons rice wine vinegar
6 tablespoons sunflower oil
2 teaspoons chilli sauce (optional)

Make the dressing by placing all the ingredients into a screw-topped jar. Add salt and pepper and shake vigorously until emulsified. Set aside while you cook the fish.

Make three diagonal slashes across the side of each fish. Brush with olive oil and season with salt and pepper. Heat a ridged chargrilling pan, or heat the grill. Brush the griddle with a little olive oil to prevent the fish from sticking. Place the fish on the griddle and cook for 5 minutes each side. Serve hot, drizzled with the dressing.

Seared tuna on a bed of spinach and asparagus

Tuna is full of beneficial fish oils, good for preventing heart disease and soothing a tired, inflamed body.

SERVES 2
Vinaigrette dressing (see page 312),
    made with lemon or lime juice
12 asparagus spears, steamed
12 cherry tomatoes,
    preferably yellow and red
450 g/1 lb baby spinach,
    cleaned thoroughly
1 avocado, cut into small pieces
1 garlic clove, finely chopped
freshly grated nutmeg
4 basil leaves, finely chopped
2 x 175 g/6 oz pieces of very
    fresh tuna
dash of olive oil
salt and freshly ground black pepper
lime wedges, to serve

First make the vinaigrette dressing and set aside.

Preheat the grill while you prepare the asparagus, tomatoes, spinach and avocado. Toss them together with the garlic, nutmeg and basil.

Brush the tuna with a little olive oil and sprinkle with salt and pepper. When the grill is very hot, cook the tuna for 1–2 minutes on each side – if it is overcooked it is no better than tinned tuna.

While the second side of tuna is cooking, toss the salad with the dressing and place on the plates. Put the seared tuna on top of the salad, garnish with a lime wedge and serve immediately.

Skate with black butter

Skate is an easily digestible source of protein, which helps build your strength.

SERVES 4–6
900 g/2 lb skate
½ lemon, sliced
1 onion, sliced
1 bay leaf
6 peppercorns
6 parsley stalks
salt
85 g/3 oz butter
1 tablespoon white wine vinegar
1 tablespoon chopped fresh parsley

Rinse the skate and wipe dry. Place in a deep frying pan and cover with 300 ml/½ pint water. Add the lemon, onion, bay leaf, peppercorns, parsley stalks and salt. Bring to the boil, cover and simmer for 25 minutes.

Using a slotted spoon, remove the fish and keep warm.

In a small saucepan, heat the butter and allow to brown, but not scorch. Remove the pan from the heat and stir in the vinegar and parsley. Pour over the skate and serve at once.

Caribbean casserole

You could use a combination of salmon, cod, halibut, or just one type of fish.

SERVES 6–8
1 teaspoon salt
2 green (unripe) bananas,
    sliced into 1 cm/½ inch rounds
4 onions, chopped
3 garlic cloves, finely chopped
2 tablespoons olive oil
½ teaspoon cayenne pepper
½ teaspoon chopped fresh thyme
2 potatoes, chopped
2 sweet potatoes, chopped
¼ small head of cabbage, chopped
12 tablespoons chopped fresh parsley
2 x 400 g/14 oz cans tomatoes, or 450
    g/1 lb fresh tomatoes, chopped
300 ml/10 fl oz fresh vegetable stock
450 g/1 lb uncooked prawns, rinsed,
    shelled and deveined
450 g/1 lb fish fillets, cut into chunks
lime or lemon slices and flat-leafed
    parsley or coriander, to garnish

Dissolve the salt in enough water to cover the sliced bananas. Soak the bananas in the water for 15 minutes.

In a large saucepan, sauté the onions and garlic in olive oil until the onions are soft. Add the cayenne and thyme and sauté for a couple more minutes. Add the potatoes, sweet potatoes, cabbage, parsley, tomatoes and stock. Bring to a simmer and cook for 15 minutes.

Add the bananas, prawns and fish. Simmer gently for 10 minutes or until the fish is opaque. Add more stock, water or tomato juice if the stew is too thick. Season to taste and serve hot, garnished with lime or lemon and a sprinkling of herbs.

Chicken, artichoke and sage pizza

Here's one suggestion for a pizza topping; you could also try roasted onions with cheese and walnuts; roasted peppers, onions and courgettes; tomato sauce and sardines or salami, to name but a few.

SERVES 4

pizza dough (see page 328)
a little olive oil
1 small buffalo mozzarella cheese, thinly sliced
8 cooked fresh or tinned artichoke hearts, sliced
225 g/8 oz cooked chicken, cut into small pieces
finely chopped fresh sage
salt and freshly ground black pepper
fresh shavings of Parmesan cheese

Preheat the oven to its highest temperature and put a baking sheet (large enough to hold the pizza) in to heat up.

Roll out the risen pizza dough to form a circle about 30 cm/12 inches in diameter. Drizzle a little olive oil over the dough and top with slices of mozzarella, artichokes, pieces of chicken and chopped sage. Season with salt and pepper.

Place the pizza on the preheated baking sheet and bake for about 15–20 minutes – or about 6 minutes in a wood-burning stove.

Shave some fresh Parmesan on top before serving.

Chicken rissoles

These rissoles are a good way of using up cooked chicken – and they're very popular with children. For a crunchy finish, you could use crushed cornflakes to coat the rissoles. They can be served with rice or mashed potato, baked beans, ratatouille or green vegetables. They can also be eaten Middle Eastern style, wrapped in unleavened bread and dunked in a yoghurt and mint raita.

SERVES 4

450 g/1 lb roast chicken meat
200 g/7 oz canned chickpeas (half a can), drained
1 small onion, roughly chopped
1 garlic clove, roughly chopped
2 teaspoons chopped fresh sage
175 g/6 oz wholemeal breadcrumbs
1 egg, beaten
salt and pepper

Using a mincer or food processor, finely mince together the chicken, chickpeas, onion and garlic. If you don't have a mincer I suggest you finely chop the chicken, crush the chickpeas with a fork and mix with the onion and garlic. Add the sage and about 50 g/2 oz of the breadcrumbs. Mix well and use enough of the beaten egg to bind the mince without it becoming too sloppy. Season to taste.

Spread the remaining breadcrumbs on a large baking sheet. Taking a handful of mince at a time, roll it in the breadcrumbs until it is completely coated.

Fry in a small amount of oil in a frying pan or grill until the coating turns golden brown. Serve at once.

Grilled spiced chicken

Chicken is a very lean protein, making it ideal if you are following a healthy low-fat diet. Plain chicken can become a little monotonous, so here is a good way to add a little spice to your life! This chicken is also delicious in sandwiches, or stuffed into warm pitta breads.

SERVES 4

4 chicken breasts, skinned
½ teaspoon ground cinnamon
½ teaspoon ground cumin
½ teaspoon ground allspice
½ teaspoon dried thyme
½ teaspoon freshly grated nutmeg
1 teaspoon demerara sugar
2 garlic cloves, crushed
1 shallot or small onion, finely chopped
½ tablespoon white wine vinegar
1 tablespoon virgin olive oil
½ tablespoon fresh lime or lemon juice
1 chilli, finely chopped (optional)
salt and freshly ground black pepper

Using a sharp knife, cut small slits in the chicken breasts, which will allow the marinade to penetrate the meat.

Mix all the remaining ingredients together in a bowl, making a thick paste. Add the chicken and, using your hands, rub the marinade all over the chicken and inside the slits. Cover and leave to marinate for at least 4 hours, preferably overnight.

When ready to cook the chicken, brush lightly with oil and place under a preheated hot grill. Cook for about 10 minutes on each side. Test that the chicken is cooked through by piercing it with a skewer: the juices should run clear. Serve at once with rice.

Chicken in a walnut cream sauce

A delicious way to eat dairy products, this could be made even richer by using all cream instead of half yoghurt and half cream. It is delicious served on a bed of spinach, which provides iron.

If you have some of this left over it can be transformed into a delicious soup. Whizz it in a blender with a little fresh chicken stock until smooth. Serve with wholegrain rolls.

SERVES 4
4 large chicken breasts, skinned
50 g/2 oz butter
8 sprigs of tarragon, leaves only
125 ml/4 fl oz double cream
125 g/4 oz natural yoghurt
a dash of white wine
125 g/4 oz chopped walnuts
lemon juice
salt and freshly ground black pepper

Slice the chicken into 1 cm/¹⁄₂ inch strips. Melt the butter in a shallow frying pan and add the chicken and tarragon. Cook, stirring frequently, until the chicken has slightly coloured, about 3 minutes.

Pour in the cream, yoghurt and wine and leave to simmer and thicken for 8–10 minutes. Add the walnuts and season to taste with a dash of lemon juice and a little salt and freshly ground black pepper. Serve at once, with steamed spinach. Wild rice is very good with this.

Almond chicken

Almonds are a good source of calcium and magnesium, for healthy bones and teeth. This dish is very quick and easy and just goes to show that you don't need ready-made sauces for a speedy supper.

SERVES 4
4 chicken breasts or legs, skinned
2 tablespoons olive oil
1 onion, finely chopped
1 large garlic clove, finely chopped
250 g/9 oz natural yoghurt
2 heaped tablespoons ground almonds
salt and freshly ground black pepper

Slice the chicken into 1 cm/¹⁄₂ inch strips. Heat the oil in a shallow frying pan, add the onion and garlic and cook gently until soft.

Increase the heat, add the chicken and cook, stirring frequently, until the chicken has slightly coloured, about 3 minutes.

Turn the heat down and stir in the yoghurt and almonds. Simmer for 8–10 minutes. Season to taste and serve at once, with a salad or a selection of fresh vegetables.

Grilled chicken with rosemary

A quick, tasty way to cook chicken, a good lean protein food. Serve on toasted focaccia, with a green salad and tzatziki, the yoghurt, garlic and mint dressing.

SERVES 4
4 chicken breasts
4 sprigs of rosemary
4 small or 2 large garlic cloves, sliced
1 tablespoon olive oil
salt and freshly ground black pepper
lemon juice

Preheat the grill to very hot.

Slice a pocket in each chicken breast and insert a sprig of rosemary and some garlic in each pocket. Brush with a little olive oil and grill, turning once or twice, until the chicken is cooked through.

Remove the main stalk of rosemary, but leave in some of the smaller leaves. Slice the chicken breasts and serve hot or cold, with toasted focaccia, salad and tzatziki.

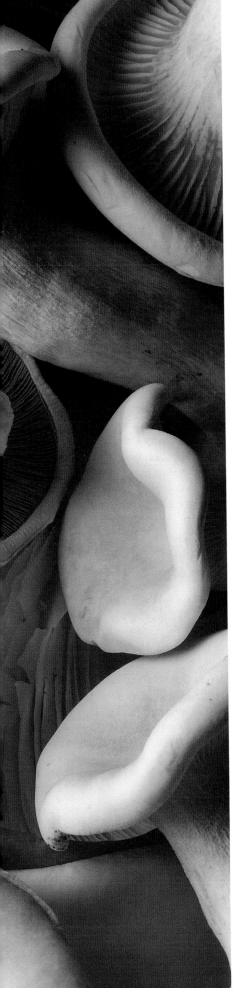

Venison with blackcurrants and redcurrants

Venison is relatively low in fat and high in flavour. In Tuscany venison is often cooked with myrtleberries, small, blue, slightly tart berries. Here I have used black and redcurrants, which are both rich in vitamin C.

SERVES 4
4 venison steaks
300 ml/10 fl oz red wine
4 tablespoons blackcurrants
1 tablespoon cracked black pepper
1 red onion, finely chopped
2 tablespoons chopped garlic
1 small bunch of parsley,
    finely chopped
salt and freshly ground black pepper
a dash of olive oil
2 tablespoons port
50 ml/2 fl oz beef stock
12 wild mushrooms
3 tablespoons redcurrants

Marinate the venison for 10 minutes in the red wine, with 3 tablespoons of the blackcurrants, the cracked pepper, onion, garlic and parsley.

Remove the venison from the marinade and pat it dry. Season with salt and pepper. Heat the olive oil in a frying pan, add the venison and seal over a high heat, turning once. Remove from the pan and set aside

Strain the marinade and add to the pan in which you cooked the venison. Add the port, stock, the remaining blackcurrants and the mushrooms. Boil the liquid until it reduces and thickens slightly. Return the venison steaks to the sauce to heat through, then serve at once, with the redcurrants.

Corned beef hash

Here's a quick, nourishing supper. It is very easy to make, especially if you have any potatoes left over from a previous meal. It is high in iron and protein, making it a good dish if you're recuperating from an illness.

SERVES 4–6
1 tablespoon olive oil
1 large onion, chopped
1 garlic clove, finely chopped
2 tins of corned beef, cut into chunks
4 potatoes, peeled, sliced and boiled
400 g/14 oz can of baked beans
400 g/14 oz can of chopped tomatoes
1 teaspoon ground coriander
1 tablespoon tomato purée
salt and pepper

Heat the oil in a large, deep frying pan and sauté the onion and garlic. Add the corned beef and brown a little. Add the potatoes and fry for a few minutes until the potatoes start to brown.

Add all the other ingredients and sauté, stirring constantly, until thoroughly heated through.

Serve hot, with homemade tomato sauce (see page 313).

Persian lamb with apricots and rice

This is an excellent way to encourage children to eat meat, and it goes well with spinach, giving you a double boost of iron. This dish is also very good the day after it is made. Warm it up in a low oven, or the rice will dry up.

SERVES 4–6

25 g/1 oz butter
½ tablespoon olive oil
1 onion, finely chopped
2 garlic cloves, finely chopped
450 g/1 lb lean lamb, cubed
salt and pepper
½ teaspoon ground cinnamon
½ teaspoon crushed coriander seeds
2 tablespoons seedless raisins
125 g/4 oz dried apricots, preferably
   unsulphured Hunza apricots
fresh lamb or vegetable stock
450 g/1 lb long grain rice

Melt the butter and oil in a large sauté pan, add the onion and garlic and cook gently until soft and golden. Increase the heat, add the lamb and brown lightly on all sides. Season with salt and pepper, then stir in the spices, raisins and apricots. Fry for a minute or two, stirring constantly to avoid sticking.

Pour in just enough stock to cover the lamb and fruits, cover the pan and simmer for about 1½ hours. Stir at regular intervals to ensure that the lamb is not sticking.

After 1½ hours the meat should be very tender and well flavoured with the fruit and spices. If the liquid is a little thin, strain it off into another saucepan and boil it until it becomes slightly thicker. Pour it back over the meat, taste and adjust the seasoning if necessary.

Boil the rice in salted water, adding a lump of butter if you like. After 10 minutes the rice should be almost, but not quite cooked. Drain off any surplus water, then arrange the rice in alternate layers with the meat in a heavy pan, beginning and ending with rice. Put a doubled cloth or piece of muslin over the top, then cover with a tightly fitting lid. Set over a very low heat for 15–20 minutes. The rice will be tender and succulent, having absorbed some of the meat sauce.

Potato, ham and spinach layer

All-in-one dishes are good for family suppers, as you only need a salad or a selection of fresh vegetables to accompany them. They are also good for sneaking ingredients into reluctant eaters, such as ham into children who claim not to like meat. This meal is very comforting, perfect for days when you need to wind down. It also keeps well until the next day, so is ideal for busy people.

SERVES 3–4

450 ml/15 fl oz milk
4 peppercorns
small bunch of fresh sage
50 g/2 oz butter
1 large onion, sliced thinly into rings
2 garlic cloves, finely chopped
50 g/2 oz plain flour
150 g/5 oz natural yoghurt or cream
225 g/8 oz ham off the bone, sliced
3 large potatoes, sliced

450 g/1 lb leaf spinach,
   washed carefully
¼ teaspoon freshly grated nutmeg
2 large slices of wholemeal bread,
   made into crumbs

Preheat the oven to 200°C/400°F/Gas 6.

Heat the milk in a small saucepan, together with the peppercorns and about three sage leaves. Remove from the heat and leave to infuse for 20 minutes.

Meanwhile, heat the butter in a large saucepan and fry the onion and garlic until translucent and turning slightly golden. Add the flour and stir for 1 minute. Remove from the heat and add the strained infused milk a little at a time, stirring constantly to avoid lumps. Bring the sauce to the boil, stirring constantly, and boil until thick. Remove from the heat and add the yoghurt or cream – be careful how much you use as the sauce should still be thick enough to coat the potatoes.

In a large ovenproof dish, arrange layers of ham, potatoes, sauce and spinach, grating a little nutmeg over each spinach layer. Finish with a layer of sauce and cover with the breadcrumbs and a sprinkling of finely chopped sage.

Place in the oven and cook for 30–40 minutes, until the potatoes are soft (test by piercing them with a sharp knife). Serve hot.

Variation
Use sheets of lasagne instead of potatoes.

Pizza dough

You can freeze the uncooked pizza bases and cook from frozen with a topping of your choice.

MAKES FOUR 30 CM/12 INCH PIZZAS
450 g/1 lb plain flour, either white or wholemeal
25 g/1 oz fresh yeast dissolved in a little warm milk
1 teaspoon salt
about 300 ml/½ pint hand-hot water (not too hot, otherwise it will kill the yeast)

Sift the flour on to a work surface and make a well in the middle. Pour the dissolved yeast into the well, then add the salt and mix together with your fingers. Gradually add the warm water, kneading all the time so that you end up with a pliable, soft dough. Continue kneading until the dough is light, smooth and very elastic. Divide into four balls and place them on a floured surface, cover and leave to rise in a warm place for about 1 hour. The dough should double in size.

Preheat the oven to its highest temperature and put a baking sheet (large enough to hold the pizza) in to heat up.

Roll each risen dough ball out to form a circle about 30 cm/12 inches in diameter. Drizzle a little olive oil over the dough and add your chosen topping. Bake in the hot oven for 15–20 minutes. If you are lucky enough to possess a wood-burning stove, your pizza should only take about 6 minutes.

Oat muffins

This is not gluten-free, but oats are lower in gluten than wheat. If you cannot get sorghum flour (look in health food shops) you can use wheat, rice or buckwheat flour.

MAKES 10
200 ml/7 fl oz lukewarm water
½ teaspoon caster sugar
1½ teaspoons dried yeast
150 g/5 oz fine oatmeal
150 g/5 oz sorghum flour
¼ teaspoon salt
1 tablespoon olive oil

Place half the water in a bowl and add the sugar and yeast, whisking to incorporate as much air as possible. Cover the bowl and leave for 10 minutes in a warm place.

Sift the oatmeal, flour and salt into a bowl and pour the yeast mixture, oil and remaining water into a well in the centre. Mix all the ingredients together to form a dough. Knead on a floured surface and then transfer to a bowl. Cover with a damp tea towel and leave in a warm place to rise, for about 1 hour, until almost doubled in size.

Turn the dough out and knead briefly. Divide into ten pieces and roll into balls. Place the balls on a board, sprinkle with flour, cover with the tea towel and return to a warm place to rise for a further 45 minutes.

Bake in a preheated oven (200°C/ 400°F/Gas 6) until they are golden brown, about 20–25 minutes. Alternatively you could cook them in a lightly oiled, heavy-based frying pan for about 5 minutes each side, until brown. Serve warm.

Soft bread

In this and the three recipes that follow I use tartaric acid to help give the bread a good texture. It is available from pharmacies in large tubs, but if you cannot get it, you can substitute extra cream of tartar.

Gluten-free breads are best served hot; if not warm from the oven, serve toasted.

MAKES A 450 G/1 LB LOAF
1 large banana
125 g/4 oz tofu
1 egg
150 ml/5 fl oz milk
150 g/5 oz rice flour
50 g/2 oz cornflour
25 g/1 oz soya flour
1 teaspoon bicarbonate of soda
1 teaspoon cream of tartar
½ teaspoon tartaric acid
pinch of salt
1 teaspoon sugar
1 tablespoon olive oil
50 g/2 oz sesame seeds for sprinkling

Preheat the oven to 190°C/375°F/ Gas 5.

Liquidize the banana, tofu, egg and milk.

Mix the dry ingredients (apart from the sesame seeds) and fold in the purée and the olive oil.

Line a 25 cm/10 inch square, 3 cm/1 inch deep tin with baking parchment and pour in the batter. Sprinkle the sesame seeds on top and bake for 35 minutes, or until a skewer inserted into the centre comes out clean.

Tip
All these breads can be cooked in a frying pan, covered with the lid. You need to turn the bread frequently.

Taste good

Buckwheat bread

Gluten-free bread.

MAKES A 450 G/1 LB LOAF
100 g/3½ oz grated carrot
150 ml/5 fl oz water or milk
1 egg
100 g/3½ oz buckwheat flour
100 g/3½ oz rice flour
1 teaspoon bicarbonate of soda
½ teaspoon cream of tartar
¼ teaspoon tartaric acid
pinch of salt
25 g/1 oz sugar
1 tablespoon vegetable oil

Preheat the oven to 220°C/425°F/ Gas 7.

Liquidize the grated carrot, milk and egg.

Mix all the dry ingredients together and fold in the carrot purée and the oil.

Line a 25 cm/10 inch square, 3 cm/1 inch deep tin with baking parchment and pour in the batter. Bake for 35 minutes, or until a skewer inserted into the centre comes out clean.

Potato bread

This gluten-free bread is lovely served with soups or made into sandwiches while still warm from the oven.

MAKES A 450 G/1 LB LOAF
85 g/3 oz peeled potato
150 ml/5 fl oz milk
1 egg
50 g/2 oz cornflour or cornmeal
100 g/3½ oz rice flour
1 teaspoon bicarbonate of soda
1 teaspoon cream of tartar
1 teaspoon tartaric acid
pinch of salt
1 teaspoon sugar
1 tablespoon olive oil

Preheat the oven to 220°C/425°F/ Gas 7.

Cook the potato until soft, then drain and liquidize. Add the milk and egg and liquidize again.

Mix all the dry ingredients together and fold in the potato purée and the olive oil.

Line a 25 cm/10 inch square, 3 cm/1 inch deep tin with baking parchment and fill with the mixture. Bake for 35 minutes, or until a skewer inserted into the centre comes out clean.

Variation
Add 2 crushed garlic cloves or some chopped fresh herbs (such as parsley, tarragon, dill) to the potato.

Rice bread

Gluten-free bread.

MAKES A 450 G/1 LB LOAF
1 large apple
1 egg
150 ml/5 fl oz water or milk
100 g/3½ oz rice flour
100 g/3½ oz potato flour
25 g/1 oz soya flour (optional)
1 teaspoon bicarbonate of soda
½ teaspoon cream of tartar
¼ teaspoon tartaric acid
pinch of salt
1 teaspoon sugar
1 tablespoon vegetable oil

Preheat the oven to 220°C/425°F/ Gas 7.

Liquidize the apple, egg and milk or water.

Mix all the dry ingredients together and fold in the apple mixture and the oil.

Line a 25 cm/10 inch square, 3 cm/1 inch deep tin with baking parchment and pour in the batter. Bake for 35 minutes, or until a skewer inserted into the centre comes out clean.

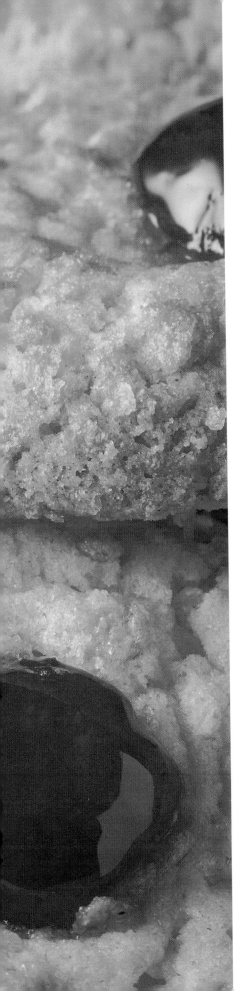

Melting moments

These biscuits were always cooked to perfection by my Auntie May. A lovely between-meal nibble, they literally melt in a moment!

MAKES ABOUT 16 BISCUITS
85 g/3 oz caster sugar
100 g/3½ oz butter, softened
½ beaten egg
150 g/5 oz self-raising flour, sifted
crushed cornflakes
glacé cherries, halved

Preheat the oven to 190°C/375°F/ Gas 5.

Cream the butter and sugar until light and fluffy. Beat in the egg and stir in the flour.

Divide the mixture into 16 balls (about the size of golf balls) and roll in the crushed cornflakes. Place well apart on a greased baking sheet, as the biscuits will flatten as they cook, and place half a glacé cherry on top of each ball. Bake for 20–25 minutes, until the biscuits are golden brown. Leave to cool before devouring.

Raspberry bars

These are delicious as biscuits, but they can also be served with ice cream or even warm with custard. Made with wholemeal flour, they are a good source of B vitamins.

MAKES ABOUT 16 BARS
225 g/8 oz plain wholemeal flour
pinch of salt
2 teaspoons baking powder
2 teaspoons mixed spice
125 g/4 oz butter
150 g/5 oz caster sugar
1 tablespoon golden syrup
1 large egg, beaten
225 g/8 oz good-quality raspberry jam

Sift together the flour, salt, baking powder and mixed spice. Cream the butter and sugar until pale and fluffy. Gradually beat in the syrup and egg, a little at a time. If the mixture starts to curdle, beat in a little flour. Gradually fold in the flour and mix thoroughly to form a dough. Leave to chill for about 20 minutes.

Meanwhile, preheat the oven to 180°C/350°F/Gas 4. Grease and line a shallow 30 x 18 cm/12 x 7 inch tin.

Break up the dough and press half into the tin. Spread the jam over the dough, then press the remaining dough on top. Bake for 30 minutes. Leave in the tin to cool slightly before cutting into bars.

Apple flapjacks

Flapjacks are an excellent snack biscuit. Although they do contain sugar, the fibre from the oats helps to slow the absorption of sugar into the body. The apple purée helps to make the flapjacks soft.

MAKES 6–8

2 large Bramley apples,
   peeled and cored
juice of ½ lemon
150 g/5 oz butter
85 g/3 oz brown sugar
85 g/3 oz black treacle
   or golden syrup
225 g/8 oz porridge oats
½ teaspoon ground cinnamon
pinch of salt

Preheat the oven to 190°C/375°F/ Gas 5.

First make the apple purée by slicing the apples into a small saucepan with the lemon juice and a dash of water. Bring to the boil, cover and simmer for 10 minutes or until the apple is soft. Using either a hand blender or a fork, mash the apple to a soft purée.

Melt the butter, sugar and treacle or syrup in a saucepan, but be careful not to let the mixture boil. Stir in the oats, cinnamon and salt and mix well.

Press half the mixture into a 20 cm/8 inch sandwich tin. Spread the apple purée on top, then cover with the remaining flapjack mixture and bake for 25 minutes, or until golden brown. Remove from the oven and mark into slices, but leave to cool before attempting to remove from the tin.

Fruit and malt loaf

This malt loaf is rich in fibre, along with calcium from the dried fruits. It is best made a day before you want to eat it, if you can resist it, as it becomes even more moist and gooey overnight, in a sealed tin. It is perfect for afternoon snacks or lunch boxes.

MAKES A 1 KG/2¼ LB LOAF

1 tablespoon malt extract
1½ tablespoons golden syrup
3 tablespoons milk
225 g/8 oz wholemeal self-raising
   flour
50 g/2 oz sugar
25 g/1 oz plump raisins or sultanas
25 g/1 oz dried figs, chopped
25 g/1 oz dried pears, chopped
1 egg, beaten

Preheat the oven to 160°C/325°F/ Gas 3. Grease a 1 kg/2 ¼ lb loaf tin and line with baking parchment.

Put the malt extract, syrup and milk in a small heatproof bowl and warm over a saucepan of hot water

Sift the flour into a bowl, adding any bran residue in the sieve. Mix in the sugar and dried fruit.

Add the malt mixture to the dry ingredients and mix well. Stir in the beaten egg.

Pour into the prepared loaf tin and bake for about 1 hour, until springy to the touch. Leave to cool before slicing.

Banana and coconut loaf

Wholemeal flour adds fibre, so the energy from the bananas and sugar is released slowly and steadily. The cake can be served cold for lunch or an afternoon snack, or warm with a spoonful of yoghurt.

MAKES A 1 KG/2¼ LB LOAF

225 g/8 oz self-raising wholemeal
   flour
¼ teaspoon bicarbonate of soda
50 g/2 oz butter (or soya margarine if
   you are unable to tolerate lactose)
2 eggs
50 g/2 oz brown sugar
4 tablespoons milk (cows', sheep's,
   goats' or soya)
3 ripe bananas
4 tablespoons roasted coconut flakes

Preheat the oven to 180°C/350°F/ Gas 4. Grease a 1 kg/2 ¼ lb loaf tin.

Place all the ingredients apart from the coconut flakes in a food processor and process for a few minutes. Pour the mixture into the loaf tin and sprinkle the coconut flakes on top.

Bake for about 1–1¼ hours, or until a skewer inserted into the centre comes out clean. Turn the cake out of the tin and leave to cool on a wire rack or, if you like a really moist, 'gooey' cake, place it in a cake tin as soon as it comes out of the oven and seal with an airtight lid. By allowing the cake to cool in its own steam, the top becomes moist.

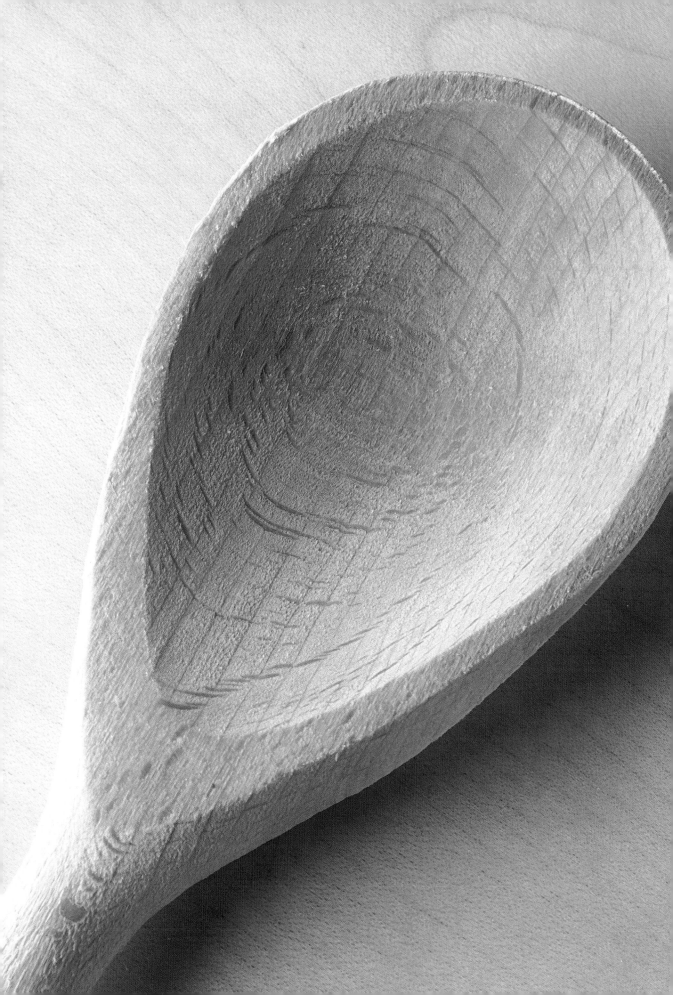

Chocolate and orange brownies

These fabulous, moist brownies are made with wholemeal flour, which slows down the absorption of sugar into the body. With the dates this is, amazingly, a high fibre treat that could be served as a snack or a dessert, with ice cream.

MAKES 16
70 g/2½ oz butter
50 g/2 oz good-quality (85% cocoa solids) chocolate
50 g/2 oz caster sugar
70 g/2½ oz self-raising wholemeal flour
pinch of salt
2 eggs, beaten
½ teaspoon vanilla essence
juice and grated zest of 1 orange
25 g/1 oz chopped dried apricots
25 g/1 oz chopped dates

Preheat the oven to 180°C/350°F/ Gas 4. Grease and flour a 20 cm/8 inch square shallow tin.

Melt the butter and chocolate together in a bowl over a saucepan of hot water and stir in the sugar.

Sift the flour and salt into a bowl and stir in the chocolate mixture, beaten eggs and the remaining ingredients. Beat the mixture until smooth, then spoon into the prepared tin. Bake for about 35 minutes.

Leave in the tin to cool slightly before cutting into squares.

Fruit mountains

This is a fun way to coax children into eating fruit. You could make star or other shaped biscuits, and children can help with cutting out the biscuits.

SERVES 8
225 g/8 oz plain flour
225 g/8 oz butter
125 g/4 oz icing sugar
drop of vanilla essence
2 egg yolks
150 g/5 oz fromage frais
150 ml/5 fl oz double cream, whipped
225 g/8 oz mixed berries (such as raspberries, strawberries, blueberries, redcurrants)

Put the flour, butter, icing sugar, vanilla and egg yolks in a food processor and process for a short burst, until just mixed, then stop. Be careful not to overbeat, otherwise the mixture will toughen. (Alternatively, sift the flour into a bowl and lightly rub in the butter, using your fingertips. Stir in the icing sugar, vanilla and egg yolks, until just mixed.)

Press the mixture together lightly, then wrap in cling film and chill in the refrigerator for 30 minutes.

Preheat the oven to 190°C/ 375°F/Gas 5. Lightly grease a baking sheet. Roll out the dough to about 5 mm/¼ inch thick. Cut out 5 cm/ 2 inch rounds or other shapes and bake for 6 minutes. Leave to cool on a wire rack.

Mix together the fromage frais and whipped cream. Put a spoonful of the cream mixture on each biscuit. Top with a spoonful of berries and dust with icing sugar. Serve at once.

Peach, plum and blackcurrant strudel

Strudels are a good way to persuade children and people with a poor appetite into eating fruit. You could use apples, apricots or pears, along with berry fruits

SERVES 6
225 g/8 oz Victoria plums
4 peaches
small punnet (125 g/4 oz) of blackcurrants
juice of ½ orange
3 large sheets of filo pastry
15 g/½ oz butter, melted
grated zest of 1 lemon
2 tablespoons caster sugar
85 g/3 oz flaked almonds

Preheat the oven to 190°C/375°F/ Gas 5.

Remove the stones from the plums and peaches, and take the tips off the blackcurrants. Place the fruit in a saucepan with the orange juice and bring to the boil. Reduce the heat, cover and simmer for 10–15 minutes, until the fruits are soft, but not too mushy. If there is a lot of liquid in the pan, remove the fruit with a slotted spoon and set aside.

Lay the filo pastry on a work surface one sheet at a time, brushing each one with melted butter. Place the cooked fruit along the centre and sprinkle with the lemon zest, sugar and half the almonds. Fold in the sides and roll up the filo sheets to form a parcel, curving the ends slightly to form a crescent shape. Brush with melted butter and sprinkle the remaining almonds on top. Place on a buttered baking sheet and bake for 30–40 minutes. Serve warm or cold.

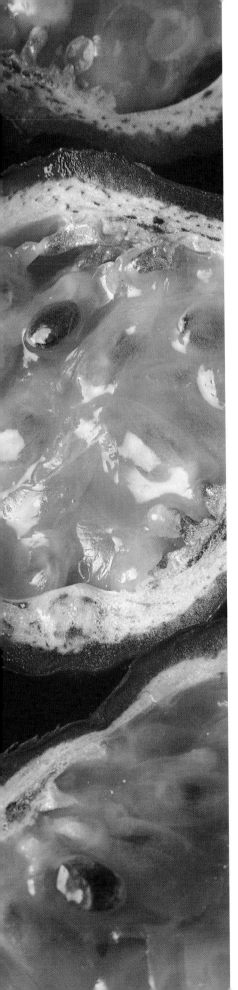

Strawberry and passionfruit fool

Enjoy this dessert for its aphrodisiac powers – or its vitamin C and beta-carotene content!

SERVES 6
5 passionfruit
70 g/2½ oz unsalted butter
100 g/3½ oz caster sugar
2 eggs, well beaten
125 ml/4 fl oz double cream, or half cream and half thick Greek yoghurt
225 g/8 oz ripe strawberries
sprigs of mint to decorate

Halve the passionfruit and scoop out the pulp into a heatproof bowl. Add the butter and sugar. Place over a saucepan of simmering water, ensuring that the water doesn't touch the base of the bowl. Cook over a medium heat, stirring, until the butter melts, then add the beaten eggs. Cook the mixture for about 10–15 minutes, stirring often, until it thickens considerably. Rub through a sieve, leave to cool, cover and chill.

Whip the cream until thick but not too stiff, then fold into the passionfruit mixture. If you are using half cream and half yoghurt, fold the remaining yoghurt into the mixture at this stage.

Slice the strawberries neatly, reserving a few for decoration, and fold into the passionfruit mixture. Spoon the fool into tall glasses and decorate with a few whole straw-berries and perhaps a little sprig of mint. Chill until ready to serve.

Ginger pineapple

Here's a novel way of serving fruit, with zingy flavours and virtually no fat – unless you serve it with vanilla ice cream! Halved peaches, nectarines or apricots could be used instead of the pineapple slices.

SERVES 6
1 fresh pineapple
1 teaspoon ground ginger
juice of 1 lemon

Cut the pineapple into 2 cm/¾ inch slices and cut off the skin. Lay the slices on a grill pan covered in kitchen foil. Mix the ginger with the lemon juice and, using a pastry brush, drizzle the juice over the pineapple slices. Leave to marinate for 2–3 hours.

Preheat the grill, and grill the pineapple until slightly golden brown. Alternatively, wrap each pineapple slice in foil and place on a hot barbecue for 2–3 minutes.

Fruit kebabs

Poached pears

In summer these kebabs can be barbecued; in the winter they can be cooked under a very hot grill or in a chargrilling pan on top of the stove

It's a simple but unusual way to serve fruit. Let your children help to make the kebabs and they will be even more eager to eat them.

ALLOW ABOUT 125 G/4 OZ OF FRUIT FOR EACH PERSON
Choose seasonal fruits for the best flavour (such as strawberries, peaches, pineapple, mango, pears, tangerines, bananas)

Slice the fruits into similar-sized chunks, but don't make them too small. Arrange the pieces of fruit in colourful patterns, then thread them on to the skewers, allowing about six pieces for each skewer.

Preheat your barbecue or grill pan. If you are using a chargrilling pan you may like to use a small knob of butter to prevent the fruit from sticking. Cook the kebabs until the edges of the fruits are starting to turn golden brown.

Serve warm, with yoghurt to dip the fruit into if you like. For very young children you should remove the fruits from the skewers.

Variation

For older children or adults you could flambé the kebabs by pouring over a small amount of Cointreau in a warmed spoon, setting light to the liqueur as you pour it. As the liqueur burns the alcohol evaporates, leaving just its lovely flavour.

Besides being a great dinner party dessert, this is designed to appeal to elderly people and children, since poaching the pears makes them soft and easy to eat. You could serve them whole, or you could slice the poached pears and layer them in a glass with yoghurt, cream or custard. A ginger biscuit is a delicious accompaniment.

SERVES 4
1 orange
½ lemon
8 ripe pears, peeled
500 ml/16 fl oz water
525 ml/17 fl oz white wine
200 g/7 oz caster sugar
1 vanilla pod

Cut the orange and half of the lemon into thin slices and remove the pips.

Place the pears in a large stainless steel or stoneware cooking pan. Pour the water, wine and sugar over the pears and add the vanilla pod (there should just be enough liquid to cover the pears). Add the orange and lemon slices.

Bring the liquid to the boil, then reduce the heat, cover with a lid and simmer for 20–30 minutes, depending on whether your pears are small and ripe, or a little larger than normal. You must not allow the pears to boil, as fierce heat will damage the pear flesh and will also cause the syrup to brown. Turn off the heat and leave the pears to cool in their own syrup.

When the pears are cold, remove them from the liquid, using a slotted spoon. Gently peel the pears and place in a glass bowl; add the orange and lemon slices and strain the syrup over them. Cover and chill for at least 8 hours.

You could use double the quantity of pears, keeping half in the refrigerator for a couple of days; ideal for an after school or after work snack or a quick dinner party dessert.

Blackberry ice cream

It is well worth making your own ice cream, for its purity of ingredients and wonderful flavour. This blackberry ice cream is light, yet rich in vitamins C and E and high in fibre. To make the dessert lower in fat and calories you could replace the cream with thick natural yoghurt.

SERVES 6
400 g/14 oz fresh or frozen blackberries
100 ml/3½ fl oz cold water
200 g/7 oz caster sugar
juice of 2 lemons
300 ml/10 fl oz double cream, or thick natural yoghurt

Purée the blackberries with the water in a liquidizer for 3 minutes. Pass the resulting juice through a fine sieve into a large bowl; you may need to coax the juice through using the back of a wooden spoon. Add the sugar and lemon juice and mix well.

Meanwhile, whip the cream in a separate bowl until it leaves a thick ribbon trail, being careful not to overbeat, otherwise it will be difficult to fold into the juice. (Alternatively, if you are using thick yoghurt, just ensure that it is smooth.) Fold the cream or yoghurt into the blackberry syrup and place in an ice-cream maker for 15–20 minutes, until the ice cream is smooth and starting to freeze. Transfer to a rigid plastic container and freeze.

Take the ice cream out of the freezer 5 minutes before you want to serve it, to allow it to soften slightly.

Fruit dreams

This is a fruity variation on baked alaska; it makes a perfect dessert for a birthday or dinner party.

SERVES 6
500 ml/16 fl oz good-quality ice cream
about 450 g/1 lb soft fruit (such as raspberries, blueberries, strawberries, or blackberries, gooseberries, plums)
dash of Cointreau (optional)
4 egg whites
225 g/8 oz caster sugar

Put a piece of baking parchment on a baking sheet. Divide the ice cream into four portions, place on the baking sheet and shape into little disks. Place in the freezer for about 40 minutes.

Mix the soft fruits together and add a dash of Cointreau if you are making this for adults. (If you are using blackberries, gooseberries or plums, stew lightly, then strain to remove any excess juice.)

Preheat the oven to 220°C/ 425°F/Gas 7.

Whisk the egg whites with 50 g/ 2 oz of the caster sugar until stiff. Lightly fold in the remaining sugar.

Spoon the fruit mixture over the ice cream, then gently cover with the meringue, mounding it into an igloo shape and making sure it completely covers the fruit and ice cream. I like to leave the meringue in rough peaks. Immediately place in the hot oven for 4–5 minutes to brown the top of the meringue. Serve at once.

You can also make this as one large igloo.

Minty berries

The juicy freshness of the berries (which should be seasonal and newly picked for the best results), combined with the refreshing mint syrup, is a perfect way to get a good dose of vitamin C and fibre. Children can help you prepare the fruit, but be careful when you are making the syrup, as boiling sugar is extremely hot.

SERVES 6
250 g/9 oz sugar
500 ml/16 fl oz water
juice of 1 lemon
a good handful (15 g/½ oz) of roughly chopped mint leaves
1 kg/2½ lb mixed berries (such as blackberries, strawberries, raspberries, blueberries, redcurrants)
mint leaves to decorate

To make the syrup, put the sugar and water in a small saucepan, bring to the boil and simmer until the sugar dissolves, then stir in the lemon juice. Put the mint in a heatproof bowl, pour over the hot syrup and leave to cool. Strain, discarding the mint leaves.

Clean the berries thoroughly and place in a serving bowl; you could arrange them neatly, but I think they look best all jumbled up together. Pour the syrup over the fruit and chill for at least 5 hours.

Decorate with some roughly chopped mint leaves.

Sweet pastry

MAKES A 22 CM/9 INCH TART
175 g/6 oz plain white flour
40 g/1½ icing sugar
100 g/4 oz cold unsalted butter,
    cut into small pieces
1 egg, separated
2 tablespoons iced water

Put the flour, icing sugar and butter in a food processor and whiz until the mixture resembles crumbs. Alternatively, sift the flour and sugar into a bowl and rub in the butter, using your fingertips. Add the egg yolk and 2 tablespoons of iced water. Whiz very briefly (or mix lightly) until a dough forms, adding a little more water if necessary. Turn out and knead lightly, then wrap in foil and chill in the refrigerator for 30 minutes, to allow the pastry to rest.

Preheat the oven to 190°C/375°F/Gas 5. Roll out the pastry to line a 22 cm/9 inch diameter, loose-bottomed tart tin. Line with baking parchment or greaseproof paper and weigh down with baking beans, then bake 'blind' for about 10 minutes or until the pastry is firm. Remove the paper, brush the pastry with the lightly beaten egg white and return to the oven for a further 5–10 minutes or until pale golden brown. Remove from the oven and leave to cool a little before filling.

Apricot cream tart

The presence of apricots and cream make this dessert not only delicious, but also high in calcium, so it is good for healthy bones and teeth.

SERVES 6–8
750 g/1 lb 10 oz fresh apricots,
    stoned, or tinned apricots in
    natural juice, drained
50 g/2 oz caster sugar
juice of ½ lemon
25 g/1 oz butter
sweet pastry case (see left),
    baked blind
grated rind and juice of 1 orange
150 ml/5 fl oz double cream
25 g/1 oz demerara sugar
flaked almonds to decorate

Chop the apricots into quarters and mix with the sugar and lemon juice. Gently melt the butter in a large saucepan and add the apricots. Cook gently for about 15 minutes, until the apricots start to soften and the butter and sugar caramelize.

Using a slotted spoon, lift out the apricots and place in the pastry case. Add the orange rind and juice to the pan with the apricot syrup and cook for about 25–30 minutes, until the juice is thick and syrupy. Remove from the heat and add the cream, stirring continuously. The cream mixture should thicken slightly.

Spoon over the apricots and sprinkle some demerara sugar and flaked almonds on top. Place under a hot grill for 2–3 minutes, until the almonds start to turn brown.

Variation
Use 750 g/1 lb 10 oz apples, peeled, cored and sliced, instead of apricots.

Raspberry and lime tart

Raspberries set in a creamy lime filling are a wonderful way to get your daily vitamin C. The tangy fruits help kickstart the taste buds and will tempt even the most jaded palate.

SERVES 6–8
4 eggs
125 g/4 oz caster sugar
finely grated zest and juice of 5 limes
900 ml/1½ pints double cream
sweet pastry case (see left),
    baked blind
325 g/12 oz raspberries
icing sugar to dust
a few raspberries and mint leaves
    to decorate

Preheat the oven to 180°C/350°F/Gas 4.

Beat the eggs and sugar together until thoroughly blended. Beat in the lime zest and juice, then the double cream, and beat until smooth.

Place the pastry case, still in its tin, on a baking sheet and arrange the raspberries on the pastry. Carefully pour the lime custard over the raspberries and return the tart to the oven. Cook for 30–35 minutes, until the custard is just set in the centre. Serve warm or cold, dusted with icing sugar and decorated with a few raspberries and mint leaves.

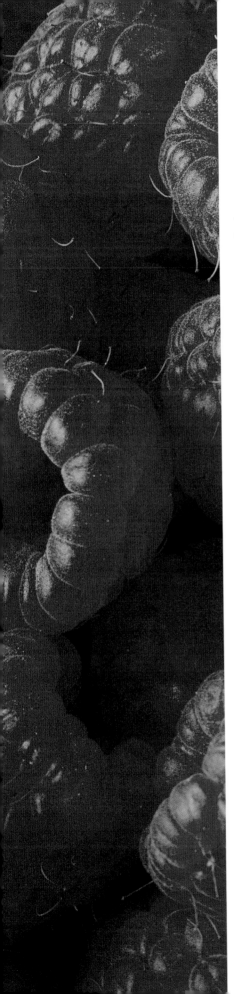

Raspberry fool

Low in sugar, high in fibre, this is a delicious alternative to the fruit yoghurts you can buy which are often full of sugar, preservatives and other additives. It can also be frozen and served instead of bought ice cream.

SERVES 4–6
275 g/10 oz fresh or frozen
    raspberries
225 g/8 oz plain fromage frais
125 g/4 oz Greek yoghurt
mint leaves to decorate

Reserve a few raspberries for decoration and purée the rest in a food processor. Push the purée through a sieve to remove the seeds.

    Mix the fromage frais and yoghurt together. Stir in the raspberry purée, making sure it is well mixed. Chill for about 1 hour.

    Serve decorated with fresh raspberries and mint leaves.

Variation
Reserve more of the raspberries and layer the yoghurt mixture with the whole raspberries.

Baked bananas

Perfect comfort food – or a romantic dessert – as it is really soft and sweet on the palate, and bananas provide fibre and potassium.

You can bake the bananas with just the lemon juice and serve with a spoonful of crème fraîche, ice cream or vanilla custard, or you can do as I have and add some spices.

SERVES 4
4 ripe bananas
1 teaspoon ground allspice
½ teaspoon ground cinnamon
½ teaspoon freshly grated nutmeg
3 tablespoons lemon juice
a handful of flaked roasted almonds
    or coconut flakes (optional)

Preheat the oven to 180°C/350°F/ Gas 4. Lightly butter an ovenproof dish. Slice the bananas lengthways and lay in the dish.

    Mix the spices together and sprinkle over the bananas. Sprinkle with the lemon juice and almonds or coconut flakes if using.

    Bake for 10–15 minutes. You may need to turn them occasionally to prevent the bananas from sticking. Decorate with roasted almond flakes and serve hot.

Variation: Flambéed bananas
Gently heat a couple of tablespoons of rum, pour over the bananas and light with a match at the table. Children love flambéed desserts, and you needn't worry about the alcohol or its calorific effect – it evaporates off, leaving just its flavour.

Golden harvest pudding

This steamed pudding is very rich and soft. The fibre within the fruit and cereals helps slow down the release of sugar into the body.

SERVES 4–6
85 g/3 oz self-raising wholemeal flour
85 g/3 oz wholemeal breadcrumbs
150 g/5 oz dried fruit (such as apricots, figs, raisins, sultanas)
85 g/3 oz sugar
85 g/3 oz shredded suet or melted butter
a little milk
butter for greasing
2 tablespoons golden syrup

Sift the flour into a bowl, add the breadcrumbs, dried fruit, sugar and suet or melted butter, with enough milk to give a sticky consistency; do not make it too dry.

Butter a 900 ml/1½ pint pudding basin and add the golden syrup. Spoon in the pudding mixture, leaving space for the pudding to rise. Cover with baking parchment and foil, tying them tightly around the rim of the basin.

Steam over boiling water for about 1¼ hours if using butter, or 1¾ hours if using suet. Serve hot with custard.

Baked egg custard

This is my mother's favourite comfort food; it is very nutritious as both milk and eggs – especially the yolks – are packed with vitamins and minerals.

SERVES 6
15 g/½ oz butter, plus a little for greasing
600 ml/1 pint milk
strip of lemon rind
2 eggs
2 egg yolks
1½ tablespoons caster sugar
freshly grated nutmeg

Preheat the oven to 180°C/350°F/Gas 4. Butter a 900 ml/1½ pint pie dish.

In a saucepan, bring the milk and lemon rind to just below boiling point, then remove from the heat. Using a fork, beat the eggs, yolks and sugar in a bowl until well mixed but not frothy.

Pour the hot (but not boiling) milk over the eggs, stir well, then strain the custard into the pie dish. Dot the custard with tiny flakes of butter, and sprinkle with nutmeg.

Set the dish in a deep roasting tin, pour in about 3 cm/1 inch of cold water, and bake the custard for about 35 minutes or until the top is golden brown and set. Serve warm or cold.

Variations
Cook in 6 individual ramekins for about 25 minutes.

You could also slice fresh fruits such as apricots, peaches or goose-berries into the dish before pouring in the custard.

Apple and oat crumble

Although not totally gluten free, this contains less gluten than a traditional crumble, so it's ideal if you can tolerate a small amount of gluten. Oats and apples are high in fibre to help clear the blood of unwanted cholesterol.

SERVES 6
100 g/3½ oz medium oatmeal
50 g/2 oz caster sugar
50 g/2 oz unsalted butter
4 Bramley apples, peeled, cored and sliced
6 dried figs, diced
2 tablespoons soft brown sugar
1 teaspoon ground cinnamon

Preheat the oven to 230°C/430°F/Gas 8.

Put the oatmeal in a bowl with the sugar, and rub in the butter. Put the prepared fruit into an ovenproof dish. Sprinkle with brown sugar and cinnamon, then sprinkle with the crumble mixture. Bake until golden brown. Serve warm.

Baked apples stuffed with apricots and figs

Cooking apples are perfect for this high fibre dessert, but you may find that children prefer eating apples, since they are slightly sweeter.

SERVES 4

4 cooking apples
250 ml/8 fl oz apple juice
4 tablespoons chopped apricots
4 tablespoons chopped dried figs
a little ground cinnamon
1 tablespoon honey
dash of Cointreau (optional)
25 g/1 oz butter

Preheat the oven to 180°C/350°F/Gas 4.

Core the apples and prick the skins with a fork to stop them from exploding in the oven. Put the apples in an ovenproof dish and pour the apple juice around them. Mix the apricots and figs with the cinnamon and honey and fill the centre of each apple. Top each apple with a dash of Cointreau and a knob of butter.

Bake for about 40–50 minutes, until the apples are golden brown and soft to the touch. Serve with ice cream, custard or crème fraîche.

Lemon-scented chilled rice pudding

This is a great way to boost your calcium intake. In summer it is delicious with fresh raspberries, blackberries or strawberries. Alternatively you could leave out half the lemon zest and mix in some chopped banana or dried fruits.

Rice pudding – hot or cold – also makes a perfect gluten-free breakfast.

SERVES 4

85 g/3 oz short-grain rice
375 ml/12 fl oz milk
1 vanilla pod
grated zest of 2 lemons
a little caster sugar
150 ml/5 fl oz double cream
    or thick natural yoghurt

Place the rice, milk, vanilla pod and lemon zest in a saucepan. Bring to the boil, then reduce the heat and simmer for 15–20 minutes, until the rice is swollen and soft. Sweeten to taste and leave to cool.

Mix the cream or yoghurt into the cooled rice and chill thoroughly before serving.

Pecan and apricot pie

This is a real treat, far superior to most shop-bought versions. It is high in calories, but a small slice can be an aphrodisiac. You will also be getting beta-carotene from the apricots and zinc from the eggs and pecan nuts.

SERVES 6–8

25 g/1 oz butter, softened
175 g/6 oz brown sugar
3 large eggs, beaten
175 ml/6 fl oz maple syrup
1 teaspoon vanilla essence
1 teaspoon salt
6 fresh apricots, halved and stoned, or canned apricots in natural juice, well drained
125 g/4 oz pecan nuts
175 g/6 oz sweet pastry case (page 337), baked blind

Preheat the oven to 200°C/400°F/Gas 6.

Beat the butter and sugar together and beat in the eggs, a little at a time. Beat in the maple syrup, vanilla essence and salt.

Arrange the apricots and pecans neatly in the pie case and pour the mixture over the top. Bake for 40 minutes, until the mixture is almost firm to the touch. Leave it to stand for about 15 minutes and it will set a little more.

Serve warm or cold, with a spoonful of crème fraîche to cut the sweetness if you like.

Chilled lemon cake

One of my favourite childhood treats, this is a delectable dessert; the lemon flavours cut the sweetness, giving a tangy yet creamy sensation. It is a high-energy pudding that's light on the palate. Be aware that this recipe uses uncooked eggs.

SERVES 6–8
6 good-quality trifle sponges
50 g/2 oz butter
50 g/2 oz caster sugar
2 eggs, at room temperature, beaten
grated zest and juice of 2 lemons
300 ml/10 fl oz double cream, whipped until stiff, or thick Greek yoghurt
thin slices of lemon and mint leaves to decorate

Line a small loaf tin with kitchen foil or baking parchment. Split the sponges horizontally and use a third of them to line the bottom of the tin.

Cream the butter and sugar together until light and fluffy. Gradually add the beaten eggs, beating well after each addition. Add the lemon zest and juice; don't worry if the mixture looks as if it has curdled. Pour half the mixture over the sponges.

Add another layer of sponges, then the remaining lemon mixture, and finish with a layer of sponge.

Cover with foil or baking parchment. Place a weight on top of the dessert and leave in the refrigerator for at least 4 hours.

Turn out of the tin and peel off the foil or paper. Spread with the whipped cream or thick yoghurt and decorate with lemon slices and sprigs of mint.

Berry fruit compote

Keep this fruit mixture in the fridge for a quick nutritious snack. Serve it with yoghurt, cream, ice cream or porridge. Have fun making up your own combinations of seasonal and dried fruit.

SERVES 4
450 g/1 lb mixed fruit (blackberries, blueberries, raspberries, halved and stoned plums, dried apricots)
150 ml/5 fl oz water
1 cinnamon stick
grated zest of 1 orange
mint leaves (optional)

Put the fruit, water, cinnamon and orange zest in a saucepan and simmer for 20 minutes. Remove the cinnamon stick and chill. Some shredded mint could be added before serving; this would be especially good if you have used raspberries.

Fig and orange boats

Children's parties are often piled high with artificially coloured and sweetened cakes and jellies. Here's a healthy, high fibre alternative.

Look in your supermarket or health food shop for dried figs that have not been sugar-dipped. Many garden leaves are suitable for the sails, but don't pick poisonous leaves, or any that have been sprayed or treated with chemicals. In any case, they should be washed carefully to remove dirt. Make sure that children don't eat the leaves or cocktail sticks!

MAKES 16 BOATS
4 juicy oranges
12 dried figs
16 cocktail sticks
16 small garden leaves

Cut the oranges into quarters. Using a sharp knife, remove the flesh, reserving the orange skins. Cut the pith from the outside of the oranges and discard. Holding the orange quarters over a bowl to catch the juice, cut the oranges into small pieces, discarding the pips and dropping the chunks of orange into the bowl as you go.

Chop the figs roughly and add to the bowl with the oranges. Mix well and leave for 2–3 hours, to allow the figs to swell in the orange juice.

When the figs are juicy and plump, place the orange skins on a serving plate and fill each 'boat' with pieces of orange and fig.

Make sails for the boats by threading each leaf on to a cocktail stick, then placing a cocktail stick in the centre of each orange boat.

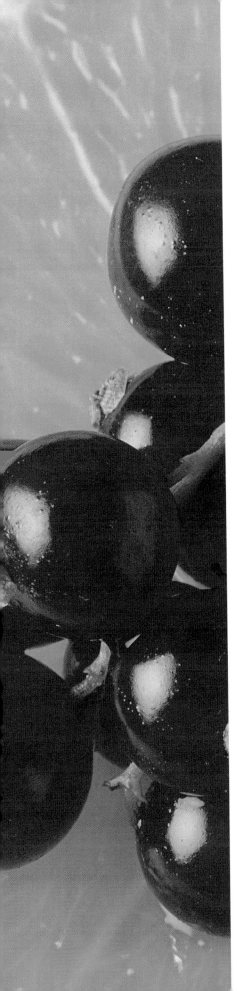

Energizing fruit shakes (Smoothies)

These refreshing and revitalizing drinks can be made with various combinations of fruits, such as oranges, grapefruit, peaches, apricots and other seasonal fruits, with or without added yoghurt. Try adding a few baked fruits or a spoonful of puréed fruit, as these give a slightly different texture and rounded taste. Simply purée all the ingredients in the liquidizer until smooth, then chill. Here are some ideas to start with.

1 mango (skin and stone removed), the juice of 1 lime, 275 g/10 oz natural yoghurt

85 g/3 oz strawberries, 85 g/3 oz raspberries, 400 g/14 oz low-fat fromage frais

juice of 2 large oranges (strained), ½ teaspoon clear honey, pinch of ground ginger, 200 g/7 oz natural yoghurt, 200 ml/7 fl oz cold milk

Strawberry and passionfruit tropical punch

This fruit shake can revitalize a tired body. is a lovely drink for children when they come home from school, and it is equally good for elderly people who need an energizing drink that is easy to swallow. To boost the calorie content you could add single cream instead of or as well as the coconut milk. Natural yoghurt will lower the calorie content.

MAKES 2 GLASSES
20 passionfruit, or 1 ripe mango, or 10 large juicy grapes
10 fresh strawberries, washed and hulled
2 teaspoons coconut milk
1 tablespoon lemon juice

Cut the passionfruit in half and scoop the flesh into a blender. If you are using mango, slice along the stone and scrape all the flesh off the stone and skin into a blender. Cut the grapes in half, discarding the pips, and add to the blender.

Add the remaining ingredients and blend well. Chill before serving.

Lemon and lime fizz

Try this as a zingy alternative to plain mineral water. It is also a good drink to serve children instead of sugary and additive-loaded squashes.

MAKES 6 GLASSES
3 lemons
600 ml/1 pint boiling water
1 tablespoon peeled and grated
  fresh ginger
50 g/2 oz sugar
juice of 3 limes, strained
6 slices of lemon
6 slices of lime
ice cubes
600 ml/1 pint sparkling mineral
  water, chilled

Pare the rind thinly from one lemon. Put the rind into a heatproof jug, pour the boiling water over it and add the ginger and sugar. Stir well, cover and leave to infuse for 1 hour, to allow the full flavours to develop.

Meanwhile, squeeze the juice from all of the lemons and strain into a serving jug. Add the lime juice, then strain in the infused ginger liquid and stir. Add the lemon and lime slices and the ice to the jug. Top up with the mineral water. Serve in tall glasses.

Orange blossom tea

In southern Morocco there are many orange orchards. When the orange trees blossom they collect the petals and extract the essential oil, which is used to make a delicious hot drink. I have found that orange blossom water is a good alternative to the oil.

This is perfect as an after-dinner drink. It cleans the palate and facilitates digestion, and is caffeine-free.

Pour boiling water into a mug. Add 1 teaspoon of orange blossom water and a pinch of finely ground cardamom. Sweeten to taste with sugar or honey.

Ginger tea

This recipe is one of my favourites for calming an upset stomach. Caffeine-free, it can be served hot or iced.

SERVES 4–5
900 ml/1½ pints water
4 cardamom pods
½ stick of cinnamon
3 cm/1 inch piece of fresh ginger
pinch of saffron strands
1 teaspoon ground almonds

Put the water in a saucepan and add the remaining ingredients. Bring to the boil and leave to simmer for 3 minutes to allow the spices to infuse into the water.

Strain the tea before serving, either hot or chilled with ice cubes. If you like you can add chunks of pineapple and slices of orange to the chilled version.

Index

glucagon 27, 123, 194, 228
glucose 25
Glucose Tolerance Test (GTT) 192
gluten sensitivity 122, 177, 178, 180–2
    see also *wheat, intolerance*
gluten-free food 181–2
glycogen 27, 124
gout 281, 287
gums 93
gut bacteria 41–2, 47, 90, 100, 137, 148,
    154–5, 175, 200–1, 242, 257

H
haemoglobin levels 38, 104–5, 275
haemorrhoids 152, 213
hair 37, 38, 103–5
hair loss 104–5, 223
hangover cures 50
hay fever 100, 185
headaches 130, 165–71, 185
health drinks 72
heart disease 27, 28, 32, 33, 41, 46, 48,
    49, 63, 66, 110, 111, 218, 220, 221, 252,
    253, 259, 269
    gut bacteria and 47
heartburn 156
helicobacter pylori 159, 243
hepatitis 48, 292
herbal teas and tisanes 35, 51, 130, 171
herbs 53–4
hiatus hernia 34, 156
histamines 171, 174
hives 98
hormone replacement therapy (HRT)
    174, 218, 219, 220, 221, 253
hormones
    growth promoting 57
    hormonal problems 96, 100, 111,
    125, 197
    and nausea 146
    sex hormones 31, 49, 91, 161,
    162–3, 251
    sleep inducing 120, 128, 162
    stress hormones 16, 145, 151, 155
    see also *hormones* by name
hydrogenated vegetable oils 32–3, 70, 99
hygiene 78–80, 210, 232, 245
hyperglycaemia 273
hyperlipidaemia 251, 253
hypertension 15, 45, 69, 170, 220, 221,
    259–63
hypoglycaemia 191–5, 228, 272
hypothalamus 15

I
ice cream 71, 210, 269, 270
illness
    and diabetes 272
    recuperation from 119, 134

immune system 38, 46, 47, 133–7, 173, 299
impotence 162, 163, 207, 221
incontinence 226
indigestion 17, 134–5, 155–8, 212,
    213, 293
infertility 111, 214–15
insomnia 213
    see also *sleep*
insulin 27, 121, 123, 145, 166, 191, 194,
    195, 265–6
intestines see *bowels; colon*
iron 43–4, 56, 57, 285
    and anaemia 275–9
    children and 23, 43
    folic acid and 39
    immune system and 134
    iron stores 103, 104–5
    iron deficiency see *anaemia*
    old age and 228
    and pregnancy 43, 209
    sources of 43–4, 277
    supplements 279
irradiated food 73
irritability 173, 275
irritable bowel syndrome 15, 28, 41, 44, 47,
    63, 100, 148, 197, 242, 268, 275, 277

J
jaundice, gall-stones and 289
joint problems see *arthritis*

K
kidneys
    migraine headaches 166
    problems 69, 259
kidneys (offal)
    pregnancy and 44
    source of iron 44, 277
    source of selenium 238
    source of vitamin A 37, 44
    source of zinc 45

L
lactose 171, 174, 178, 179–80
laxatives 148, 149, 151–2, 153, 226
libido 45, 54, 161, 162
    loss of 31, 45, 49, 111, 162, 221, 223
    see also *sex*
listeria 79–80, 210
liver
    alcohol and 49, 124
    bile production 289, 292
    cancer of the 243
    cholesterol and 251–2, 254
    cirrhosis 49
    hypoglycaemia and 192
    in middle age 221
    migraines and 170
    raised liver enzymes 292–3

liver (offal)
    pâtés 23, 209, 210
    pregnancy and 209, 277
    source of iron 44, 277
    source of selenium 238
    vitamin D and 41
    vitamin A and 37, 44, 97, 209
    zinc and 45
lysine 105

M
mad cow disease see *BSE*
magnesium 44, 90, 93, 134, 136, 200, 219
manganese 91, 207
manicures 105
margarines 32–3, 37, 41, 254
massage 105, 133, 282
ME 119
meats 80, 105, 113, 210
    B vitamins and 38, 57, 58
    beef 57–8
    lamb 56–7
    lean 23, 45, 46, 161, 209, 254
    and migraines 169
    pork, ham and bacon 58–9
    sausages 58–9
    source of iron 44, 56, 123, 275, 277
    source of zinc 45, 56, 58, 135
    see also *poultry*
medications
    alcohol and 48
    and arthritis 281–2
    for colds 136
    dementia patients and 230, 233
    and depression 139, 141, 142, 143
    and folic acid 39, 207, 285
    hypoglycaemia and 192
    for indigestion 155
    and liver complaints 292
    nausea and 146, 249
    old age and 226, 227–8
    potassium and 45
    sleep and 129
    tiredness and 125
meningitis 137, 165
menopause 217–22
    bone mass and 89
    and cholesterol 253
    migraines and 166
menstruation see *periods*
migraines 48, 130, 165–71
    see also *allergies*
milk 59
    babies and 176
    calcium source 42–3, 90
    indigestion and 158
    protein source 30
    sensitivity to 102, 178, 179–80, 271
    vitamins and minerals 37, 38, 41–3, 46

Acknowledgements

Jim Ainsworth, Jamie and Lyn Falla, Lucy Holmes, Eve McLeod, Katingo and Anthony Giannoulis, Neil Benson, John Cohen, Helen Gourley, Jamie Harrison, Simon Majumdar, Naji, Jill and Jack Halabi, Margaret, Simon, Cat and Mark Vinton, Kirstin Romano, Julian Alexander, Tom Cussen, Ann Marie Clarke, Paul Clarke, Laura Marriott, Susan Haynes, Jess Koppel, Emily Hare, Lyn Rutherford, Maggie Ramsay, Victoria Blackie, Dr Martin Scurr, Andrew Barr, Terry Gibson, Judy, John, Mark and Meg Morrison, Liz and Bernie, Brian Price, Herman Smeding, Juliet Cousins, Chris Rose, Mum and Dad, Dr Hugh Rushton, Gloria Thomas, Patricia and Daniel Michelson, Tim Adkin, James and Angelika Richards, Matt Lawrence

Support groups and useful addresses

Association of Spina Bifida and Hydrocephalus
Asbah House, 42 Park Road
Peterborough, Cambs PE1 2UQ
Tel: 01733 555988

British Diabetic Association
10 Queen Anne Street, London W1M OBD
Tel: 0171 323 1531

British Dietetic Association
7th Floor, Elizabeth House
22 Suffolk Street, Queensway
Birmingham B1 1LS
Tel: 0121 643 5483

British Rheumatism & Arthritis Research Council
Copeman House, St Mary's Court
St Mary's Gate, Chesterfield S41 7TD
Tel: 01246 558033

Coeliac Society
P O Box 220, High Wycombe
Bucks HP11 2HY
Tel: 01494 437278

Hyperactive Children's Support Group
71 Whyke Lane, Chichester
West Sussex PO19 2LD
Tel: 01903 725182

MENCAP
123 Golden Lane, London EC1Y ORT
Tel: 0171 454 0454

Migraine Trust
45 Great Ormond Street, London WC1N 3HD
Tel: 0171 831 4818

Multiple Sclerosis Society
25 Effie Road, London SW6 1EE
Tel: 0171 610 7171

National Childbirth Trust
Alexandra House, Oldham Terrace
London W3 6NH
Tel: 0181 992 8637

National Eczema Society
Tavistock House North, Tavistock Square
London WC1H 9SR
Tel: 0171 388 4097

Rococo
321 King's Road, London SW3
Tel: 0171 352 5857
(Sell and deliver fine chocolates, including some with low sugar and high cocoa bean content)

The Soil Association
86 Colston Street, Bristol BS1 5BB

Vegetarian Society
Parkdale, Dunham Road, Altrincham
Cheshire WA14 4QG
Tel: 0161 9280793

YAPP&RS (Young person's support group for Parkinson's disease)
Emma Benyon, Church Farm
Burcham Newton, King's Lynn, Norfolk
Tel: 01485 578 603